Fixing the Poor

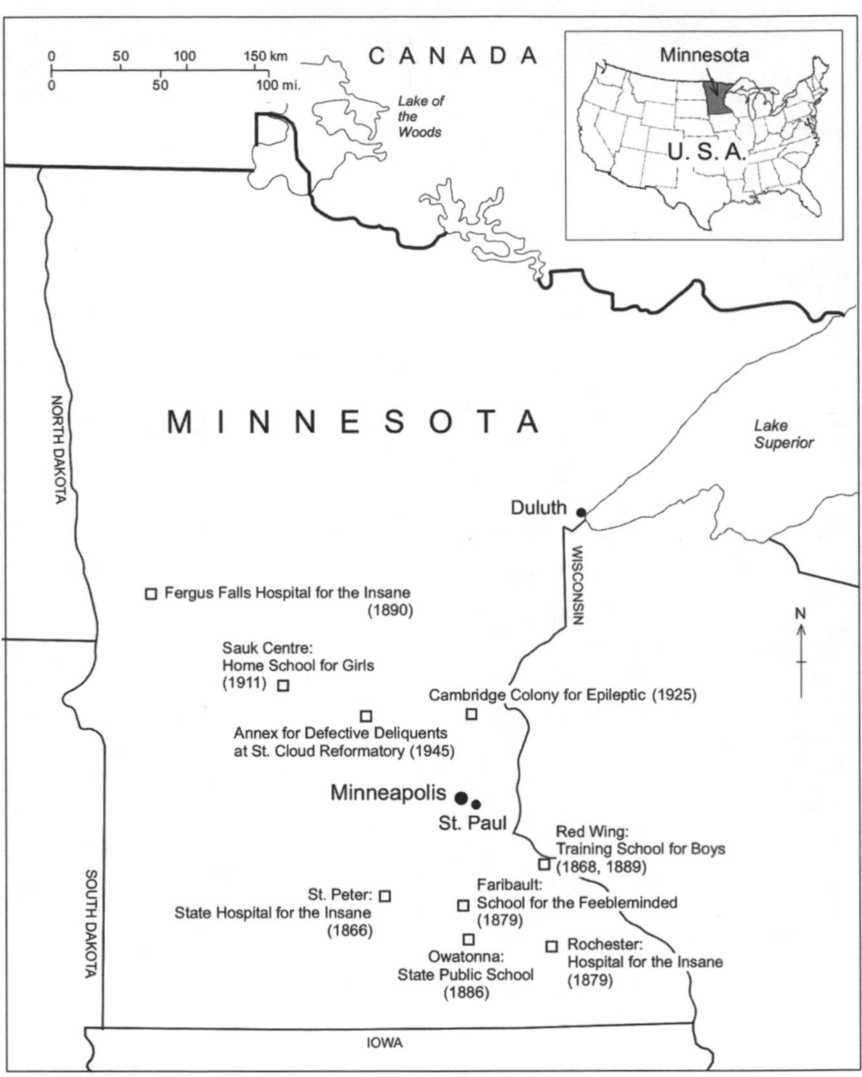
0 50 100 150 km
0 50 100 mi.
CANADA
Lake of the Woods
Minnesota
U.S.A.
MINNESOTA
NORTH DAKOTA
Lake Superior
Duluth
WISCONSIN
Fergus Falls Hospital for the Insane (1890)
N
Sauk Centre: Home School for Girls (1911)
Cambridge Colony for Epileptic (1925)
Annex for Defective Deliquents at St. Cloud Reformatory (1945)
Minneapolis
St. Paul
Red Wing: Training School for Boys (1868, 1889)
SOUTH DAKOTA
St. Peter: State Hospital for the Insane (1866)
Faribault: School for the Feebleminded (1879)
Owatonna: State Public School (1886)
Rochester: Hospital for the Insane (1879)
IOWA

FIXING THE POOR

Eugenic Sterilization and Child Welfare in the Twentieth Century

MOLLY LADD-TAYLOR

Johns Hopkins University Press
Baltimore

Printed in the United States of America on acid-free paper
9 8 7 6 5 4 3 2 1

Johns Hopkins University Press
2715 North Charles Street
Baltimore, Maryland 21218-4363
www.press.jhu.edu

Library of Congress Cataloging-in-Publication Data

Names: Ladd-Taylor, Molly, 1955– author.
Title: Fixing the poor : eugenic sterilization and child welfare in the twentieth century / Molly Ladd-Taylor.
Description: Baltimore : Johns Hopkins University Press, 2017. | Includes bibliographical references and index.
Identifiers: LCCN 2017007360 | ISBN 9781421423722 (hardcover : alk. paper) | ISBN 1421423723 (hardcover : alk. paper) | ISBN 9781421423739 (electronic) | ISBN 1421423731 (electronic)
Subjects: LCSH: Involuntary sterilization—United States—History—20th century. | Sterilization (Birth control)—United States—History—20th century. | Eugenics—United States—History—20th century. | Mentally ill—Government policy—United States—20th century. | Poor—Government policy—United States—20th century. | MESH: Sterilization, Involuntary—history | Mentally Disabled Persons—history | Intellectual Disability—history | Eugenics—history | Vulnerable Populations | Human Rights Abuses—history | History, 20th Century | Minnesota
Classification: LCC HV4989 .L24 2017 | DDC 363.9/7—dc23
LC record available at https://lccn.loc.gov/2017007360

A catalog record for this book is available from the British Library.

Frontispiece: Carolyn King

CONTENTS

ACKNOWLEDGMENTS

I have been working on this book for the entire lives of my now-adult children, and in that time I have accrued many debts. My first debt is to the archivists and librarians who facilitated my research: David Klaassen and Linnea Anderson of the Social Welfare History Archives, the Inter-Library Loan department of Scott Library, and the staffs of the American Philosophical Society, the National Archives, and the Minnesota Historical Society. At the Minnesota Historical Society, I am especially grateful to Debbie Miller, who supported this project at its beginning, and Ellen Jaquette, who helped me at the end.

I have also benefited from the generous financial support of the Social Sciences and Humanities Research Council of Canada (SSHRC), the Burroughs Wellcome 40th Anniversary Award in the History of Medicine or Science, the Hannah Institute for the History of Medicine (now Associated Medical Services, Inc.), the Minnesota Historical Society, and York University.

Portions of this book have been published elsewhere in a different form and are reprinted here with permission. Early versions of my main arguments appeared as "Coping with a 'Public Menace': Eugenic Sterilization in Minnesota," *Minnesota History* 59 (Summer 2005); "The 'Sociological Advantages' of Sterilization," in *Mental Retardation in America: A Historical Anthology*, ed. Steven Noll and James W. Trent Jr. (New York University Press, 2004); and "Fixing Mothers," in *Child Welfare and Social Action*, ed. Jon Lawrence and Pat Starkey (Liverpool University Press, 2001). Part of chapter 5 was published in Paul A. Lombardo's *A Century of Eugenics in America: From the Indiana Experiment to the Human Genome Era* (Indiana University Press, 2011), and part of the conclusion appeared as "Contraception or Eugenics? Sterilization and 'Mental Retardation' in the 1970s and 1980s," *Canadian Bulletin of Medical History* 31 (2014). I am grateful to the editors and publishers of these works.

Thanks to funding from SSHRC and York University, I was privileged to have a village—or perhaps county is a better metaphor—help me with various aspects of the project. Julia Mickenberg, Andrea Sachs, and Kim Heikkila, then graduate students at the University of Minnesota, got the research off to a good start. Liz O'Gorek, Chelsea Bauer, and Disa Clifford helped me at the project's end. In between, I received assistance from Katie Bausch, Becky Beausaert, Katina Deischel, Jason Ellis, Laila Haidarali, Eva Kater, Cindy Loch-Drake, Crystal Luxmore, Elaine Naylor, Liza Piper, Jason Reid, Sara Stratton, Lindsey Tashlin, and Joseph Tohill; Carolyn King and Byron Moldofsky, who did the maps; and Charis Wahl, who read the manuscript at a critical juncture. I am especially grateful for the research support and companionship of the four former York students who accompanied me to Minnesota: Katie Bausch, Laila Haidarali, Eva Kater, and Liza Piper. Liza Piper transcribed and analyzed the sterilization database and tracked down the Supreme Court cases; her contribution to this project was vital.

Since I began working on this book, a flourishing scholarship on eugenics, the history of childhood, and disability history has kept me interested, inspired, and humble. I have benefited from the work of too many people to mention them all here, but I would like to give special thanks to the co-panelists whose critical comments, encouragement, and, in some cases, friendship sustained me through this journey: Johanna Schoen, Erika Dyck, Alexandra Minna Stern, Leslie Reagan, Susan L. Smith, Janet Golden, Franca Iacovetta, Paul Lombardo, Claudia Malacrida, Kim Nielsen, Steven Noll, and Amy Samson. Brianna Theobald generously shared her research notes and scholarship on the sterilization of Ojibwe women. At Johns Hopkins University Press, Jacqueline Wehmueller, Matthew McAdam, and Jeremy Horsefield guided the book to completion.

My thinking about eugenics and disability has been informed by the important work of community activists and eugenics survivors. At the beginning of the project, Molly Woehrlin and Robert J. Levy shared their impressions of Faribault's sterilization program, and I was fortunate to meet Rick Cardenas and the Remembering with Dignity team at an early stage of their gravestone restoration project. In the 2010s, I had the pleasure of participating in the Living Archives on Eugenics in Western Canada project, a SSHRC-CURA project led by Robert A. Wilson at the University of Alberta, which brought together academics, community workers, and eugenics survivors. I have also benefited from the impressive digital project on the history of developmental disabilities in Minnesota, sponsored by the Minnesota Governor's Council on Developmental Disabilities (and launched after I completed most of my research). Readers are encouraged to check out this extraordinary resource: http://mn.gov/mnddc/past/index.html.

I could write a book on how not to write a book, and I am grateful to the many friends and colleagues who supported me over the years. In the Twin Cities, I was sustained by the generosity and warmth of Elaine Tyler May, Jennifer Gunn, and Neal Holtan. Neal read the entire manuscript and offered invaluable advice. I am also grateful to my colleagues and friends in the History Department at York University, especially Bettina Bradbury, Stephen Brooke, Boyd Cothran, Patricia Di Benigno, Michele Johnson, Rachel Koopmans, Sean Kheraj, Kathryn McPherson, Anne Rubenstein, Marc Stein, and Bill Wicken. I could never have finished this book without Ann Braude, who took me in at a difficult time and, toward the end of the project, took me up into the mountains to prove we are strong. Ann's superb editing skills, incisive commentary, and friendship shaped this book in crucial ways.

My family and friends in Toronto helped me make it through these past few years. Franca Iacovetta, Ruth Mandel, Beth Savan, Lindsey Tashlin, and Stacey Whyne Berman provided great company and much-needed support. Kathryn McPherson, Michele Johnson, Andrea Davis, Bettina Bradbury, and Anne Rubenstein read the entire manuscript several times, helped me sharpen my arguments, and pressed me to think harder about what I was really trying to say. More importantly, our walks, movie nights, and rich conversations kept me going. Last but certainly not least, Bill Wicken pushed me to work on the book every day, took his metaphorical red pen to the entire manuscript, and helped me understand the importance of the data. We work with words, but words cannot express what all of you have meant to me.

I have spent a lot of time thinking about the heartbreak of child removal and sterilization, and writing this book has been a constant reminder of my good fortune. During the years I have been working (and not working) on this book, Disa, Julian, and Timothy Clifford have grown into wonderfully kind, thoughtful, and engaged adults. I am blessed that they are in my life. This book is for my children, with love.

NOTE ON TERMINOLOGY AND NAMES

In this book, I use words that readers may find offensive, such as *feebleminded, defective*, *moron*, *insane*, and *retarded*, regularly and without quotation marks. Disability rights groups justifiably criticize the use of these hurtful words and the tendency to turn supposed attributes into nouns (for example, by not speaking of individuals with disabilities, but of "the disabled" or "the feebleminded" as a class). Yet no other phrasing so vividly conveys the scientific and cultural assumptions behind state eugenics policies and sterilization laws. *Feebleminded* and *defective* are also more expansive than present terms, like *intellectual disability*, because they include people whose differences would now be seen as cultural, socioeconomic, or psychological in origin.

Throughout this book, I follow the terminology used by public officials and experts at the time. Thus, the early chapters focus on the feebleminded, but the subject of chapter 6 is mental retardation. Persons confined to the Minnesota School for the Feebleminded (which itself went through numerous name changes) are called inmates, patients, or residents, depending on the time period. The shifting terminology reveals how attitudes toward persons with intellectual disabilities and concepts such as normality and disability have changed over time.

For consistency's sake, I use the colloquial Minnesota School for the Feebleminded (without a hyphen) or Faribault School when referring to the institution where most of the state's sterilizations were performed. The Faribault School underwent eight formal name changes between 1879, when an experimental School for Imbeciles was authorized within the Minnesota Institute for the Deaf, Dumb and Blind, and 1998, the year the Faribault Regional Center closed. During the period covered in this book, its name included School for Idiots and Imbeciles (1881), School for Feeble-Minded (1885), School for Feeble-Minded and Colony for Epileptics (1906), Minnesota School and Colony (1949), and Faribault State School and Hospital (1955). The Minnesota Historical Society holds the institution's archives under the name Faribault State School and Hospital (FSSH), so I use that name in the notes.

Out of respect for the privacy of the affected families and to comply with Minnesota State Archives requirements, I have invented pseudonyms for the sterilized and allegedly feebleminded individuals discussed in this book, except when their names already appear in the public record (for example, in court cases). A key to my pseudonyms has been deposited at the Minnesota Historical Society.

INTRODUCTION

"I am in the place where they keep the feeble minded at Faribault. They won't let me out of here if I don't get sterilized." So began Minnesota writer Meridel Le Sueur's 1935 short story, "Sequel to Love," about a young woman resisting state-sponsored sterilization. The unnamed narrator became trapped in the welfare system when she got pregnant out of wedlock. Social workers took her baby away, gave the young mother an intelligence test, and sent her to the state institution to be sterilized. Although the girl's father hired a lawyer to keep her out of the institution, social workers said she liked men too much and should not have another baby. They pressured her to consent to sterilization, but the girl was defiant. She insisted on staying in the institution with the "cracked ones" rather than submit to an operation she saw as "a sin and a crime." At the end of the story, she remained "locked up here with the feeble minded."[1]

Few people today would defend the sterilization policy described in Le Sueur's story, but between 1907 and 1937 thirty-two US states passed laws resulting in the sterilization of more than 63,000 Americans. In Minnesota, the site of Le Sueur's story, at least 2,350 people, nearly 80 percent of them women, were sterilized. Today, many critics emphasize the connection between US eugenics laws and the forced sterilization of thousands in Germany and the occupied territories, suggesting that American policies were similar to Nazi crimes. "The eugenics movement was a shameful effort in which state government never should have been involved," Virginia governor Mark Warner declared in the first of seven official state apologies. "We must remember . . . past mistakes in order to prevent them from recurring." Yet how did eugenic sterilization become a social policy? Despite more than two decades of scholarship, a single explanation still prevails in most popular and many scholarly accounts: elite experts infatuated with eugenic science manipulated state power to sterilize people who were pronounced unfit because of their race, ethnicity, and class. The broad consensus against sterilization has carried a deeply cynical lesson: beware of experts, and beware of government power.[2]

This book tells a different story. Tracing the social history behind Le Sueur's fictional critique, this book analyzes eugenic sterilization as part of one state's public welfare system. It focuses not on the worst eugenics abuses, but on the best-case scenario, a state where surgical sterilization was voluntary (at least on paper) and administered within a progressive child welfare system that continues to win national praise. Le Sueur's story, which was based on the experiences of women the author met as a Depression-era journalist and written from the perspective of a supposedly unfit mother, makes no mention of a Nazi-like quest for racial purity; in fact, there is no reference to eugenics ideology at all.[3] The protagonist is victimized as much by poverty and the boyfriend who left her as she is by social workers and the state. Le Sueur's main concern is how sterilization and the threat of sterilization were used to discipline working-class women's lives. This book, like her short story, situates eugenic sterilization within a broad set of social welfare policies that aimed to solve the problems of poverty, sex, and single motherhood by "fixing" the poor. While eugenics-inspired fears of the menace of the feebleminded clearly enabled the passage of Minnesota's sterilization law, I argue that the policy's actual design and administration over the years were equally shaped by a longer-term concern with limiting the state's financial responsibility for the poor; the fear that poor women who got pregnant out of wedlock deepened poverty in their own generation and transmitted deprivation to the next generation was not new. When eugenic sterilization is examined from a social welfare perspective, it appears less like a deliberate plan for genetic improvement than a mundane and all-too-modern tale of fiscal politics, troubled families, and deeply felt cultural attitudes about disability, welfare dependency, sexuality, and gender.

This volume is a social history of one state's sterilization program from the point of view of those who imposed it and those who experienced it. As such, it focuses as much on the implementation of sterilization as a social welfare policy as it does on eugenic ideas. Minnesota enacted its eugenic sterilization law in 1925, and in some accounts the campaign for that law is where the story of sterilization begins. In fact, the policy was rooted in a set of ideas and administrative arrangements that began in the 1880s and were written into the child welfare laws passed in the 1910s. The sterilization program peaked during the New Deal of the 1930s, but the operations continued in reduced numbers at least until the law was changed in 1975. Studying sterilization as a social welfare measure, and interrogating its relationship to local governments' efforts to keep welfare expenditures low, helps us understand why sterilization arose as a social policy and why it persisted long after "eugenics" went out of fashion. Although it is tempting to zero in on the offensive pronouncements of past eugenics propagandists, our society still struggles with the problem that sterilization was intended to solve: the welfare of the nation's poorest and most vulnerable citizens. This book examines Minnesota's program of sterilizing the "feebleminded" from the policy's conceptual origins in the late nineteenth century to its official end in the 1970s, asking a series of question arising from Le Sueur's story. How did eugenic sterilization develop as a social policy, and where does the surgical "fix" of sterilization fit in the twentieth-century welfare system as a whole? Who was considered feebleminded and designated for sterilization? How were specific sterilization decisions made? Above all, how did eugenic sterilization become routine?

There are three other themes of Le Sueur's story that are vital to understanding sterilization as a social welfare policy. The first is sterilization's place in the child welfare system. Eugenics arose in tandem with the Progressive Era child-saving and moral reform movements. Middle-class reformers, especially women, sought to extend middle-class ideas about sexual morality, proper home life, and "normal" child development to people like Le Sueur's narrator, a young working-class girl swept off her feet by a boy who promised her the good life. Yet Le Sueur's portrait of the child welfare system is scathing. A prenatal clinic gave the girl advice but nothing to eat. Social workers forced her to breastfeed the baby and then took it away, "saving" the child by having it raised by someone else. The heartbreak of child removal and family breakup is rarely mentioned by scholars of eugenics, but it was a defining aspect of US sterilization (and welfare) policy and central to Le Sueur's poignant critique.

The ordeal of institutionalization is another theme of this book. Sterilization was one component of a comprehensive welfare–eugenics policy in which permanent segregation in a total institution was the ultimate threat. Le Sueur's short story illustrates this vividly: sterilization was the "price of freedom" from the state institution. Yet most critics of eugenics, including Le Sueur, treat surgical sterilization as worse than endless detention in a state institution, and most official apologies focus only on sterilization.[4] Although the protagonist in Le Sueur's story resists eugenics by choosing institutionalization over sterilization, few people actually made that choice. Le Sueur's story downplays the awfulness of indefinite incarceration and the true cost of resistance to sterilization.

The images of disability that saturate Le Sueur's story underscore a final theme of this book: interrogating the concept of feeblemindedness used to justify both segregation and sterilization. I examine how and why feeblemindedness was constructed as a social problem and how the attribution of disability legitimized the infantilization and mistreatment of nonconformists, the chronically poor, and people of color. Le Sueur, like many critics of eugenics, highlights the injustice of sterilization by emphasizing the inaccuracy of the feebleminded label. Readers are told more than once that the narrator was not dumb, her baby was "awful bright," and she should not have been locked up with the "cracked ones" who moaned and moaned all night. As the title "Sequel to Love" implies, Le Sueur viewed sterilization—and indeed the designation of feeblemindedness itself—as an unjust punishment for female sexual desire.[5] In contrast, this book complicates our understanding of how the designation of feeblemindedness was constituted. It explores how and why certain people were labeled feebleminded and targeted for sterilization, while others with very similar demographic profiles and behaviors were not. *Fixing the Poor* is both an analysis of the cultural concepts of disability used to justify eugenic segregation and surgery and a social history of persons who were labeled defective, committed to state guardianship, and sterilized.

Rethinking Eugenic Sterilization

In standard accounts of eugenics in America, compulsory sterilization was the logical result of an ideological crusade to improve the genetic quality of the human race. *Eugenics*, a term invented in 1883 by the British statistician Francis Galton from the Greek *eu* + *genēs*, meaning "well born," was defined by the American Charles Davenport in 1911 as the "science of the improvement of the human race by better breeding." A popular cause in Progressive Era America, eugenics was animated by race, class, and sexual anxieties about social and economic change, while also reflecting an optimistic faith in science, rational planning, and state action. Eugenics is often portrayed as an elitist ideology aligned with Nazi racial hygiene, and critics emphasize its broad acceptance among academic experts, philanthropists, and middle-class reformers who saw themselves as fit and defined the unfit as "other" in terms of their race, ethnicity, and class. According to one best-selling account, the American campaign to create a master race victimized urban immigrants, poor white "trash," blacks, Mexicans, Jews, criminals, alcoholics, the mentally ill, and "anyone else who did not resemble the blond and blue-eyed Nordic ideal the eugenics movement glorified."[6]

In the past few decades, a growing body of scholarship has rejected the simplistic association between eugenics and the most egregious Nazi policies and explored the ways that eugenics reflected and reworked popular and scientific ideas about race, gender, disability, and modernity itself. As the historian Frank Dikötter wrote in 1998, eugenics was "not so much a clear set of scientific principles as a 'modern' way of talking about social problems in biologizing terms." The most exciting twenty-first-century scholarship presents eugenics as a cluster of social and scientific ideas about human improvement which traveled the globe, took a different form in different regional and national contexts, and constituted a vital component of modernization and nation building. I build on this scholarship, as well as new literature on disability history and children's studies, to explore the development and implementation of eugenic sterilization as a "child welfare" policy in one locale.[7]

Eugenicists themselves divided their work into two distinct strategies. "Positive" eugenics, such as marriage counseling and better baby contests, encouraged the fit to have more children, while "negative" eugenics aimed to reduce the proportion of the population that was considered unfit. In the United States, most historians agree, positive eugenics was largely limited to education or propaganda, while negative eugenics policies, such as immigration restriction, antimiscegenation laws, and legislation mandating the institutional segregation and surgical sterilization of so-called defectives, had the most legislative success. Many states based their sterilization policies on a model law written in 1914 by Harry Laughlin, superintendent of the nation's premier eugenics research institute, the Eugenic Record Office (ERO) in Cold Spring Harbor, New York. The model law aimed to prevent the procreation of "socially inadequate" individuals —such as the feebleminded, insane, epileptic, inebriate, and criminalistic—by sterilizing people with "inferior hereditary potentialities, maintained wholly or in part by public expense." While much has been written about eugenicists' capacious understanding of inferior hereditary potentialities, the important second part of the phrase, "maintained wholly by public expense," has been largely overlooked.[8] This book aims to rectify that omission.

Many Americans today see eugenics and sterilization as synonymous, but the linkage between eugenics and sexual surgery was never fixed. Sterilizations could be, and often were, authorized on therapeutic or penal as well as "eugenic" grounds. For example, therapeutic, or medically necessary, sterilizations were (and are) performed to remove cancerous tumors or uterine fibroids or when pregnancy would endanger the mother's life. Doctors at the turn of the century also performed castrations, hysterectomies, vasectomies, and tubal ligations as treatment for what they considered serious medical conditions, such as dementia praecox (schizophrenia), manic depression, homosexuality, and excessive masturbation. Sterilizations could also be performed for contraceptive purposes. Indeed, sterilization became a leading form of birth control after legal restrictions on contraception were relaxed. By the 1970s, one-third of US couples reported that they had chosen to be sterilized. Yet coercion was ever present, as several highly publicized lawsuits made clear, and many poor women of color were threatened with the loss of welfare benefits or medical care if they did not "consent" to be sterilized. Sterilization could also be a punishment for crime. Indeed, the earliest advocates of sterilization, writing amid the white supremacist terror campaigns of the late nineteenth century, promoted castration as a way to punish sex criminals and protect innocent women and children from the imagined black rapist. The United States Supreme Court outlawed sterilization as a punitive measure in *Skinner v. Oklahoma* (1942), but until then several states permitted sterilization (by castration, vasectomy, or tubal ligation) of "habitual" criminals, rapists, child molesters, and sexual perverts. Therapeutic and punitive rationales for coerced sterilization were just as influential as eugenic ones in the early twentieth century, and scholars' exclusive focus on eugenic justifications can be misleading. Moreover, regardless of the legal rationale for surgery, sterilizations were often ordered for what were essentially institution-management reasons, such as controlling unruly inmates or reducing overcrowding by facilitating a patient's release.[9]

To complicate matters further, most eugenicists initially opposed sterilization. Even those who became the leading proponents of compulsory sterilization, such as Charles Davenport and California eugenicist Paul Popenoe, initially questioned the efficacy of sterilization for eugenic purposes and assumed that permanent segregation in a custodial institution was the best way to prevent the "unfit" from reproducing. Only in the 1920s did advances in surgical techniques, improvements in due process and legal procedures, and a vigorous pro-sterilization campaign convince eugenicists and policy makers alike that compulsory sterilization was a viable policy, more cost-effective and humane than segregation (since sterilized persons could be released from the institution).[10]

The notorious Supreme Court decision *Buck v. Bell* (1927) was the turning point. Prior to that ruling, which upheld the constitutionality of a Virginia statute based on Laughlin's Model Sterilization Law, eugenic sterilization was highly controversial, and most state sterilization laws had been struck down by the courts or were rarely enforced. After *Buck*, "opposition to sterilization seemed to melt away." The story of the case is well known. It centered on seventeen-year-old Carrie Buck, a "white feeble-minded woman," who was committed to the Virginia Colony for Epileptics and Feeble Minded a few months after giving birth to an illegitimate child. The Virginia Colony superintendent described the Buck family as part of the "shiftless, ignorant, and worthless class of antisocial whites of the South." Carrie's mother, who was considered promiscuous, was an inmate of the same institution, and her baby Vivian, after a brief examination, was pronounced feebleminded too. To the court, Carrie's family history was proof that her feeblemindedness was hereditary and that she was a "probable potential parent of socially inadequate offspring." They determined that Carrie's own welfare, and the welfare of society, would be aided by her sterilization. As Justice Oliver Wendell Holmes Jr. declared in a chilling and often-quoted decision, "It is better for all the world, if instead of waiting to execute degenerate offspring for crime or to let them starve for their imbecility, society can prevent those who are manifestly unfit from continuing their kind. . . . Three generations of imbeciles are enough."[11]

Buck made compulsory eugenic sterilization lawful in the United States, fusing sterilization and eugenics in the public mind. Although public reaction was muted, subsequent legal critics have described *Buck* as one of the worst decisions of the Supreme Court. In making this case, they have bolstered a compelling but one-dimensional narrative in which powerful eugenics experts convinced the government to sterilize people who were "perfectly normal both mentally and physically" and labeled unfit for no other reason than that they were trapped at the "bottom of the nation's economic and social hierarchies." Legal historian Paul A. Lombardo has demonstrated that Carrie Buck was a woman of average intelligence labeled promiscuous and therefore feebleminded because she bore a child out of wedlock after being raped. Eugenics experts "manufactured evidence to fit the state's case against Carrie Buck," and her own lawyer colluded with the state against his client. Carrie and her sister were terribly poor and lacking in education, another historian explained, but they were "clearly able and intelligent." Carrie "came from the sort of family the eugenicists wanted to put in the spotlight," writes journalist Adam Cohen; "she was not a threat to society, but its victim."[12]

The narrative of overzealous experts victimizing innocent women has also shaped the popular and scholarly literature on postwar sterilization abuse. The coerced sterilization of poor African American, Latina, and indigenous women in the 1970s did not usually take place under eugenics statutes, but the fact that most of the operations were performed under the auspices of federally funded family planning programs is sometimes taken as proof that sterilization was a deliberate policy of racial genocide, a neo-eugenic plan to reduce the birth rate of poor women of color. In this account, pro-sterilization activists working with and within Planned Parenthood and federally funded family planning agencies imposed their bigoted notions of reproductive fitness on poor black communities and forcibly sterilized many thousands of women. While this narrative is not wrong, it is incomplete, and that incompleteness can be distorting. The emphasis on the harm done by family planning programs masks the limited economic and reproductive options of poor women and overlooks the more mundane mechanisms of race and class inequities: the fiscal politics of Medicaid, the structure of hospital funding, a punitive child welfare system, and racialized concepts of intellectual disability and mental retardation. It also creates a misleading contrast between a supposedly enlightened "us" of today and a prejudiced eugenicist "them."[13]

This book draws on scholarship in gender, sexuality, and disability history to tell a more complicated story. It emphasizes the centrality of normative sexual and gendered behaviors in eugenic notions of reproductive fitness while also interrogating the concept of mental deficiency which justified eugenic commitment and sterilization. In the 1920s and 1930s, young white "sex delinquents" were the chief targets of state eugenics programs because experts and the lay public alike considered mental deficiency a plausible explanation for young women's moral delinquencies and uninhibited sexual behavior. In the postwar years, African American welfare mothers became the focus, reflecting concerns over illegitimacy, rising welfare costs, and the supposed pathology of poor black families. Reform schools for delinquent girls operated as a pipeline to eugenics in the interwar years, while county welfare departments served that role in the 1960s. In both eras, delinquency and dependency (that is, sex and welfare) were the driving concerns, but "defectiveness," the presumption of disability, was the connecting thread. Rather than dismissing allegations of low mentality or pathology as spurious, scholars can use the social construction of disability as an analytic frame to explore the persistence of welfare–eugenics practices in the post–civil rights era of ostensible racial equality and colorblindness. Even so, as historian Joanna Schoen reminds us, poor women of color were never a homogenous group, and sterilization did not have the same meaning for all. Economic hardship and a lack of access to legal birth control and abortion can make it difficult for historians to distinguish coerced "eugenic" sterilization from women's reproductive choice.[14]

The history of eugenic sterilization also intersects with the history of children and youth. The legal and administrative foundation for sterilization in Minnesota was laid in the 1917 Children's Code, a much-praised package of laws that modernized the state's child welfare apparatus and significantly improved the status of illegitimate children, even as it legalized the compulsory eugenic commitment of so-called defectives. Scholars have begun to examine the eugenics work of child welfare reformers, but few have interrogated how maternalist reformers often described the feebleminded sex delinquents they targeted for sterilization as children in need of protection, rather than simply disparaging them as innately inferior stock. Many women targeted for sterilization *were* young, and reformers thought they were protecting them from the stresses of parenting, while also protecting the unborn from being raised by an incompetent parent. Yet many so-called feebleminded Minnesotans were also child-like in a legal sense, for regardless of age they were wards of the state, permanent children who were deprived of the right to vote, own property, marry without the state's permission, and make their own medical decisions in exchange for the state's "protection." Moreover, sterilized feebleminded women often lost more than the right to procreate; they also lost the opportunity to raise children they already had. Carrie Buck had her daughter Vivian taken away. Although *Buck v. Bell* was a precedent-setting case pertaining specifically to sterilization, scholars' narrow focus on the surgery obscures the heartbreak of child removal. Examining sterilization through a child welfare lens puts the policy of "negative" eugenics in new light.[15]

The conceptual and administrative linkages between feeblemindedness and childhood also illuminate the changes to eugenics and disability policies in the postwar years. They explain why social worker Mildred Thomson, who administered Minnesota's sterilization program for nearly thirty-five years, was an early supporter of the parent movement and facilitated the 1950 creation of the National Association for Retarded Children (NARC; now The Arc), winning praise from disability advocates. From the nineteenth century, when evolutionary theory defined racialized and feebleminded persons as representing the childhood of the race, to post–World War II characterizations of "mentally retarded" citizens as perpetual children who never grew up, concepts of childhood and feeblemindedness were entwined.[16]

A fuller understanding of sterilization practice also necessitates "bringing the state back in" to the history of eugenics. Eugenic ideas received support internationally and across the political spectrum, but as sociologist Véronique Mottier points out, the precise purpose and implementation of actual policies were shaped by the specific institutional design of states. Administrative structures and individual bureaucrats played an important role in the creation of social policies. As the fine-grained state-level analyses by Johanna Schoen, Alexandra Minna Stern, and others demonstrate, eugenics practices and even eugenics theories developed at the state and local level; they did not simply originate with East Coast eugenics leaders, such as Charles Davenport and his associates at the ERO, nor did they spread fully formed across the country. An overemphasis on the theories and motivations of nationally prominent eugenicists obscures the manifold aims of state sterilization programs and how they were shaped by local leaders and preexisting institutional structures. It also makes it difficult to understand the considerable variation in the timing and intensity of sterilization policies. Nearly thirty years passed between the first state sterilization law (in Indiana in 1907) and the last, enacted in Georgia toward the end of the New Deal. In the end, thirty-two US states legalized eugenic sterilization at some point, but eighteen did not, and the number of recorded sterilizations ranged from thirty (in Arizona) to twenty thousand in California.[17]

The individuals targeted for sterilization and the procedures for making sterilization decisions also varied from state to state. Although male prisoners were the intended targets of the first sterilization law in Indiana, 60 percent of sterilization patients in California were classed as insane (their numbers almost equally divided between men and women). The racial profile of the sterilized population also varied across space and over time. In Virginia and North Carolina, southern states with particularly aggressive sterilization programs, the initial focus on white sex delinquents shifted dramatically in midcentury, when African Americans became the principal targets. In California, institutionalized persons with Spanish surnames were 3.5 times as likely to be sterilized as the institutionalized population as a whole. In Minnesota, by contrast, supposedly feebleminded white women like Le Sueur's narrator accounted for nearly two-thirds of all sterilizations, and the number of sterilizations dropped markedly and permanently during World War II. Scholars often attribute these differences to individual actors and to the class, race, and ethnic prejudices that shaped their understanding of inherited degeneracy. This book argues that numerous other factors, including fiscal considerations, administrative structures, a statute's construction and how local judges interpreted it, and the wishes of family members, were equally important. Even the chief administrator of Minnesota's eugenics law was so bothered by the apparent arbitrariness of feebleminded commitments and sterilizations in the 1930s that she conducted a study. But she found no consistent criteria for eugenic judgments, only the capricious cruelty of eugenics practice.[18]

The variation in state sterilization laws and practices is not incidental; it was constitutive of US sterilization policy as a whole. A fuller understanding of "eugenic" sterilization, then, requires an exploration of the intricacies of state-level policies and procedures and routine administrative practices at the state and local level. This book is a contribution to that project.

Eugenics and Welfare in US History

The affinities between eugenics and the welfare state have received a great deal of scholarly attention. Both ideas developed at about the same time in the late nineteenth century, were centrally concerned with the health and betterment of the population, and were based on the premise that individual interests were secondary to the collective good. As Gunnar Broberg and Nils Roll-Hansen demonstrated in their study of sterilization in Scandinavia, eugenics was an essential feature of the modern welfare state. Yet when news of the sterilization practices of Scandinavian social democracies came to light in the 1990s, they ignited a firestorm. Critics of social welfare entitlements used Sweden's aggressive sterilization program to denounce the welfare state as a Nazi-like program of social engineering, while writers on the left critiqued the racial concerns and surveillance techniques they considered intrinsic to modern states. The issue, however, was not simply a "too powerful" state. Rather, the expansion of welfare entitlements added a practical economic motive for eugenics. Since "inferior" people were key beneficiaries of social programs, Véronique Mottier observes, "limiting the numbers of 'weeds' in the national garden therefore appeared as a rational means of reducing welfare costs." Many policy makers and administrators who disagreed with eugenicists' hereditarian views supported the surgical fix of sterilization because it was cheaper than long-term financial support.[19]

In this book I use the term *welfare* to refer not to the planned welfare state entitlements associated with European social democracy or even the New Deal, but to America's miserly, locally based system of public assistance for the poor. The historian Michael Katz has described the United States as a "semiwelfare" state because benefits are not universal and ideological resistance to state-funded social programs remains strong. In contrast to European welfare states, US practice has been marked by local variation, a blurred boundary between public and private agencies, and a sharp division between social insurance entitlements and means-tested public assistance. Sterilization laws, which operated within state-level public welfare systems, had much in common with public assistance. As we shall see, the eugenic and welfare functions of sterilization policy overlapped when the object of eliminating the so-called unfit converged with keeping taxes and relief costs low, yet at times the welfare goal of providing assistance to the poor and the eugenics goal of reducing their numbers collided.[20]

Let me step back and define "the poor." While poverty has been pervasive throughout US history, the last third of the nineteenth century witnessed a growing distinction between the condition of being poor, an acknowledged fact of life for many people, and dependency on public relief, which was increasingly stigmatized and seen as a moral flaw. This book focuses on the dependent poor. I am particularly concerned with the "defective, dependent, and delinquent classes," a term introduced in a special schedule of the 1880 census by Frederick Wines and elaborated in the 1890s by sociologist Charles Henderson. The "defective, dependent, and delinquent" label was eventually superseded by "socially inadequate," the term preferred by eugenicists and written into a number of sterilization laws, but it still echoed in post–World War II constructions, such as the "culture of poverty" and "underclass." In all these formulations, the problem of dependency was the central concern.[21]

At the administrative level, state sterilization programs were shaped by two fundamentals of US welfare practice rooted in English poor law: local responsibility and the distinction between deserving and undeserving poor. From the Elizabethan Poor Law of 1601 until the 1900s, the smallest unit of government —the parish, township, or county—was charged with the care of the poor. Family members were obliged to support their destitute relatives, but local governments had the ultimate responsibility; they were required by law to support their economically dependent residents. Under Minnesota law, a resident was someone who had lived in a community for one year. At the turn of the twentieth century, most localities fulfilled their poor-relief obligations through indoor relief, and needy residents were usually placed in an institution, such as a poorhouse or poor farm. Outdoor relief, the public provision of food, coal, or other assistance to the poor in their own homes, was rare; officials believed that such assistance whet recipients' appetite for more relief and weakened their self-respect. Indoor relief, in contrast, provided shelter and a firm hand. It thus became the policy of choice both for the "worthy" poor, who were considered genuinely needy through no fault of their own, and for the "unworthy" paupers, whose destitution was allegedly caused by their own vice, intemperance, or immorality. Poorhouses required able-bodied residents to work and, in theory, taught them good habits of industry and morality. They also kept the hungry from starving, removed "ugly" disabled beggars and alcoholics from mainstream society, and were supposed to be so unpleasant that they deterred other poor people from applying for public relief. In practice, poorhouse conditions varied from locality to locality. Especially in rural communities with a low tax base, they were often rundown, vermin-infested farmhouses without indoor plumbing or protection from fire, where children lived alongside adults with mental health problems and contagious diseases. It is not surprising, then, that a "fear of the poorhouse became key to sustaining the work ethic in nineteenth century America," and that a crusade against gruesome poorhouse conditions captured the imagination of child welfare reformers.[22]

State governments took on more public welfare responsibilities in the late nineteenth century, as the boom-and-bust industrializing economy intensified poverty and an increasingly mobile population made the provision of poor relief too costly and complicated for small counties or towns. In the 1880s, many states, including Minnesota, created state boards of charities to standardize local relief practices and expenditures. Most also established specialized state institutions for poor people with distinct needs—orphans, juvenile delinquents, the deaf and blind, the mentally ill, and the so-called feebleminded. The Minnesota School for the Feebleminded was established at Faribault in southern Minnesota in 1879, and the Minnesota State Public School, a residential institution for dependent and neglected children, opened in Owatonna, just twenty miles away, seven years later. In the appropriate institution, it was believed, innocent children would be separated from hardened adult paupers and criminals who might corrupt them, and people with intellectual disabilities could live with "their own kind." Yet while placement in a reformatory, mental hospital, or orphanage was temporary for most people, for individuals labeled defective institutionalization became an end in itself.[23]

Despite the state's growing welfare role, poor relief largely remained a local responsibility. County poorhouses constituted the principal form of public relief until the 1930s, and counties also paid part of the cost of supporting indigent residents at the state institutions. Aid to Dependent Children, a state program to keep poor women and children out of poorhouses which became federal policy in 1935, was mostly financed and administered at the county level. Even after the federal government began to provide unemployment insurance and social security during the New Deal, public assistance for so-called unemployables remained paltry and locally run. As a result, the practice of sending vagrant strangers out of town—or simply refusing to pay for indigents whose legal residency was in dispute—remained an important part of welfare practice into the 1930s. In Minnesota, county judges and welfare workers used any tool at their disposal, including eugenic commitment, to keep local relief costs low, reduce the number of babies born to unwed mothers or welfare-dependent families, and shift a portion of the financial responsibility for destitute residents from the county to the state.

The distinction between deserving and undeserving poor formed another basis of US eugenic sterilization programs. Cost-conscious relief administrators had long distinguished between the blameless or "worthy" poor, who were widowed or elderly, and the "unworthy" paupers, whose misery and dependence on public relief were supposedly due to their own laziness, intemperance, or degeneracy. For most of US history, persistent poverty was viewed as a religious or moral failing, but from the 1870s onward it was increasingly seen through the lens of biology and viewed as hereditary or innate. Social scientists and charity officials, drawing on the popular science of evolution and degeneration, assumed that immoral behavior and a degraded environment could trigger anatomical changes that might be passed down to subsequent generations and cause reversion to a less civilized state. Yet the distinction between deserving and undeserving was fluid, at least for whites. Most charity reformers believed that degeneration could be reversed by clean living and a better environment. The descendants of paupers and criminals still had a chance to become the worthy poor.[24]

Such hopefulness faded in the early twentieth century, as French naturalist Jean Baptiste de Lamarck's theory of the inheritance of acquired characteristics was displaced by the genetic theories associated with the Austrian monk Gregor Mendel. Eugenicists such as Charles Davenport applied Mendel's laws to human heredity and determined that pauperism, criminality, and feeblemindedness were genetic traits unaffected by the environment and inherited in a predictable pattern. The practical impact of this new theory of heredity should not be overstated, however, for whether their failures were considered environmental or genetic, poor women classed as "bad" mothers were often prevented from raising their own children and transmitting their unfitness to their young.

While the distinction between deserving and undeserving poor has been a near constant in US history, who counts as deserving or undeserving has changed over time. It is no coincidence that the eugenics movement took off in the Progressive Era, just as maternalists and child welfare reformers attempted to bring a new group, innocent children, into the ranks of the deserving poor. Sociologist Viviana Zelizer argues that the economic and sentimental value of children underwent a profound transformation between the 1870s and 1930s. Childhood came to be seen as a period of dependency to be cherished and protected, and the expectation that children should contribute to the family economy was replaced by the ideal of the "economically 'worthless' but emotionally 'priceless' child." This "sacralization" of children's lives contributed to dramatic changes in welfare policy. For most of the nineteenth century, no special consideration was given to poor children, but the twentieth century was known as the "century of the child," in which children became the most deserving of the deserving poor. Reformers campaigned against child labor, undertook to remove innocent children from poorhouses and jails, where they might be harmed or corrupted by adults, and sought to ensure that every normal child had a stable home and a mother's love. They established juvenile courts, child health clinics, and mothers' pensions (also known as Aid to Dependent Children, or welfare), as well as enacting compulsory school laws and crusading against alcohol and vice.[25]

Progressive Era child welfare reforms reshaped the social experience of children and the relationship between families and the state. Juvenile courts and mothers' pension administrators monitored women's housekeeping abilities and children's school attendance and attempted to standardize child-rearing practices and sexual morality in poor people's homes. Child health clinics and graded schools imposed new standards of "normal" child development. The imposition of middle-class ideas about home life and morality on poverty-stricken families affected all working people, but it also inadvertently sharpened the distinction between the deserving and undeserving poor. This distinction was apparent at the first White House Conference on the Care of Dependent Children, hosted in 1909 by President Theodore Roosevelt, where two hundred prominent child welfare reformers passed a set of resolutions that reflected the emerging consensus that institutions were bad for most children and governments should assume some responsibility for children's well-being. The delegates differed on whether assistance to children should come from public relief or private charity, but all agreed that "home life is the highest and finest product of civilization," and that dependent mothers and children should be counted as deserving poor. "Children of parents of worthy character . . . and children of reasonably efficient and deserving mothers who are without the support of the normal breadwinner should, as a rule be kept with their parents. . . . Except in unusual circumstances, the home should not be broken up for reasons of poverty, but only for considerations of inefficiency or immorality." The White House Conference thus defined most dependent children as innocent and worthy of aid but kept those whose mothers were deemed immoral or inefficient—because of race, disability, or poor literacy or English language skills—within the undeserving poor. Progressive reformers thus created two strands of child welfare policy: one for the innocent and (newly) deserving children who were dependent and delinquent and another for youth viewed as undeserving or "defective." This two-track system shaped child welfare policies in the 1910s and 1920s and would be written into the fiscal and administrative structures of the New Deal welfare state.[26]

Local courts were a vital part of this bifurcated state-building process. Municipal courts administered an interconnected system of criminal and welfare policies that legitimated state intervention in working-class families, enforced the male-breadwinner role, and advanced the "regulatory enterprise of welfare as a *mode of governance*." In doing so, local courts created what historian Michael Willrich calls a "eugenic jurisprudence, the aggressive mobilization of law and legal institutions in pursuit of eugenic goals." The development of the juvenile court was central to this process in Minnesota. By the time the eugenic sterilization law was passed in 1925, juvenile courts already had jurisdiction over delinquent and dependent children under the age of eighteen, and probate courts, which acted as juvenile courts in rural counties, could commit "defectives" to state guardianship without the approval of parent or kin. As civil courts in Minnesota and elsewhere incorporated professional expertise and diagnostic categories such as feeblemindedness into everyday judicial practice, local judges gained unprecedented power to identify and control potential paupers and criminals *before* they became a welfare burden or committed a crime. In the era of eugenic jurisprudence, the legal rights of the potential troublemakers were set aside.[27]

Studying State Sterilization Laws: The Case for Minnesota

Recent scholarship on both eugenics and welfare has emphasized the importance of place. Although eugenics and child welfare were global movements, tangible policies developed in specific political-institutional contexts and were often implemented by local actors who did not always act in concert with the larger movements' stated aims. When compared to the more aggressive and better-known programs in California, Virginia, and North Carolina, for example, Minnesota's sterilization program seems relatively restrained. Minnesota did not target young children or teenagers, and operations were only performed on individuals already committed to state guardianship as feebleminded or insane. At least 2,350 Minnesotans were sterilized, but as will be discussed in chapter 4, even when Minnesota's sterilization program was at its peak, the state only ranked eighth in the number of sterilizations reported per 100,000 people. The unremarkable quality of Minnesota's sterilization program makes it especially worthy of study. The tendency to focus on the racist intent and impact of sterilization programs makes states like North Carolina seem the norm, but prior to 1945 more sterilization operations were performed on poor whites in midwestern states like Minnesota than in all the former Confederate states combined.[28] A case study of Minnesota expands our understanding of the spectrum of sterilization programs.

Minnesota's example also gives us tools to understand the overlooked role of welfare and bureaucracy in sterilization practice. As mentioned above, Minnesota's eugenic sterilization program operated within a child welfare system and program of legal guardianship for people with intellectual disabilities which won national praise. As late as 1962, President John F. Kennedy's Panel on Mental Retardation commended Minnesota's guardianship program as a model for other states.[29] Explaining this apparent paradox is a central objective of this book. It is also why a history of eugenic sterilization in Minnesota must begin in the 1880s, nearly forty years before the founding of the Minnesota Eugenics Society (MES) and the enactment of the state's sterilization law, and why it must extend long after the eugenics movement waned. Although Minnesota's sterilization law was signed in 1925 by a Republican governor who prided himself on cutting taxes and government spending, nearly half of Minnesota's recorded sterilizations were performed in the late 1930s, when a left-wing Farmer–Labor government was in power. Sterilizations continued after Republicans regained the statehouse in 1939 and only dropped off during World War II because of a shortage of medical personnel. Minnesota, unlike southern states, reported little sterilization in the 1950s and 1960s. But the law remained on the books until 1975.

The distinctive administrative structure of Minnesota's sterilization program allows us to begin to untangle eugenics rhetoric from the routine implementation of sterilization as a child welfare policy. Most sterilized Minnesotans were feebleminded "sex delinquents," unmarried mothers like Le Sueur's narrator, or older women with large families thought to be a burden on the welfare system; the men tended to be sex offenders considered a threat to the innocent child. Although most state officials assumed that "mental deficiency" was inherited, their chief concern was the "dependent" poor—in the present, even more than the future. Indeed, those who designed and implemented the sterilization law touted its economic and institution-management benefits more than its eugenic goals. Some even saw sterilization as a way to bring some feebleminded women into the ranks of the deserving poor—or, at least, into the ranks of those deemed harmless enough to live and work outside an institution. Just as juvenile courts and mothers' pensions allowed *delinquent* and *dependent* children to stay out of jail and avoid the state orphanage, eugenic sterilization was thought to benefit *defective* "children" by letting them live and work outside the institution under an expanding network of social work surveillance and supervision.

Minnesota's rural economy and tradition of Populist activism also challenge the simplistic notion that eugenics policies were supported mostly by urban elites. At the turn of the twentieth century, the state's economic growth was spurred by three rural industries—farming, lumbering, and mining—and the population stayed largely rural until World War II. Although the majority of Americans were city dwellers by 1920, nearly 56 percent of Minnesotans still lived in the country, and 37 percent were farmers. As late as 1950, nearly 20 percent of Minnesotans still lived on farms. This sizable rural population shaped Minnesota's political culture. Although the Republican Party dominated the executive branch, except during the Depression, popular anger at wealthy bankers, railroad magnates, mine owners, and middlemen fostered an unusually successful farmer–labor alliance. From the 1890s, when the fiery Minnesota Populist Ignatius Donnelly penned the preamble to the famous Omaha Platform of the new People's Party, to the turbulent 1930s, when Farmer–Labor governor Floyd Olson insisted that it was the government's responsibility to relieve the suffering of the people, populism reverberated through Minnesota politics. At the same time, the Populists' insistence that "wealth belongs to him who creates it" carried a message for those at the bottom as well as the top of the economic scale. Few Minnesotans expressed any sympathy for people who were disabled or dependent, or for the paupers, defectives, "Indians," and "white trash" they thought would not (or could not) work. The Populists' producer mentality was woven into the fabric of Minnesota politics and reinforced the distinction between the deserving and undeserving poor. Even socialist writer Meridel Le Sueur drew a distinction between her unwed-mother narrator, who was wrongly diagnosed as feebleminded, and the "cracked ones" who really did have feeble minds.[30]

Finally, Minnesota's large German and Scandinavian populations (considered racially superior "Nordics" by some eugenicists) complicate the conventional eugenics-equals-scientific-racism paradigm. Some Minnesota eugenicists did speak about preventing the degeneration of the superior white race, and the feebleminded label did reflect, to some extent, the "tainted whiteness" of those considered sexually impure or from the wrong ethnic or racial background. Yet while nationally prominent eugenicists accentuated the supposedly low mentality of American Indians and African Americans, there is no evidence that sterilization administrators in Minnesota focused on any particular racial or ethnic group. The state's black population, located mostly in the Twin Cities, was very small, and although Minnesota was one of the most "foreign" US states in the early twentieth century, the evidence suggests that immigrants were sterilized in proportion to their population. In 1900, nearly three-quarters of the state population were immigrants or the children of immigrants, mostly from Germany and Scandinavia. As late as 1930, more than one-half of Minnesotans still were foreign born or had at least one foreign-born parent, and despite increasing numbers of southern and eastern Europeans, an astonishing 34 percent of Minnesotans were of German, Norwegian, or Swedish birth or parentage. The anti-immigrant views expressed by eugenicists in other states were clearly a nonstarter in Minnesota, where Norwegians and Swedes were a powerful political force.[31]

This is not to say that ethnic prejudice and racial discrimination were muted. German Minnesotans were subjected to a fierce and sometimes violent Americanization campaign during World War I, the smoldering racism against the state's relatively small African American communities exploded into public view when three black men were lynched in Duluth in 1920, and Minneapolis was dubbed the "capital of anti-Semitism in the United States" in the 1940s. While there is no denying the racist discourse of national eugenics leaders, Minnesota's sterilization program peaked in the 1930s, after the racially tinged diatribes about the menace of the feebleminded were supplanted by ethnically based and often anti-Semitic allegations of disloyalty and communism.[32] The development and everyday operation of Minnesota's sterilization program owed less to abstract ideas about preventing the degeneration of the white race than to practical concerns with keeping relief costs low by controlling dependency, delinquency, and sex.

Given Minnesota's sizable indigenous population and the conceptual link between eugenics and scientific racism, one might reasonably assume that Native Americans were specifically targeted for sterilization. In support of this assumption, one could point out that Minnesota's eugenics program began in the 1880s, when the expropriation of indigenous lands was ongoing, and came to a formal end in the 1970s, when a nationwide scandal about mass sterilization in Indian Health Service (IHS) hospitals was brewing. Yet although I identified nine women sterilized in the 1930s as indigenous, I found no evidence of a targeted eugenics campaign. Some "Indians" were sent to the Minnesota School for the Feebleminded, but the sterilization medical records do not list race or tribal status, and there are few references in the state archives to the eugenic sterilization of indigenous women or men. Enforced poverty and child removal, rather than medical intervention, seem to have characterized Minnesota's "eugenics" policy toward indigenous communities well into the 1930s. Health conditions on the reservations were appalling, and death rates from diseases such as tuberculosis were high. This finding is consistent with eugenics programs in Virginia and North Carolina, which initially targeted whites but focused on blacks after World War II, and the Canadian province of Alberta, where First Nations and Métis communities were specifically targeted only in the final years of the eugenics program, which ended in 1972. Those jurisdictions, unlike Minnesota, had aggressive eugenic sterilization programs well into the 1960s. Minnesota authorized few eugenic surgeries after World War II.[33]

The relative absence of Anishinaabe or Dakota women and men from the Minnesota sterilization records speaks to a central argument of this book: the importance of fiscal politics and administrative routines. Minnesota's sterilization law applied only to feebleminded or insane wards of the state, whereas most people living on reservations were wards of the *federal* government. Since relief was a local responsibility (even during the New Deal), county judges and welfare boards had an economic incentive to commit the nonindigenous dependent poor to state guardianship—while denying any responsibility for tribal members on the grounds that they fell under the jurisdiction of the federal Indian Service. Jurisdictional disputes were complex, but in spite of some important welfare interventions in the 1930s, most Ojibwe in northern Minnesota had little access to white-dominated hospitals and health services until the postwar period, after routine eugenic sterilizations declined. When allegations of sterilization abuse in IHS hospitals came to light in the mid-1970s, they exposed the depressing persistence of racism, America's miserly welfare politics, and culturally biased ideas about unfit mothering and children's social needs. Under the law, however, these were "contraceptive" sterilizations. They were not performed under the state's eugenics law, and they are beyond the scope of this book. Further research on coerced sterilization in indigenous communities is urgently needed.[34]

Documenting Sterilization

Since the 1990s, the courageous testimony of sterilization survivors has reshaped scholars' thinking and writing about eugenic sterilization. Survivors such as Canada's Leilani Muir have told their personal stories of involuntary medical procedures and systemic abuse in the public institutions, and they have demanded formal apologies and recompense from state and provincial governments. Individuals once labeled mentally defective and forced to spend much of their lives in a state institution have demonstrated their ability to live and work independently and become valuable members of society.[35] Yet the eugenics survivors whose stories are known today mostly came of age after World War II. We know surprisingly little about the larger numbers of individuals who were labeled unfit and sterilized in the interwar period, when eugenics was mainstream and social workers openly pushed for sterilization. This book is an attempt to reconstruct some of their histories.

Documenting eugenic sterilization in any period presents unique methodological problems because it requires uncovering information that many people would prefer to remain secret. State and county officials, worried about lawsuits or bad publicity, may have "lost" or destroyed records. Persons touched by eugenics policies, either directly or as a member of an affected family, were often unable, unwilling, or too ashamed to let their stories be known. Numerous operations were performed outside the law by private and state-employed physicians, and an untold number went unrecorded. The actual number of eugenic sterilizations performed in Minnesota is undoubtedly much higher than the 2,350 listed in most historians' reports. That number comes from a 1963 report by the pro-sterilization Human Betterment Association in California, and the law remained on the books for another twelve years.[36]

The difficulties of documenting the surgeries performed under Minnesota's eugenic sterilization law are compounded by the decentralized nature of the state's child welfare system. Although some states established eugenics boards that authorized (and recorded) sterilizations, the Minnesota law applied only to individuals already committed to state guardianship by a probate judge. The state's three-step eugenic sterilization procedures—judicial commitment, institutionalization, and finally surgery—involved numerous steps by agents from a variety of professional backgrounds working at different levels of government. The sterilization process began at the local level, when a school official, police officer, or child welfare worker first identified an individual as possibly feebleminded or insane. A probate judge decided whether the person met the legal definition of feeblemindedness (or insanity) and whether to commit him or her to state guardianship or a psychiatric hospital. The State Board of Control, a three-person panel appointed by the governor, functioned as guardian of the "feebleminded ward" and decided whether he or she should be institutionalized. Then, a panel composed of the superintendent of the School for the Feebleminded, a psychologist, and a Board of Control representative decided whether the individual should be sterilized. Although the Board of Control issued the final authorization for surgery, a family member had to provide written consent. In cases of insanity, the law required consent from the patient. Specific sterilization decisions in Minnesota were thus shaped by numerous individuals and an assortment of factors, including local law enforcement and welfare needs, concerns about overcrowding in the state institution, electoral politics (for the probate judges were elected officials), and family dynamics.

It is impossible to recover the life stories, viewpoints, or even the names of most individuals sterilized under Minnesota's eugenics law, but we can learn a great deal about officials' reasoning from the published reports and internal correspondence of the Minnesota School for the Feebleminded and other state institutions, and we can catch glimpses of the men and women who were sterilized. To better understand who was sterilized and why, I compiled a database of the Faribault State School and Hospital's Record of Sterilization Cases, which listed the first thousand eugenic surgeries performed at the institution hospital, and I attempted to trace sterilization patients as they proceeded through the welfare system. I compared the medical record of sterilization cases with the admissions registers of the Faribault School, case files from the Home School for delinquent girls, county welfare board minutes, and the records of several state mental hospitals. Although the story I have been able to reconstruct is partial, it reveals much about the varied meanings of feeblemindedness, the routine treatment of individuals classed as mentally deficient, the troubling nature of the state's power over children and vulnerable adults, and state-sanctioned violations of human rights.

Both the incompleteness of the historical record and the importance of historical research on eugenics were brought home to me in an e-mail correspondence I had a few years ago with the great-niece of "Edna Collins," an allegedly feebleminded woman whose sterilization at age eighteen I wrote about in *Minnesota History*. My correspondent, an architect, had been researching her family and recognized the description of Edna's mother, a polio survivor said to have a "crippled arm." In a series of e-mails, she told me about the impressive educational and professional accomplishments of a family whose "stock" had been considered bad. I learned the unsettling information that Edna's mother had nine children, but only five grandchildren. My correspondent noted that Edna's case file showed that her "acting out," the main symptom of her supposed feeblemindedness, developed after she was molested by an elderly man when she was nine or ten years old. She also told me that her great-uncle had been sterilized. This last point was startling news, since I had no record of his surgery. I combed through my files again and again. Perhaps, I thought, Edna's brother was sterilized at Faribault, but an accidental or intentional clerical error kept his surgery out of the record books. Perhaps he was sterilized at a different facility, where records were never kept (or were kept at a different location so I never found them). Or perhaps, as we later concluded after finding his descendants, Edna's brother had not been sterilized at all. My correspondent's side of the family simply assumed that he had the operation because he spent part of his youth at Faribault, and the family had drifted apart. Plainly, the impact of Minnesota's eugenics program went far beyond the actual surgery. Individuals and entire families were mortified and stigmatized; family ties were broken. "That Minnesota took away the possibility of there being more people like my grandfather, I can't even describe the feeling," my correspondent wrote. "I now understand better why my grandfather left Minnesota as soon as he could and returned only twice the rest of his life."[37]

This book traces Minnesota's eugenic sterilization program for the "feebleminded" from its origins at the end of the nineteenth century until its official end in the 1970s. Chapter 1 explores the twin foundations of Minnesota's sterilization law in the eugenics and child welfare movements prior to 1917. The chapter begins with a review of nineteenth-century welfare policy and then proceeds to the Minnesota School for the Feebleminded at Faribault, where Superintendent A. C. Rogers, a nationally prominent expert on mental deficiency and eugenics, advanced the idea that fertile feebleminded women were a menace to society and should be placed under state guardianship and segregated for life. It then moves to Minneapolis, where child welfare reformers established community services and a juvenile court that extended state authority over poor families. The chapter ends with the 1917 Children's Code, which liberalized policies for delinquent, dependent, and illegitimate children but authorized the compulsory institutionalization of so-called defectives and provided the legal and administrative foundation for Minnesota's sterilization law. Chapter 2 examines state welfare officials' growing support for a sterilization law following the enactment of the Children's Code, as well as the bitter conflict between the hard-line MES and the welfare-oriented State Board of Control. The very public dispute between the eugenics society and the state officials who actually wrote and administered Minnesota's sterilization law underscores the gap between hard-line eugenics discourse and everyday welfare practice.

The three middle chapters examine the routine operation of Minnesota's eugenic commitment and sterilization laws. Chapter 3 examines who was designated feebleminded and who got to decide. It analyzes the concept of feeblemindedness which justified commitment, institutionalization, and, ultimately, sterilization, but it also emphasizes the fiscal and welfare considerations that shaped specific adjudications of mental deficiency. Chapter 4 shows how surgical sterilization functioned as the "price of freedom" from the state institution and explores the developments in social casework which accompanied the policy shift away from eugenic segregation and toward community living after sterilization. Chapter 5 examines the routinization of "eugenic" institutionalization and sterilization as the state bureaucracy expanded during the New Deal and the repudiation of those practices around the time of World War II. I argue that the growing opposition to the institutionalization and sterilization of the so-called feebleminded owed as much to new ideas about social welfare entitlements as to a changed outlook on eugenics. The irony that Minnesota's Annex for Defective Delinquents opened on the grounds of a men's prison in 1945, just as the sterilization program was winding down, underscores the need to see institutionalization and sterilization as two interrelated components of a single policy.

Chapter 6 and the conclusion analyze the postwar transformations in eugenics and welfare by exploring both the changes and continuities in the state program for the "mentally retarded" after 1945. Minnesota's mental institutions came under fire in the postwar years, just as the newly formed Minnesota Association for Retarded Children (MARC) and the new field of genetic counseling began calling attention to intellectual disability in middle-class families and describing "mentally retarded" persons as perpetual children. The 1960s War on Poverty and expansion of biomedical research on mental retardation further weakened the purported connection between race, class, and intelligence. Despite the resurgence of punitive sterilization proposals targeting poor black women in the South, most Minnesota reformers in the 1960s were more concerned with combating poverty than imposing a surgical "fix" on the poor. Minnesota's sterilization law was repealed in 1975, and the Faribault Regional Center (as the School for the Feebleminded was then called) shut down in 1998. Governor Tim Pawlenty signed an official apology in 2010. By then, most Minnesotans condemned eugenics, which they now associated with southern racism and German Nazism. Yet their abstract repudiation ignored the Minnesota sterilization law on the books until the 1970s and obscured the durability of the fiscal arrangements, bureaucratic structures, and social prejudices that continue to shape the state's welfare policy.

Despite significant improvements in the legal rights of people with disabilities and a formal apology for past abuses, US welfare practice and thus the social experience of poor women and men remain much the same. Political expediency and tax-cut fervor have drastically reduced the social services and income supports available to welfare-dependent families, juvenile delinquents, and individuals with disabilities. Local courts make rulings that remove the children and curtail the parenting rights of marginalized women who might have been labeled feebleminded in another era. Youthful "sex offenders" are characterized as predators and branded for life, and the policy of eugenic segregation has a parallel in mass incarceration. The Faribault School for the Feebleminded is now a medium-security prison.[38] In exploring the welfare function of eugenics policies in the past, this book provides an opportunity to reflect on the eugenic implications of child protection and welfare practices today.

CHAPTER ONE

THE FEEBLEMINDED MENACE AND THE INNOCENT CHILD

When Mildred Thomson took up her post as director of Minnesota's Department for the Feeble-Minded in 1924, she was surprised to find that her agency was part of the state children's bureau and she would share her staff of six women with the units for dependent and neglected children, unmarried mothers, and the blind. Years later, the longtime administrator of Minnesota's eugenic sterilization law recalled that she initially found it odd that a program for feebleminded adults had emerged from the Commission on Child Welfare, but she enjoyed the tie-in with children and the opportunity to work with the bureau's female staff.[1]

Why did a program to segregate and sterilize the feebleminded operate from the state's children's bureau, and what was the impact of this administrative arrangement? The answers to these questions reveal both the deep-rooted connection between the supposed menace of the feebleminded and the idea of the innocent child and the importance of administrative structures. They also shed light on the complex relationship between eugenics and progressive child welfare reform. Many historians, pointing to eugenicists' trust in science, expertise, and governmental solutions to social problems, have analyzed eugenics as a progressive reform. Some stress the diversity and complexity of the progressive movement and emphasize the differences between child welfare reform, which assumed the malleability and potential of young children and sought to improve their environment, and eugenics, which considered poor people innately inferior and aimed to control their breeding. Others stress the inseparability of child welfare and eugenics, both of which extended state control over sexuality and reproduction and narrowed the definition of a worthy parent. The campaign for mothers' pensions, aimed at deserving mothers, and compulsory sterilization laws, which targeted the unfit, were simply two sides of the same coin. In this telling, the story of progressive welfare reform is a "dark story," a cautionary tale about reformers' arrogance and the dangers of state power.[2]

This chapter advances a somewhat different perspective. Analyzing eugenics as a public welfare policy, it places eugenic segregation and sterilization policies in the context of a long-term effort to reduce the apparent burden of the "defective, dependent, and delinquent classes," the undeserving poor who relied on public relief. In many ways, eugenics reflected a very old impulse, and it simply "tossed the mantle of science over the ancient distinction between the worthy and the unworthy poor." But eugenics policies were also linked to a new shift away from institutional settings and toward a more generalized system of surveillance in a disciplinary society. Sterilization in most states was a precondition for institutional discharge, and sterilization policy mirrored the move away from indoor relief—assistance that required the recipient to live in a public institution or poorhouse to be eligible for aid—and toward community casework and supervision. As we shall see, this shift began with progressive efforts to remove dependent and delinquent children from poorhouses and jails, but it did not extend to "defectives" until eugenic sterilization was legalized in the 1920s.[3]

The fusion of child welfare reform and eugenics also emerged from the cultural transformations in both childhood and disability which took hold around 1900. Although the idea of childhood as a distinct stage of life dates back to the eighteenth century, when philosophers such as Jean-Jacques Rousseau described children as naturally innocent and uncorrupt, it was not until the period between 1870 and 1930 that the ideal of the "economically 'worthless' but emotionally 'priceless' child" was written into social policy and extended beyond the middle class. To progressive reformers, children were impressionable and supposed to be dependent, and child-centered policies, such as the juvenile court, were necessary to shield them from corrupt adults. Innocent children, almost always imagined as white, represented the future of the nation, the possibility of human perfection, and the eugenic ideal. Yet the symbolic power of the innocent child depended on the opposing image of the wicked or "defective" child, often represented as a darkened, sexualized throwback to a primitive past. It is no coincidence that the myth of the menace of the feebleminded, which powered eugenics policy making, arose in tandem with the imagined vulnerability of the innocent child. Neither image would have had as much power without the other.[4]

The link between feebleminded menace and innocent child did not rest at the level of discourse alone. As the existence of a department for the feebleminded within Minnesota's children's bureau suggests, the dynamic tension between these two ideas was also built into the policies and administrative structure of the emerging welfare state. This chapter explores the origins of this bifurcated child welfare policy, which established the state's responsibility for the care and support of "innocent" dependent and delinquent children while also asserting its control over "defectives" defined as a public menace. I follow three different but intersecting groups of welfare reformers as they worked to dismantle the amorphous concept of the "defective, delinquent, and dependent classes," which had dominated welfare thinking in the late nineteenth century, and to redefine dependent and delinquent children—but not defectives—as part of the deserving poor. A. C. Rogers, the superintendent of the Minnesota School for the Feebleminded, developed a scientific rationale for the permanent segregation of "defectives" by defining feeblemindedness as a burden and a menace and established the custodial institution for the feebleminded as a site of eugenics–welfare control. Meanwhile, a different but overlapping group of mostly urban reformers created the social welfare infrastructure needed to "protect" dependent and delinquent youth living in their own homes. Minneapolis judge Edward F. Waite led the efforts to establish and consolidate the state's legal authority over poor children, first in his role as a juvenile judge in Hennepin County and then as the Child Welfare Commission's chair. The Women's Welfare League of Minneapolis, an elite group of "maternalist" reformers, helped establish the moral regulations and social services that made it possible to monitor sexually delinquent girls—and, in the 1920s, sterilized feebleminded women—living in the community.

By 1917, Minnesota reformers with different but complementary agendas had transformed an unwieldy set of charity initiatives that treated chronically poor people of all ages as one degenerate mass—the defective, dependent, and delinquent classes—into a two-track child welfare policy. One track reflected a new optimism and new opportunities for dependent and delinquent children, who were now defined as the deserving poor. The other track was reserved for so-called defectives, who remained undeserving—and institutionalized. The two tracks were closely connected; indeed, delinquents and dependents might not have been given a second chance in the community had not the harsher institutional treatment continued for the rest. The two tracks were officially bound together in 1917 with the passage of Minnesota's Children's Code, the crowning achievement of the state's child welfare movement and the foundation of its eugenic sterilization law.

Unfit and Undeserving in the Nineteenth Century

When the British scientist Francis Galton coined the word *eugenics* in the 1880s, the United States was in the midst of a great economic upheaval. Spectacular industrial growth had turned the United States into a global power, but it also brought financial panics, cyclical unemployment, and a series of agrarian crises that intensified poverty for many Americans and upset time-honored ideas about the deserving and undeserving poor. The growth of cities and the rise of wage labor had led to unparalleled migration, industrial accidents, and periodic dependency that disrupted families and heightened both the vulnerability and resentments of the poor. The customary local mechanisms of poor relief—families, soup kitchens, charities, churches, and poorhouses—were inadequate to the task. Urban elites faced both a humanitarian crisis and a problem of social control.[5]

The growing visibility of urban poverty and a series of bitter labor disputes led in the 1870s and 1880s to a new welfare strategy, scientific charity, a remarkably mean-spirited effort to reduce relief costs and fix the character of the poor. As public begging, tramping, and relief applications increased, charity reformers assumed that too-generous assistance was weakening the character of the recipient and encouraging fraud. First in eastern cities and then across the country, they created charity organization societies to combat pauperism and dependency by systematizing charitable giving and restricting access to public relief. In the view of these charity reformers, only a truly scientific approach, based on careful investigation, coordination among relief agencies, and "friendly visits" to recipients, would ensure that aid was morally uplifting and only went to the deserving poor. In the National Conference of Charities and Correction (NCCC), a professional association founded in 1874, charity organizers, public welfare officials, institution superintendents, and religious reformers had a forum in which to discuss the causes of dependency, how to make welfare administration more efficient, and the problems of the "defective, dependent, and delinquent classes." Through the NCCC, the proponents of scientific charity shaped the philosophies and practices of welfare officials across the nation.[6]

Most scholarship on charity reform focuses on cities, but the theory of scientific charity also resonated in the "frontier" state of Minnesota, where the very idea of poor relief, which was funded from property taxes paid by struggling farmers, clashed with the ideal of the self-sufficient pioneer. Although Minnesota Territory became a state in 1858, white settlement had been slow until the mid-1870s, when railroad construction and the forced removal of indigenous communities intensified lumber production and agricultural development. The state's population tripled between 1870 and 1890. Wheat farming and, later, dairying dominated the fertile lands of the Southeast and West, especially after the lumber industry's decline. In the North, the development of the Mesabi Iron Range in the 1880s and 1890s made Minnesota one of the nation's leading iron producers, as well as a hotbed of labor radicalism. Immigrant labor was vital to Minnesota's economic development, as it was to economic growth across the nation. By the 1890s, nearly one-third of state residents were European immigrants, mostly from Germany, Norway, and Sweden.[7]

Even though Minnesota's economy was booming, most of the state's residents were rural and poor. Work was seasonal, and a volatile wheat market, high railroad freight rates, and low prices kept many farmers in a deficit position and strained the resources of local communities traditionally responsible for relief. Minnesota's first poor law, enacted in 1864, made the counties responsible for supporting indigent residents whose families could not care for them. The county commissioners, as superintendents of the poor, were empowered to levy poor taxes, build poor farms and workhouses, bind out minors as apprentices, and drive indigent nonresidents—the undeserving poor—out of their community. (As explained earlier, legal residency for welfare purposes was established at one year.) Although the state provided some assistance for disasters, such as the devastating grasshopper plagues of the 1870s, most aid was local, parsimonious, and limited to those considered truly needy and deserving. At the height of the grasshopper crisis, Minnesota governor John Pillsbury reminded supplicant farmers that "poverty and deprivation are incidents of frontier life at its best" and averred that state-level aid to the weak would merely drain the resources of the more self-reliant farmers and lead the unscrupulous to "habitual beggary." The secretary of Minnesota's Board of Charities, Reverend Hastings Hart, similarly believed that people who drink from the "stream of public relief acquire an insatiate appetite for it," and that pauperism was caused by the "excessive disbursement" of relief.[8]

This miserly localism did not go unchallenged. Populists and labor radicals across the Midwest urged the state and federal governments to restrict the power of corporations and take responsibility for stimulating the economy and relieving poor people's poverty and distress. In the preamble to the People's Party's famous Omaha Platform of 1892, Minnesota's Ignatius Donnelly forcefully denounced the wealthy bankers and railroad magnates who amassed great fortunes by stealing the "fruits of the toil of millions" and called for a graduated income tax, public ownership of the railroads, and political reforms that would put government back in the hands of the "plain people." At the same time, the Populists shared charity reformers' antipathy toward the "pauper and criminal classes of the world." They thought of themselves as the deserving poor and, like urban elites, worried about society's drift into "physical degeneracy and mental imbecility." Populists stressed the urgency of economic and social reforms to make the world a "fit abode" for superior people such as themselves.[9]

Widespread poverty and unrest led to intense discussions at the NCCC and an increasing reliance on the natural and social sciences to explain and resolve the problems of the "defective, dependent, and delinquent classes." The growing influence of social science and evolutionary theory can be seen in three important texts. The first and best known is Richard Dugdale's famous *"The Jukes": A Study in Crime, Pauperism, Disease and Heredity* (1877), the first eugenics family study and the prototype for similar studies sponsored in the 1910s by the ERO. Dugdale, a prison reformer, traced the lineage of six relatives he found in a rural New York jail back seven generations and determined that over the course of seventy-five years, this one family had produced some 1,200 prostitutes, thieves, paupers, and beggars, costing New York State $1,308,000 in relief costs, trials and imprisonments, and lost revenue. *"The Jukes"* was one of the first studies to use statistics to chart the economic and social costs of bad heredity and one of the first to conceptualize the undeserving poor by means of evolution science. It reflects the powerful influence of French biologist Jean Baptiste de Lamarck's theory of the inheritance of acquired characteristics, which held that the damaging effects of (for example) alcoholism and venereal disease could be transmitted to subsequent generations. Dugdale believed that the manifestations of inherited degeneracy did not always take the same form—thus, insanity in one generation could produce pauperism or criminality in the next, sexual immorality could produce idiocy, and so on—and he further believed that the effects of a bad inheritance could be reversed through public health reform, early childhood education, and a better moral environment. "The tendency of heredity is to produce an environment which perpetuates that heredity; thus the licentious parent makes an example which greatly aids in fixing habits of debauchery in the child," he explained; "the correction is change of environment." Yet although Dugdale himself believed in possibilities of environmental reform, his frightening depiction of inherited degeneracy had a much greater impact. According to Nicole Hahn Rafter, "'*The Jukes*' gave the nascent eugenics movement a central confirmational image." The picture of an inbreeding rural family too lazy to look for work and living in a hovel epitomized the supposedly innate unfitness of poor "white trash."[10]

While Dugdale traced inherited degeneracy in one family over several generations, Frederick Wines's special schedule of the 1880 census provided a sobering statistical snapshot of its prevalence at a single point in time. Wines, a Protestant minister, secretary of the Illinois Board of Public Charities, and one of the NCCC's founders, used census data and physicians' responses to questionnaires to count "unfortunates" in institutions and, for the first time, outside of them as well. His 1880 *Report on the Defective, Dependent and Delinquent Classes of the Population of the United States* reached two disturbing conclusions: the ratio of "idiots" and "insane" to the general population was substantially higher than in the 1870 census, and the vast majority of defectives received no institutional care.[11]

Wines created the alliterative "three Ds" by combining seven overlapping groups of "unfortunates"—the insane, idiotic, blind, deaf and dumb, homeless children, paupers, and criminals—into a single metaclass of "defective types of humanity." He justified treating the seven groups as one on the grounds that they were essentially the same. Like Dugdale, he believed that whether the deficiency took one form or another was simply a matter of chance, writing, "There is a morphology of evil which requires to be studied."[12]

Despite Wines's moralistic language, his chief concern—like Dugdale's—was the burden on the public purse. The cost of caring for orphans, criminals, the insane, and the feebleminded absorbed a sizable share of tax revenues, Wines pointed out, and his census schedule was meant to tally the "wrong side of the balance sheet in making up the national account." In contrast to the regular census, which enumerated wealth and property, Wines's schedule calculated the tax burden that "civilization" had to bear. As historian Michael Katz points out, Wines's decision to group poor people from a variety of circumstances into one "metaclass" of defectives, and his assumption that their dependency was due to hereditary inferiority rather than structural factors such as seasonal employment, provided a scientific rationale for parsimonious relief policies and inexpensive institutional care. At the same time, Wines, like Dugdale, held a Lamarckian optimism about the prospects for environmental reform. His faith in the value of "preventive work among children" led him to support the juvenile court and other child welfare reforms.[13]

Dependency was also a central concern of Charles Richmond Henderson's popular sociology textbook, *Introduction to the Study of the Dependent, Defective and Delinquent Classes* (1893). Henderson, like Dugdale and Wines before him, used science and harsh eugenicist language to make the case for environmental reform. Henderson described the three Ds in eugenic terms, as " 'outcast' survivals of an imperfect past race . . . unfit to endure the strain of modern competition," but he too was principally concerned with pauperism, which he described as a contaminating influence, "the nest out of which all loathsome diseases of body and soul are hatched." In Henderson's view, paupers were social parasites who attached themselves to other members of the community and lived at their expense, weakening themselves in the process. Yet like Dugdale and Wines, he saw the solution to the interrelated problems of dependency, defectiveness, and delinquency in education, environmental reform, and Christian charity.[14]

Minnesota officials participated in these national discussions, and they responded to the growing concern about the "defective, delinquent, and dependent classes" with three lines of attack. The first was administrative: they tried to impose order, fiscal prudence, and state supervision over what they saw as a chaotic and too-generous system of relief. This emphasis on administration was in some ways a rational response to the stunning arbitrariness of locally administered relief. In the 1870s and 1880s, the state legislature passed more than twenty laws concerning the administration of relief. Some established the township as a community's primary relief authority, while others reasserted the county system. (The township system was preferred by those who thought that a smaller jurisdiction would make it easier to identify the undeserving, but the county system had the advantage of a larger tax base.) Since counties (or townships) funded and administered their own welfare systems, the everyday lives of poor Minnesotans varied tremendously. Arbitrariness and inequity lay at the foundation of public relief.[15]

State officials also tried to assert their control over state-funded public institutions. The first step to state authority came in 1883, when the legislature established an all-volunteer State Board of Corrections and Charities, which

Hastings Hart headed. Then, in 1901 the legislature created the State Board of Control, with three salaried members appointed (and, if necessary, removed) by the governor for overlapping six-year terms. The Board of Control was given full supervisory authority over nine of the state's charitable and penal institutions, including the School for the Feebleminded, and partial financial control over several others. Its mandate was to improve managerial efficiency, reduce expenditures, standardize record keeping, and eliminate "local influences and politics" from the institutional administration. The board was remarkably successful and uncontroversial, and its power and influence grew along with the state's population. In 1917, the Children's Code extended its authority beyond institutions, and the Board of Control became the state's central welfare agency.[16]

Minnesota officials' second strategy for controlling costs and arresting degeneracy focused on children. Henderson had argued that indiscriminate almsgiving was pauperizing for adults, but he believed that children were "proper objects of charity, since they are helpless . . . [and] youth is plastic." As Hastings Hart explained, "Environment, rather than heredity, controls the destiny of the normal child." He and other reformers believed that hereditary conditions such as feeblemindedness condemned a few children to lifelong dependency, but that a good environment would overcome bad heredity in the vast majority of cases, and even children of "questionable parentage" could develop into useful members of society. When Minnesota established separate state institutions for delinquents (1868), defectives (1879), and dependents (1886), it began the process of separating children from their unfit parents and untangling the three Ds.[17]

The 1886 creation of the State Public School for Dependent and Neglected Children is particularly important in this regard: it defined dependent children as the deserving poor and separated them from delinquents and defectives. Located in Owatonna, a prosperous farm community in southern Minnesota where well-to-do families usually needed an extra hand, the state school was conceived as a "temporary home" for youngsters under the age of sixteen who were adjudged dependent or neglected and "in suitable condition of body and mind to receive instruction." The children became wards of the state and lived in family-style cottages until they were placed out to work or adopted. The State Public School was not a penal institution and the children were not delinquent, Superintendent Galen A. Merrill declared, nor did they have any "taint of mental imperfection." Rather, they were all "fit subjects to be placed in good families" once their parents had relinquished custody and the "filth of the slums" and "poor-house marks" had been washed away. In Merrill's view, parental rights had to be terminated so the children could begin life anew. The state had a "moral obligation to its innocent children who need to be protected," he proclaimed. "There are parents who are not worthy to rear citizens of this republic." By taking innocent children away from undeserving parents, welfare institutions could turn children from the "defective, dependent, and delinquent classes" into the deserving poor.[18]

Owatonna's policy of cutting children off from their families of origin was not simply a way to eliminate the influence of "unfit" parents, however. It was also an economic policy that shifted the cost of supporting dependent children from the counties to the state. Most Owatonna children were either permanently adopted or apprenticed out until they reached the age of majority and became self-supporting, so sending a child to Owatonna almost always removed him or her permanently from the local relief rolls. A childhood at Owatonna was far removed from the dependency and sheltered ideal of the middle class, and many state schoolers suffered deeply from the forced separation from their families and, in some cases, physical or psychological abuse. Still, unlike youngsters who were considered defective or (before the juvenile court) delinquent, and unlike even their own parents, children at Owatonna were defined as the deserving poor. They were released from state control when they reached the age of majority and could—and usually did—grow up to be respected citizens and parents. In the 1890s, the juvenile court movement extended that innocence and deservingness to delinquents as well. In contrast, those sent to the School for the Feebleminded remained undeserving and were supposed to be institutionalized for life.[19]

This brings us to welfare officials' third strategy for controlling the three Ds: preventing "'gutter girl[s]' like Ada Juke" from transmitting their diseases, bad habits, and physical and moral degeneracy to their young. At a time when the womanly ideal was domestic, submissive, dependent, and chaste, charity reformers tended to see any sign of female independence, immodesty, or disreputable sexual behavior—such as prostitution, out-of-wedlock pregnancy, thievery, or the presence of venereal disease—as evidence of inherited defect. They stressed the urgency of removing pauper girls from poorhouses and the streets, lest they grow up to be mothers of criminals or bear illegitimate children who would become a public charge. Importantly, these reformers strongly believed that most girls could be saved if the intervention came in time, and even the daughter of dissolute parents could become a virtuous mother herself. But they did not doubt that a few unfortunates—those afflicted with feeblemindedness, epilepsy, syphilis, or moral imbecility—would have to remain in the institution for life so that they would never become parents. "The fecundity of the feeble-minded is proverbial," a Faribault politician declared bluntly in 1887, but permanent segregation in the Faribault School would "keep those whom we cannot cure and equip for life until they are past the reproducing age, and stamp out hereditary imbecility and epilepsy right here and now."[20] In this way, what had been a single welfare strategy for dealing with the mutable "defective, dependent, and delinquent classes" divided into two increasingly separate streams: one for dependents and delinquents who had the potential to be good citizens and mothers, and another for defectives, who had to remain institutionalized.

Containing the Feebleminded Menace: A. C. Rogers and the Faribault School

Reformers talked a lot about stamping out hereditary imbecility, but eugenics policies would have had little practical consequence if the state lacked the legal power, funding, and administrative capacity to implement them. This is something Dr. Arthur Custis Rogers, the superintendent of Minnesota's School for the Feebleminded, understood very well. As director of the Faribault School from 1885 until 1917, Rogers presided over "the best planned, best equipped and in my opinion, the best managed institution for the feebleminded in the world" (to quote the famous Massachusetts superintendent Walter Fernald). Rogers was the founding editor of the *Journal of Psycho-Asthenics*, the organ of the American Association for the Study of the Feeble-Minded, and chaired the first formal eugenics organization in the United States, the subcommittee on hereditary feeblemindedness of the American Breeders' Association's Eugenics Committee. Other superintendents achieved more publicity, but Rogers was recognized by his peers as one of America's leading experts on mental deficiency and eugenics. Upon his death in 1917, his fellow superintendents mourned the loss of their "mentor and guide" and agreed that modern work with the feebleminded "owes more to him than to any other man of his time."[21]

When Rogers became superintendent of the Faribault School in 1885, the idea that the so-called feebleminded were a menace to society was just beginning to take hold. Prior to the Civil War, most institutions for people with intellectual disabilities were based on the theories of French physician Edouard Seguin, who believed that even severely disabled "idiots" would benefit from physiological education and sensory training. In midcentury, however, Seguin's optimistic belief that people with intellectual disabilities could be economically productive gave way to a more cynical view of feeblemindedness as a principal source of pauperism, prostitution, and crime. Since the "bright hopes" of early leaders had not been realized, Rogers wrote, institutions enlarged their custodial departments and abandoned plans to prepare feebleminded children for the larger world. Increasingly, they portrayed feebleminded people as a burden to their families, communities, and the state. The change in attitude did not happen overnight, however. As late as the 1870s the sponsors of the proposed school for the feebleminded at Faribault still maintained that "all human beings are capable of improvement, and even the poor imbecile is not an exception to this rule."[22] Unfortunately, their optimism would not last long.

By 1890, the Faribault School was well established as a custodial institution.

It housed 169 male and 134 female "children," equally divided between two departments: a training school for those considered capable of some instruction, and a custodial department for the "unimprovable" who had to be institutionalized for life. Residents were called children regardless of age. Admissions records and photographs poignantly capture the wide range of disabilities and nondisabilities among Faribault inmates. Some inmates had identifiable intellectual disabilities and mobility impairments. Others had visible deformities or disfigurements. Still others had no visible disabilities at all. Many were epileptics, and many were women in their childbearing years, whose offspring supposedly posed a burden on the state. By 1910, the Faribault School had 1,194 inmates and was the fifth-largest institution for the feebleminded in the country.[23]

The growth of large custodial institutions for the feebleminded coincided with the harsh new approach to public welfare. Indeed, the two developments were related, for the post–Civil War assault on outdoor relief had made it nearly impossible for poor families to support dependent and disabled relatives at home, especially in economic hard times, and anti-begging ordinances were deployed with particular vehemence against people with visible disabilities. Yet even after the depression of 1893 caused many charity workers to rethink their assumption that dependency was caused by an individual's moral failings, they still tended to see the disabled and "undeserving" poor as feebleminded. Charity officials and institution superintendents met regularly at the NCCC, and superintendents also formed their own professional organization, the Association of Medical Officers of American Institutions for Idiotic and Feeble-Minded Persons (AMO), where they developed the idea of a new welfare institution, a feebleminded colony. This new custodial institution would house feebleminded people of all ages, sexes, and degrees of disability and be economical for the state because inmates did much of the work to sustain it. Indeed, feebleminded women were prioritized as custodial cases, not only because, if left unsupervised, they might become mothers and transmit their degeneracy to the next generation or inflict a charge on the county relief rolls, but also because their labor as cooks, housekeepers, seamstresses, and caregivers was essential to the institution's daily operation.[24]

The Faribault School also bore an intriguing similarity to another late nineteenth-century "child welfare" institution, the Indian boarding school. The resemblance is unsurprising: the Faribault area had long been a site of missionary activity to the Dakota and Ojibwe communities. Faribault's first mission school, attended by indigenous and white children, opened in 1858, and missionary teacher George B. Whipple was one of the first trustees of the School for the Feebleminded. Rogers himself had been a physician and clerk at the Forest Grove Indian Training School (later the Chemawa Indian School) in Oregon prior to assuming his position at Faribault. Boarding schools for "Indians" and institutions for the "feebleminded" were both sustained by Christian humanitarians who believed that removing children from their supposedly savage (or degenerate) cultures and families would protect them from worse cruelties, including extermination. Superintendents at both types of institutions had to defend their schools—and their "children"—from skeptical and even hostile communities. They also relied on students' unpaid labor. Rogers boasted that Faribault was the first school for the feebleminded to employ the "coordinate plan" of training, and he may have adapted the idea of moving students back and forth between elementary-level schoolwork and a half day of manual training (in tasks such as sewing and carpentry) from Indian boarding schools. Rogers also recognized the students' need for controlled leisure activities, music, and dance. He played Santa Claus at the annual Christmas festival and took the "children" on regular outings, such as picnics and boat rides. In the 1890s, the Faribault School also put on theatrical productions, operated a school band, and even fielded a football team, which in 1900 defeated the local high school, 16–11.[25]

The parallels between the Minnesota School for the Feebleminded and Indian boarding schools were not lost on Henry Benjamin Whipple, Minnesota's first Episcopal bishop and one of the town of Faribault's most famous residents. A prominent missionary and the brother of the Faribault School trustee, Bishop Whipple was a staunch assimilationist and powerful critic of US Indian policy, who won national attention for his successful campaign to secure pardons for hundreds of Dakota Sioux who were threatened with execution in the aftermath of the US–Dakota War. When the AMO held its annual meeting at Faribault in 1890, Bishop Whipple was one of five hundred local citizens to join the nation's superintendents to watch the students perform a complicated three-act operetta. After the performance, which was a "great triumph," the bishop made a stirring speech that compared the Faribault School to missionary work among Indians and commended it as the "highest evidence of Christian civilization."[26]

As five hundred townspeople attending a school event suggests, Rogers was acutely aware of the need for public support. He tried to win that support by simultaneously appealing to the public's pity for unfortunate "children" and playing on their fear and contempt. He spoke regularly before church and women's groups and mounted exhibits at state fairs. He also organized the AMO's exhibits at the 1893 World's Fair in Chicago and the 1904 Louisiana Purchase Exposition in St. Louis. In an insightful article on the 1904 exposition, James Trent has noted the contrast between the AMO exhibit organized by Rogers and the better-known anthropology displays, which placed Africans, Filipinos, and indigenous North Americans—real people from allegedly primitive races—on display in living exhibits. Deaf and blind students were also put on display, so Rogers's decision to showcase student penmanship and craftsmanship, not the people themselves, is significant. The AMO display was undoubtedly designed with fee-paying families and a budget-minded public in mind, and Trent stresses the contrast between the visual presentation, which was "benign, educational, and even optimistic," and the accompanying speeches, which stressed the urgency of preventing the feebleminded from propagating their kind. Rogers did not give any of the speeches, but the exhibit as a whole reflected his dual message: the feebleminded were a menace when they were at large in the community, but they were harmless when inside the school. In the institution, the feebleminded menace could become an innocent child.[27]

Rogers's dual image of feeblemindedness as alternately childlike and menacing was a well-considered strategy to get funding from the state legislature and persuade families to pay the school fees. Public distrust of so-called degenerates was deeply entrenched, and resentment of poor taxes was as well, so superintendents had to demonstrate that public monies were well spent. Rogers had to deal with critics who saw "Fool Schools" as a waste of the taxpayer's money and viewed any assistance to the feebleminded as a dangerous attempt to reverse the law of the survival of the fittest. He made the case for indefinite institutionalization by appealing to Minnesotans' child-saving aspirations, economic concerns, and sexual and eugenic fears. Pleading for compassion for vulnerable children, he noted that "nearly all feeble-minded children suffer continually . . . from forced comparisons with normal children" and needed the "friendly protection" of a residential school; otherwise, the "continual torture" they endured would render them "callous and ugly in disposition, a helpless burden to their friends and a nuisance to the neighborhood." Rogers also appealed to economic considerations, pointing out that institutionalization relieved families of the terrible burden of caring for disabled relatives and could move them from welfare dependency to self-support. Finally, and most important for our purposes, Rogers stirred up eugenic anxieties by describing fertile feebleminded women as a "medium for the reproduction of imbecility" and underscoring the economic and social costs of prematurely discharging them. Again and again, he called for the eugenic segregation of feebleminded women during their childbearing years.[28]

Still, Rogers responded to other superintendents' growing preoccupation with eugenic surgery with caution. He was fascinated by medical research suggesting a causal relationship between diseased sexual organs and insanity, and he was energized by the claims that castration or oophorectomy could cure compulsive masturbation, which he considered both a cause and consequence of insanity and degeneration. In the early 1890s, he publicly endorsed a surgical solution to medical problems that were "plainly attributable to sexual perversion" and performed some sterilization operations. But he objected to any surgery not performed for what he considered a therapeutic purpose and urged his fellow superintendents to proceed slowly. In 1905, Rogers translated and published a

Danish article that criticized the American obsession with sterilization, adding a prefatory reminder that not every American expert favored such "radical surgical treatment." He made the *Journal of Psycho-Asthenics* a forum for debate about eugenic surgery, but he himself remained skeptical, even after 1907, when Indiana passed the first sterilization law. Rogers supported the principle of sterilization in "certain well defined cases," but he did not support the sterilization bills introduced into the Minnesota legislature in 1911 and 1913.[29]

An institution administrator above all else, Rogers insisted that segregation, not sterilization, was the best way to ensure that the feebleminded never became parents. When other superintendents got carried away discussing surgical remedies and "arousing public alarm" about the feebleminded menace, Rogers would remark coolly that the AMO needed less bluster, more scientific research, and better institutions. Ultimately, he declared, "The extension of our work will depend more upon the *kind* of *institutions* we are building than any forensic advertising." Rogers's chief goal was to make institutionalization compulsory (and permanent) upon a court order, so that fertile women and other troublesome people could be prevented from early release. "We should be able to retain those that need the protection and mothering of the institution," he declared in child-saving language that masked the cruelty of the policy. "Our aim must be the permanent custodial care and control by the mother state, not merely of a few, but of the whole class of idiots and imbeciles." In 1917, the Minnesota legislature fulfilled Rogers's policy aspirations and enacted a compulsory commitment law. Ironically, he had died three months earlier.[30]

Welfare and Eugenics: The Institution in the Community

In the early 1900s, Rogers became involved with the budding eugenics movement. From then on, his conception of feeblemindedness was shaped by the hereditarian theories of Charles Davenport, the Harvard-trained founder of the ERO in Cold Spring Harbor, New York. Davenport was one of the first US scientists to apply Mendel's theory of inheritance to human beings. He theorized that height, eye color, and even feeblemindedness were single traits, or unit characters, passed down from generation to generation in a predictable pattern. Each trait was governed by two factors (genes), and if both parents had the same gene, the trait would appear in the next generation. But if the child inherited two different genes, the offspring would manifest only one of the parental traits. A dominant trait would appear in the next generation, but a recessive trait like feeblemindedness could pass through several generations without appearing. Thus, although two feebleminded parents would definitely produce feebleminded children, the mating of a feebleminded and normal person would lead, on average, to one out of every four children being feebleminded (depending on whether the normal person carried the defective gene), and even normal-seeming parents could conceivably transmit feeblemindedness to a future generation. Although Rogers greatly admired Davenport, he did not jettison his old beliefs. He stressed the difficulty of applying Mendel's laws of averages to the human family and complained that Mendel's laws were "liable to be 'overworked' to explain manifestations that are due entirely to environment."[31]

Still, the Faribault superintendent responded enthusiastically when Davenport's ERO offered to pay the salary of a eugenics field-worker if the state of Minnesota would pay travel and living expenses. The ERO was the eugenics movement's institutional base; it published books and articles on human heredity, acted as a clearinghouse for eugenics propaganda and research, and ran a six-week summer course that eventually trained more than 250 field-workers to gather eugenic data and link eugenics researchers with superintendents across the country. In 1911, Rogers convinced the Minnesota legislature to allocate the sizable sum of $10,000 for two years of "clinical and scientific" research conducted under Rogers's direction. Saidee Devitt, a graduate of the first ERO summer training course, started work in October, and Marie Curial, a native of Anoka, Minnesota, joined her the following year. For the next five years, Devitt and Curial traveled hundreds of miles throughout southern Minnesota, battling impassable roads, late trains, and subzero temperatures to gather information about supposedly feebleminded families.[32]

Devitt's and Curial's field research in Minnesota formed the basis of *Dwellers in the Vale of Siddem* (1919), a salacious but forgettable book published by Rogers's assistant Maud Merrill two years after the superintendent died. Merrill described the book as the "true story" of the degeneracy rampant in an isolated ravine along the Root River Valley, where six brothers and sisters who settled there in the 1850s spawned generations of criminals and defectives. In fact, *Dwellers* is a hodgepodge of stories loosely drawn from Devitt's and Curial's reports and Rogers's *Journal of Psycho-Asthenics* editorials. Quotations and anecdotes are taken out of context, people who left the valley are discussed as if they still lived there, and unrelated individuals are treated as members of one degenerate family. The writing is "self-consciously 'artful' in style," Nicole Hahn Rafter observes, but "even by family studies standards, they play fast and loose with evidence."[33]

Dwellers exemplifies eugenicists' obsession with dependency—and with the high-grade feebleminded, or morons, who could pass as normal. The idiot or low-grade imbecile was not a menace to society, Rogers and Merrill opined; the real threat came from "the ne'er-do-wells, who lacking the initiative and stick-to-it-iveness of energy and ambition, drift from failure to failure, spending a winter in the poor house, moving from shack to hovel and succeeding only in the reproduction of ill-nurtured, ill-kempt gutter brats to carry on the family traditions of dirt, disease and degeneracy." The book's final chapter was titled simply "The Cost." Without providing any dollar figure, Rogers and Merrill stressed the "toll of human misery . . . and the deadening social burden of deficiency" exacted by the rural poor and underscored the terrible futility of charitable aid and fixed prison sentences, which allowed defective families to reproduce at an alarming rate. The state's efforts to care for the feebleminded, they declared, were "like trying to stamp out malaria or yellow fever in the neighborhood of a mosquito breeding swamp."[34]

If the published book was packed with the crude slurs typical of eugenics propaganda, the day-to-day interactions between the field-workers and local residents were decidedly more complex. Davenport recognized the need to establish "a friendly feeling" toward the institution and understood that the "field worker performs many of the services that usually fall under the head of purely social worker." Rogers, for his part, viewed eugenics fieldwork as a form of institutional extension work that could strengthen both the Faribault School's scientific prestige and its practical influence in the community. Prior to 1917, admission to Faribault was voluntary, at least on paper. Families could take their adult relatives out of the institution if they wanted, and to Rogers's great annoyance, many did. The field-workers' mission therefore went beyond the mere collection of eugenic information; it also involved working with Rogers, local charity officers, and parole agents to investigate and supervise paroled patients and their families.[35]

Most historians assume that poor families objected to eugenic surveillance and that fieldwork pitted the relatives of those considered feebleminded against the state. In fact, although many individuals did object to the field-workers' intrusive questions, the record suggests that others relished the chance to gossip, talk about their families, or complain about annoying relatives or neighbors. Some took pleasure in discussing the failings of their relations, especially their in-laws, and a few tried to get troublemakers sent (or sent back) to the state institution, which had a long waiting list. As superintendent, Rogers received regular entreaties from families who wanted to institutionalize a disturbed or disabled relative. Campaigns to discredit the other side of the family were common when new patients were admitted to the institution, he explained; if the patient is "brought by the father, all the troubles come from the mother's side, and if he is brought by the mother, all the troubles come from the father's side."[36]

The inseparability of eugenics fieldwork from the work of public welfare agencies is evident in the field-workers' correspondence and reports. In 1907, the legislature authorized the Board of Control to employ parole agents to supervise individuals who had been released from the state institutions and to arrange for their readmission if necessary. Devitt and Curial worked closely with the state parole agent, Mira Gray, and with county officials to investigate dependent and delinquent families. Officials in one town, for example, asked Curial to examine a feebleminded welfare mother whose allegedly feebleminded daughter had several illegitimate children. Curial obliged, telling Rogers that even though the case was not very interesting from a hereditary standpoint, it had budgetary implications for the town. If the entire family was feebleminded and some of them could be placed in the Faribault School, part of the cost of supporting them would shift from the town's relief fund to the state.[37]

At times, Devitt and Curial played the familiar "friendly visitor" social work role. Devitt told attendees at the 1914 meeting of the Minnesota Conference of Charities and Correction about her "very pleasant visit" with a poor farm wife who cared for eight children and kept her small home neat and clean, despite a difficult husband and her own epilepsy. The poor woman reportedly greeted her by saying, "I spose you are one of them rich bugs who likes to go round once in a while and see how us poor folks live. Well, come in, I'm glad to see you anyway." Devitt also described a moving encounter with a mother whose son had died at Faribault. This woman was surprised and pleased by Devitt's interest in her boy and (according to Devitt) hoped that the information she provided could help another suffering mother. It is tempting to see Devitt's apparent kindness as a ploy to obtain incriminating genetic information, but this interpretation is too simple. Historians writing in other contexts have observed that poor mothers often turned to child protection agencies, juvenile courts, health clinics, and other instruments of the state when they needed help dealing with difficult family situations or thought it could save their children's lives. It is possible that at least some of the face-to-face encounters between eugenics field-workers and the mothers of institutionalized children should be understood in this light.[38] The relationship between the field-workers and individual families was a complex amalgam, and the line between eugenics and social work was less clear than the eugenicists—and their critics—supposed.

Local people actively shaped eugenics fieldwork in Minnesota, in part because Devitt's and Curial's close working relationships with Superintendent Rogers, parole agent Mira Gray, and local welfare workers fused welfare and eugenics practice. The continuous negotiations between welfare officials and poor families, and the resulting inconsistencies and unevenness of state power, are reflected in the archival record. For example, juvenile judges had the legal power to commit dependent, neglected, or delinquent children to a "suitable" institution, but doing so was often impossible because of public opinion, lack of institutional space, or reelection concerns. Similarly, admission to the Faribault School was voluntary for adults, at least on paper, but relief recipients faced considerable pressure to institutionalize relatives who were considered feebleminded. A judge or welfare board might withhold public relief or a mother's pension until a desperate mother agreed to send her allegedly feebleminded child to the state institution. Prior to the compulsory commitment law of 1917, the Faribault School was not terribly different from a poorhouse or other welfare institution: it was a hateful place that poor families tried to avoid but also used for their own advantage when they needed it to survive during hard times. In Rogers's era, the school had many urgent applications from poor families who needed economic relief or respite care and were frustrated by the long wait for admission. In 1908 alone, the school received nearly four hundred applications beyond its capacity, more than two-thirds from "pressing cases." To meet the demand, Rogers regularly acceded to requests to make difficult cases "special," moving them to the top of the waiting list in order to expedite institutionalization.[39]

The multiple sites of eugenic authority and the complexity of family decision-making when poverty and disability were involved are poignantly revealed in the correspondence about these "special" cases. There were two main groups of special admissions. The first consisted of individuals perceived as a welfare burden. Many in this group came from hardworking but impoverished families who felt encumbered by a child or adult relative who had a disability or exhibited aberrant behavior. Often, the family had managed for years with little or no assistance, but a recent setback—job loss, illness, or simply the effects of aging—left them anxious and unable to cope. Sometimes, the parents of the prospective inmate had died, and the "feebleminded" person lived with an uncle, sister, or brother who already had a large family and could no longer support another dependent. Judges and welfare agents often viewed these families with sympathy, and many of the families looked on institutionalization with relief.[40]

The second group of special admissions consisted of "immoral" women and girls whose sexual proclivities—and possible pregnancy or venereal disease—marked them as a social menace. Many of these women's parents were dead or no longer present in their lives, so they were economically dependent on other relatives for support. They usually came to the state's attention when the family felt they could no longer control the woman's behavior or when she had a baby they could not (or would not) support. In some instances, the parents themselves negotiated with state officials to place a troublesome daughter at Faribault. Not infrequently, they changed their mind after she had been institutionalized. This was the case for Anna Grein, a pretty girl who (according to the parole agent) refused to mind her mother, had spells of laughing and crying, and was incapable of distinguishing between right and wrong in her interactions with men and boys. Anna's entire family was in distress. Her father was unemployed, her mother had heart trouble, and her sister, who was the sole support of the family, was overwhelmed. Welfare authorities scrambled to make Anna's case special, but just two days after she entered the institution, the family took her out. Rogers complained that this was not the first time authorities bent over backward to help a desperate family but were unable to do so because the parents balked when the patient said she was unhappy. In Rogers's opinion, the families of "defectives" could not understand the needs of the feebleminded child.[41]

Anna's experience was uncommon only because she was at Faribault for such a short time. Rogers's correspondence contains numerous references to other women who were admitted to the institution as special cases and then removed over his objections. (Some were eventually admitted again, a fact that Rogers took as proof of the need for a compulsory guardianship law.) In theory, institutionalization was voluntary after an individual turned seventeen and no longer fell under the jurisdiction of the juvenile court. In reality, some people spent years trying to get relatives released, either because other family members wanted the person to stay in the institution or because poor people with little education were unfamiliar with their legal rights and unable to circumvent the bureaucracy. In one instance, an eighteen-year-old woman, sent to Faribault in 1902 along with her one-month-old baby, was still in the institution in 1920, despite her mother's efforts to get her released. In another case, a man who put his pregnant seventeen-year-old daughter in Faribault to have her baby and work off the cost of hospital care complained to the Board of Control that she was still there four years later. His daughter was not a criminal, the man protested: "Just because that thing happened to her—it happens to a lot more, too—she does not belong in prison for life." When Rogers claimed that the girl was better off in the institution, her father responded that he knew in his heart that "there is no better place for anybody than home." At times, the inmates themselves wrote the Board of Control, the governor, and even the federal government about their loneliness, uncompensated labor, and emotional distress. "I am just as much human as you are," Myrna Jones told the Board of Control. "I like the same things . . . have the same feelings. I know you couldn't live for one week in my place." Erma Stewart wrote the governor that she was "as innocent as a butterfly. . . . Will you please grant me my freedom?"[42] As these examples illustrate, poor women's "immoral" behavior often led relatives to seek institutional care, but subsequent efforts to secure their release were not welcomed. To Rogers and many welfare officials, the possibility of pregnancy turned every feebleminded woman outside the institution into a social menace.

Still, the common assumption that the family represented the best interests of the feebleminded is not entirely accurate. Many people remained in the institution because their families wanted them there, and even relatives working for an inmate's release did not necessarily have the person's best interest in mind. Occasionally, parents sought the discharge of feebleminded girls so they could prostitute or sexually abuse them. More often, they wanted family members discharged so they could contribute to the household economy. As one mother stated frankly, "I am 50 years Old and Worked hard all of my life I need my Daughter to help me." Most Minnesota families relied on the economic contribution of every member, so it is understandable that they would object to a relation working without compensation in a state institution when their labor was needed at home. Still, requests for help at home were not always benign. Some people exploited the labor of "slow" family members and put them to work at the most grueling tasks. Even more commonly, people used the institution to dispose of family members who were difficult to get along with or could not earn their keep. When one inmate died following a gruesome accident that even Rogers found troubling, his mother remarked that "she was glad he was dead as he had never earned a cent in his life."[43] The dehumanizing treatment of people labeled feebleminded because they exhibited nonstandard sexual behavior, had physical or intellectual disabilities, or had a parent from the "wrong" racial or ethnic background was not simply a policy the state imposed. Chronic poverty and family dysfunction had a eugenic momentum of their own. The cruel power of eugenics did not only flow one way.

Protecting the Innocent Child: Dependency and Delinquency in the Juvenile Court

A. C. Rogers provided the intellectual justification for Minnesota's eugenics program, and the Faribault School became its institutional base. Yet the sterilization program could never have been implemented without a dramatic expansion of the state's legal and supervisory power over those living outside the institution. Ironically, this expansion of state power was not primarily achieved by eugenicists seeking to control the unfit, but by urban child welfare reformers striving to "protect" the innocent child. The child-saving movement burst onto the scene in the 1890s, bringing together a diverse coalition of reformers around three key principles: the state was responsible for the care of the dependent and neglected child; the environment, rather than heredity, determined the destiny of the "normal" child; and the family home was preferable to institutional care. Delinquent and dependent children of normal intelligence should be removed from the institution with the least possible delay.[44]

Reformers' concerns about the dangers of institutionalization reflected the influence of G. Stanley Hall, the president of Clark University and a towering figure in the new academic discipline of psychology. It is difficult to overstate Hall's impact on child welfare policy. His theory of childhood as a series of developmental stages provided a scientific rationale for a raft of child-centered policies, such as school reform and the juvenile court, and many of his students became leaders in the field of child development and intelligence testing: Henry Goddard, the director of research at New Jersey's Vineland Training School, imported the IQ test to North America and invented the term *moron*. Lewis

Terman, a psychology professor at Stanford University, worked with Goddard testing army recruits during World War I and supervised the graduate work of Maud Merrill and Mildred Thomson. Frederick Kuhlmann, the chief proponent of intelligence testing in Minnesota, was the director of research at the Faribault School and A. C. Rogers's right-hand man.[45]

Hall's ideas about child psychology were rooted in his Lamarckian understanding of heredity and the then-accepted theory of recapitulation, which held that the psychological development of every individual repeated the evolution of the human race. Hall believed that the primitive boy became a civilized man by passing through the same developmental stages as his ancestors, moving from animal to savage to civilized adult. Parents and educators should ensure that the child's environment was free of any possible cause of evolutionary arrest or degeneration and then "keep out of nature's way." Boys reveled in savagery, Hall proclaimed, and they needed to indulge their tribal penchant for idleness, roving, fighting, and predatory behavior so that these tendencies did not "crop out in menacing forms" in later years. Adolescence, however, was the most important developmental stage, a period of sexual awakening that should be carefully monitored so that young men and women did not engage in dangerous behaviors like masturbation, which would damage heredity and harm future generations.[46]

Hall's theory of child development was paradigm shifting, and it hastened the untangling of the three Ds. Delinquency in youth was no longer a sign of degeneracy or defectiveness. Instead, a "period of semicriminality" was considered essential to the healthy development of the normal boy. Delinquents were not "a separate race of beings to be differentiated from mankind generally as the lion is from the horse, nor even as the wild-cat is differentiated from the domestic Tabby," Rogers explained. Experts now understood that even youngsters from good families could become nominal criminals by following the "impulses of childhood" and taking an apple without paying for it or throwing a stone through a window. These children needed guidance, not strict punishment, for most mischief makers were "active, energetic and . . . have . . . initiative. In other words, the very children who are most apt to get into trouble among the normal minded are the ones who, under proper conditions, make the very best citizens and be [*sic*] of the most use in the world."[47]

This normalization of youthful misbehavior provided a conceptual basis for the juvenile court, first established in Cook County, Illinois, in 1899. Coincidentally, Hastings Hart, who had just left Minnesota for a position in Chicago, wrote the first draft of the new law. The juvenile court removed young offenders from the adult criminal justice system. A child accused of a crime would not be a defendant in a criminal trial that determined innocence or guilt, but would have an informal hearing in which the judge acted as a "wise and kind father" and administered constructive discipline without damaging the child's reputation or self-respect. In psychology, the court was based on Hall's theory that children were fundamentally good and a certain amount of mischief making was natural. In law, it derived from the common law doctrine of *parens patriae*, which established the state's power to protect children (and adults) legally incompetent to act on their own behalf. "The essence of the juvenile court idea," Hart later explained, was the "obligation of the great mother state to her neglected and erring children, and her obligation to deal with them as children, and wards, rather than to class them as criminals and drive them by harsh measures into the ranks of vice and crime."[48]

Minnesota enacted its own juvenile court law, modeled on the Illinois statute, in 1905. The law initially applied only to the three most populous counties (Hennepin, Ramsey, and St. Louis), but it was soon extended to the rest of the state. In the urban counties, the juvenile judge was a member of the district court, but the probate judge functioned in that capacity in the rest of the state. Thus, probate judges whose main responsibilities had been wills and estates gained substantial new power over children and (mostly working-class) families. A judge could, at his discretion, allow a delinquent child to live at home under the supervision of a probation officer. He could send the child to a "suitable" institution, authorize a permanent adoption or short-term indenture, or order a jury trial. Minnesota's juvenile court law did not give children any of the rights as adult criminal defendants, such as the right to an attorney, due process, or a jury trial. Instead, it empowered elected judges to enforce standards for home life and behavior which had little resonance with the lives of the poor.[49]

Class inequities were written into the juvenile court statute. At a time when middle-class children were supposed to be economically and socially dependent on their parents, the law defined the delinquent child as one who was too independent: anyone under seventeen who left home without parental consent, wandered the streets at night, rode the rails without permission, broke a law, patronized a saloon or gambling hall, associated with thieves or immoral persons, or used indecent language. The definition of a "dependent or neglected" child was equally class specific: anyone under seventeen who was destitute, homeless, or dependent on the public for support, habitually begged or received alms, lacked proper parental care, or lived in a house of prostitution. Children under ten could be adjudged dependent if they were begging, peddling, or entertaining on the street. The law thus defined many ordinary working-class activities and neighborhoods as detrimental to children and extended the court's jurisdiction over many families who were law-abiding but poor. Moreover, the laudable attempt to treat the "whole child" by consolidating all children's issues in a single court had the effect of eliding the distinction between dependency and delinquency and reinforcing the old association between pauperism and crime.[50]

The structural connection between dependency and delinquency became even tighter when in 1913 Minnesota again followed Illinois's lead and passed a mothers' pension law. Under this law, a juvenile judge could order a county to pay a mother up to $10 per month to support a "dependent or neglected" child under the age of fourteen if (note the inconsistency) the mother was a "proper person to have the custody of such child." The court's new role was "well outside the beaten path," Hennepin County judge Edward F. Waite recalled, for it had been given "administrative authority far beyond that commonly exercised by judicial tribunals." It was supposed to function like a welfare agency. Judges could grant allowances to deserving mothers whose dependency was caused by the husband's death, physical incapacity, or detention in a penal institution or insane asylum (but not, significantly, the School for the Feebleminded). Yet counties bore the full cost of the program, and the recipient had to have resided in the county for at least one year. Mothers' pensions thus replicated the two fundamentals of US welfare practice: local responsibility and the distinction between deserving and undeserving poor.[51]

Placing mothers' pension administration in the juvenile court was meant to distinguish aid to dependent children from poor relief, but it also reflected a new theory of the law as a quasi-administrative instrument of welfare governance. As historian Michael Willrich argues in his penetrating analysis of the Chicago Municipal Court, progressive legal theorists such as Harvard law professor Roscoe Pound rejected the established view that judges should only protect abstract individual rights or adjudicate private disputes between supposedly equal parties, arguing instead for a sociological jurisprudence that considered "social facts" and addressed "human needs." Trusting in professional expertise and the tools of social science, progressive legal reformers sought to improve the conditions of modern industrial life through administrative remedies and, in the juvenile court, ongoing supervision. The socialized courts laid the foundation for the New Deal administrative state, but Willrich points out that the new emphasis on individual treatment also fostered the rise of a "eugenic jurisprudence" and gave civil courts unprecedented coercive power. By the 1920s, even rural judges who lacked their urban counterparts' access to social science expertise concerned themselves less with individual rights than "community obligations," as they understood them, and routinely used the state's police power to protect what they considered the general welfare. In the process, safeguards for individual rights were set aside.[52]

Judge Waite had serious reservations about these developments, especially when it came to rural courts. In a 1922 article, "How Far Can Court Procedure Be Socialized without Impairing Individual Rights?," he rebuked juvenile judges for failing to distinguish between criminal and noncriminal cases and for using *parens patriae* to bypass constitutional protections such as the right to legal representation and a jury trial. For example, although hearsay was inadmissible in a regular court, juvenile judges could—and often did—rely on hearsay or gossip when sentencing children to correctional facilities or removing them from their parents' custody. When children were denied the legal rights held by adults, Waite wrote, the "state's parental power which [the judge] embodies is prostituted . . . and the juvenile court falls into suspicion and disrepute."[53]

Waite had fewer reservations about socialized court procedures ten years earlier, when all of Minnesota's juvenile courts were urban and he was on the bench. Then, he put a lot of faith in social science research and judicial fairness. Waite was deeply influenced by psychiatrist William Healy's multicausal explanations for juvenile delinquency, and like Healy, he rejected the idea of born criminality and the assumption—still popular in spite of G. Stanley Hall's research—that most delinquents were defective or feebleminded. Instead, he believed that most delinquent youth could be rehabilitated if they had a proper diagnosis and individual treatment.[54] Examination and classification were crucial to this process. In Waite's court, the first step was a medical exam, after which the doctor would prescribe eyeglasses or order a surgical procedure, if necessary. Then a social worker gathered information about school performance and the parents' occupation, marital status, religion, nationality, and lifestyle (e.g., tobacco and alcohol consumption). Finally, if intellectual disability was suspected, a psychologist would administer an intelligence test in order to "weed out the mentally defective." This last step was indispensable because rehabilitation was considered possible only when a juvenile delinquent was intellectually normal. Distinguishing between the "normally bright child, capable of aspiration and progress to real leadership," and the child who was hopelessly defective was essential to the everyday practice of the juvenile court.[55]

Concepts of disability were central to the court's classification scheme. Waite acknowledged in a 1913 speech before the American Academy of Medicine that nearly 90 percent of boys who came before his court had physical problems and 70 percent were behind in school, mainly because poor health had led to irregular attendance. But he insisted that mental deficiencies, rather than physical concerns, were "the most perplexing element in the problem of juvenile criminality" because the usual techniques of probation or punishment did not work. "Many physical causes contributing to crime may be remedied; homes may be improved and other conditions of environment made more fit for the normal development of childhood," Waite explained. "But the case of the feeble-minded child is hopeless as long as he remains in the stress of community life." Echoing eugenicist claims that every feebleminded person was a potential criminal, he said that no one was "so pathetic, so hopeless and so menacing" as the high-grade mentally defective child.[56]

Waite, the juvenile court judge and child welfare reformer, thus played an important role in furthering the myth of the menace of the feebleminded in Minnesota. "The Jukes, the Kallikaks and the Ishmaels are not confined to New York, New Jersey and Indiana," he told his medical audience; these degenerate families had spread across the country and were "an unspeakable curse to themselves and to society." The solution, he declared, was to extend the state's power over feebleminded children through mandatory medical examinations, special public school classes for the "improvable retarded," permanent institutional segregation for custodial cases, and greater power for the courts. Like Rogers, Waite proposed extending legal guardianship past the age of majority for young offenders who were "plainly incorrigible—defectives with criminal tendencies," and averred that the "breeding of imbecile and probably criminal offspring by defective and degenerate parents" should be stopped.[57] As chair of Minnesota's Child Welfare Commission in 1916–1917, Waite expanded the courts' administrative power and wrote the two tracks of juvenile court practice into the state's child welfare system as a whole: a chance in the community for dependents and delinquents who were "normally bright," and unending institutionalization for so-called defectives.

Expanding Innocence: Maternalism, Moral Reform, and the Sexually Delinquent Girl

The two tracks of juvenile court practice were deeply gendered. Waite was known as a "bully good" friend to misbehaving boys, but he and other jurists rarely extended the same tolerance to delinquent girls, who were often brought before the court on sexual charges. Perhaps Waite worried that the delinquent girl would get pregnant and become dependent on relief. Or perhaps he accepted the circular logic of eugenicists: "immoral" girls were usually feebleminded, and feebleminded girls were "almost invariably immoral." They spread venereal disease, gave birth to defective children, and inflicted a public charge. For that reason, A. C. Rogers and other superintendents believed that while "higher grade" boys could get along nicely outside the institution, "no feebleminded girl should be sent out into the community." These opinions were widely shared by juvenile judges and social reformers; even the progressive social work magazine *Survey* described the feebleminded woman at large as the "most dangerous person the state can harbor . . . the plentiful cause of cost and trouble."[58]

In the 1910s, women reformers began to challenge this double standard. Frustrated and angry that young girls were punished while the adult men who seduced and abused them went free, women activists in the Twin Cities attempted to uncouple sex delinquency and feeblemindedness. At a time when male authorities generally emphasized the dangers of female sexual desire and treated sex delinquency and mental deficiency as interchangeable, "maternalist" reformers portrayed most sexually active working girls as innocent victims of male lust and insisted that they were deserving of aid. Their goal was to give wayward girls a second chance to become respectable adults, just like delinquent boys. To that end, they established a girls-only reform school and boarding homes for wage-earning women and tried to prevent delinquency by regulating commercial amusements and campaigning against alcohol and vice. Countless young sex delinquents avoided jail or the Faribault School as a result of their efforts. But the moral regulations and community services women reformers established subjected young working-class women to new forms of surveillance.

Recent historians have analyzed the vital role maternalists played in Progressive Era campaigns for child welfare and eugenics. Historian Michael Rembis observes that elite women's conviction that they could speak "as 'universal mothers' on behalf of impoverished women and children" led many of them to support a eugenic commitment law in Illinois. In Minnesota, too, elite organizations such as the Women's Welfare League expressed a "strong protective sentiment toward the young women of the city" and used maternalist language to justify their public activism.[59]

Yet maternalism was not the only reform philosophy circulating through the state, and a concern for respectability was not just something that elite women imposed on poor working girls. Many working-class parents and unions had similar concerns. Nearly 50 percent of wage-earning women in Minneapolis lived separately from their families in 1900, and many barely earned enough to make ends meet. They lived at the boundaries of respectability and often turned to "treats" from their better-paid male counterparts to eat or partake in commercial amusements. While maternalists blamed male lust when working girls stumbled, Populists and labor radicals blamed greedy capitalists. Prostitution was a potent symbol of economic inequality, and in Minnesota the image of the promiscuous feebleminded menace was always counterbalanced by the contrasting image of the innocent country girl who moved to the city in search of work and fell prey to unscrupulous businessmen. The fluid line between respectability and immorality shaped state policy on dependency, delinquency, and eugenics.[60]

The contradictory influences of maternalism, populism, and eugenics reverberated through Progressive Era efforts at sex delinquency reform. In 1911, the same year the Minnesota legislature approved Rogers's eugenics fieldwork plan and considered (but rejected) a eugenic sterilization law, three other reform developments undercut eugenicists' claim that female delinquency and defectiveness were one and the same. The first was the submission of the Minneapolis Vice Commission's report. One of twenty-seven similar bodies across the nation, the vice commission formed after the mayor closed the city's red light district after years of toleration and appointed fifteen citizens, including Waite, to advise him on prostitution policy. Like its counterparts in other cities, the Minneapolis commission concluded that vice districts should be permanently abolished. Unlike them, it said it found no evidence of "white slave traffic" and contained virtually no reference to feeblemindedness. Instead, the commission blamed prostitution on poverty, congested living conditions, commercialized recreation, the "overwork and exploitation" of women workers, and an "intrenched spirit of materialism" which led many "daughters of the poor" to seek an "easy way" to acquire possessions. The commission vigorously defended wage-earning women from charges of immorality and praised community organizations, such as the Catholic House of the Good Shepherd, which treated fallen women "not as criminals, nor outcasts, but as human beings, who need encouragement and kindly sympathy." Yet its most concrete recommendations—better policing, regulation of commercial amusements, and public health measures to control venereal disease—expanded the state's power of surveillance over working-class women and girls.[61]

The second development, the opening of the new Minnesota Home School for Girls at Sauk Centre, reflected a similar environmentalist stance. Although the Home School would serve as a pipeline to sterilization in the interwar years, its first superintendent, Fannie French Morse, explicitly challenged long-established ideas about inherited degeneracy, as well as the newer theory of eugenics. Even the school motto, "Womanhood, Motherhood and Citizenship," was an implicit criticism of those who believed that sex delinquents were invariably feebleminded and should never reproduce. Morse scoffed at officials' obsession with heredity and mental tests. She based the Home School program instead on a belief in the delinquent girl's "possibilities; a belief in her as a normal creature; a belief in her as one needing a chance." Morse insisted that almost every sex delinquent could eventually lead a respectable married life; only the "exceptional girl" who failed to respond to Sauk Centre's regular treatment program would be considered for transfer to Faribault. As with the juvenile court, distinguishing the majority of delinquents who could be rehabilitated from the few defectives who were hopeless cases was a principal objective of individual treatment.[62]

The third event of 1911 was the formation of the Women's Welfare League of Minneapolis. A group of elite maternalist reformers, expressing alarm over the "apparent moral laxness in this city" and frustration with the conservatism of established women's clubs, combined fact-finding investigations into girls' housing conditions and recreational activities with a spirited political campaign for more female police officers and stricter regulation of movie theaters and dance halls. The league operated several boardinghouses for working girls, monitored court proceedings involving minors, and set up a citizens' network to report violations of child labor laws. Its executive also endorsed the eugenic sterilization and antimiscegenation bills introduced into the Minnesota legislature (but defeated) in 1913. The league's archives contain little information about the endorsements, which may have been a last-minute decision, as they were added in pen to typed minutes. But it is revealing that the endorsement of the antimiscegenation bill came less than three months after the legendary black boxer Jack Johnson was arrested for transporting eighteen-year-old Lucile Cameron, a white woman originally from Minneapolis, across state lines "for immoral purposes" and six weeks after the couple got married—a marriage that Cameron's mother, who still lived in the Minneapolis area, very publicly opposed. The endorsement of these eugenic policies reveals more than the executive's troubling racial prejudice; the women's refusal to accept the sexual choices of an eighteen-year-old exposes the coercive underside of maternalists' "protective sentiment."[63]

Ultimately, the welfare league's main contribution to Minnesota's sterilization program lay not in its support for eugenic legislation, but in the community-based services it developed. The boardinghouses that maternalists established for working girls in the 1910s served as a prototype for the residential clubhouses it extended to sterilized feebleminded women in the 1920s. As we shall see in the next chapter, the private-sector Women's Welfare League, not the state of Minnesota, provided the institutional base for supervising feebleminded women released from Faribault after sterilization.

In the short run, the league's most successful, or at least most sensationalized, achievement involved a very public sex crime scandal that rocked Minneapolis in 1915 and 1916. The saga began when a weekly gossip paper accused the Minneapolis Humane Society, the agency supposed to investigate allegations of child abuse, of sending "young girls who are in trouble" to jail in order to protect the reputations of the elite men "who are the cause of their condition." Then, in early 1916, Joseph Bragdon, a prominent businessman who was a Humane Society donor, was accused of sexually abusing several teenage girls. Three girls, aged thirteen to fifteen, told an investigator that "Uncle Ned," a mysterious man driving a "big green automobile," lured them to hidden places and performed unnatural acts in the bushes. The welfare league pressed the police to pursue the investigation, kept the scandal in the public eye, and crowded the courtroom to monitor Bragdon's three remarkable trials. The first trial ended in acquittal, as the key witness against Bragdon changed her story and (it was later alleged) two of the defendant's friends served on the jury. The second resulted in a hung jury. During the third trial, the three teenage witnesses ran away (likely at the behest of the defendant). When they were found and Bragdon was finally convicted and sent to jail, Minneapolis women's groups cheered.[64]

Bragdon's trial and conviction are important because they signaled a dramatic shift in the perception of the sexually delinquent girl. For perhaps the first time, the court, the press, and much of the public treated sexually active, working-class teenagers as youthful innocents and considered their court testimony credible. Even after the girls ran away "on a lark" during the third trial, the judge treated them as juveniles, not mental defectives or hardened prostitutes, and ordered them returned to the custody of Sauk Centre superintendent Fannie Morse instead of sentencing them to Faribault or jail. The girls themselves clearly experienced coercion from all sides. Yet the fact that the testimony of three so-called sex delinquents could bring down a well-connected businessman was stunning. The entire episode exposed the class tensions simmering in the city and Populist anger at the business elite. But Bragdon would not have been convicted without the righteousness and political savvy of maternalists, who insisted that the wayward girls were impressionable adolescents with the capacity to achieve respectability. Now the businessman was a menace, and the sexually delinquent teens were innocent children who deserved a second chance. The line between deserving and undeserving was shifting.[65]

The Child Welfare Commission, the Feebleminded Menace, and the Innocent Child

The mutually constitutive relationship between feebleminded menace and innocent child is strikingly evident in the 1917 *Report of the Minnesota Child Welfare Commission*, which established a new mechanism for eugenics control within an innovative child welfare system widely praised for its liberal approach to illegitimacy. Judge Waite was the driving force behind the commission. He had complained for years that the child welfare laws passed in the Progressive Era were sloppily written and either internally inconsistent or in conflict with other statutes. Similar concerns were expressed in other states. By the early 1920s, thirty-one states and the District of Columbia had expert commissions to revise and codify their state laws relating to children. The federal Children's Bureau called the commission movement "one of the most significant and hopeful developments in the child welfare field."[66]

The twelve members of Minnesota's Child Welfare Commission were appointed by Republican governor J. A. A. Burnquist in the summer of 1916, when Minnesota's progressive coalition was starting to fracture. Although prohibitionists had achieved a big win with the 1915 passage of a "county option" liquor bill, most German Minnesotans opposed the bill, and the state was further divided over farmer–labor militancy, women's rights, and the war raging in Europe. The members of the commission were clearly chosen to ensure its political credibility. Most were prominent in state politics and welfare circles. Three were women. A. C. Rogers was too sick to serve, but his influence was palpable, and several obituaries listed him as a member. Yet in a state of tremendous ethnic and regional diversity, the Child Welfare Commission was conspicuous for its homogeneity. The commissioners were all white, heavily urban, Protestant, and Republican. There was not one doctor, union leader, or minister. (There was, however, a rabbi.) There were no representatives from western Minnesota or the Iron Range, and farmers and ethnic charities were seriously underrepresented. Nevertheless, the commission was remarkably effective. While some states' commissions dragged on for years, the Minnesota group issued a report within six months, and most of its recommendations became law within the year.[67]

The commission's legislative success reflected the emerging consensus on the state's responsibility for child welfare, as well as the commissioners' acute sense of what was politically possible in Minnesota. To combat the common complaint that child welfare measures undermined the father's authority in the home, Waite pointed out in two preliminary reports that the idea of governmental responsibility for children was not new: the doctrine of *parens patriae* had long established the state as the "ultimate guardian" over those incapable of caring for themselves. In addition, he pointed out that the commission's scope was limited to those children who had "handicaps"—dependency, delinquency defectiveness, illegitimacy, or neglect—that could be remedied through legislation. Waite harshly criticized what he saw as the state's meager policies regarding the twin problems of feeblemindedness and illegitimacy. Feeblemindedness had a spiraling impact on poverty, disease, vice, and crime, he wrote, but "our state has not made an intelligent effort to prevent the propagation of the feebleminded, nor to provide adequately for their care and supervision." Minnesota should move quickly to prevent the "alarming increase of children born into the world with this tragic handicap." In contrast, Waite portrayed the child born out of wedlock as an "unoffending and helpless human being" who should be given every opportunity for a normal life. Decrying social norms that privileged men's property and the public purse over defenseless children, Waite called for new legislation to prevent the "conventionalities of society" from imposing "hardships" on the illegitimate child.[68]

The contrast between the innocent child who needed the state's care and the feebleminded menace that had to be controlled was also a major theme in the Child Welfare Commission's final report, which was submitted to the governor in February 1917. The commission affirmed the state's role as the "ultimate guardian of all children who need what they cannot provide for themselves and what natural or legal guardians are not providing" and proposed forty-three new or revised bills, which the *Minneapolis Journal* described as "radical departures, in some respect, from present methods."[69]

The commission's first and most important recommendation, and the cornerstone for all others, was administrative: it proposed to centralize authority for child welfare in the State Board of Control. The board would gain sweeping powers of legal guardianship over children committed by a judge to its care, including the authority to move inmates between institutions, such as from Sauk Centre to Faribault School, without having to seek a new judicial order.

The proposed law authorized the Board of Control to create the necessary machinery for administration (e.g., a state children's bureau) and permitted—but did not require—counties to establish their own child welfare boards, which would represent the Board of Control at the local level. With this unusual structure, the commission established a mechanism to extend the state's child welfare authority into every corner of the state, while retaining the principle of local responsibility.[70]

Several proposed bills sought to redefine dependent, neglected, and illegitimate children as "innocent and helpless" and guarantee their place in the deserving poor. The commission sought to remove the "sting" of dependency so poor children could be "adjudged dependent without reflection upon a worthy parent" and proposed expunging the offensive term *bastard* from the statute books. It endeavored to combat the "well-known evils" of baby selling or adopting a child just to get his or her labor through a strict licensing system for boarding homes, maternity hospitals, and other institutions dealing with children, as well as new legislation that made the state a party to every adoption. With the passage of the Children's Code, Minnesota became the first state to require an investigation (home study) to ensure that adoptive parents were "suitable" and the first to try to lessen the stigma of illegitimacy by sealing adoption records. Yet the same law also protected parents who adopted a "defective" child: an adoption could be annulled if within five years a youngster developed "feeblemindedness, epilepsy, insanity, or venereal infection . . . by reason of conditions existing prior to the adoption." Social workers sung the praises of Minnesota's modern adoption law, but the state's efforts to improve the lives of the majority of adopted children clearly depended on distinguishing them from a "defective" minority.[71]

Reformers praised the commission's approach to illegitimacy because it did not demean—and actually tried to protect—the illegitimate child. Prior to 1917, the state had no jurisdiction over a child born out of wedlock unless the mother initiated bastardy proceedings or the child became a public charge. Children born outside of marriage were usually poor and stigmatized, and as a result, infant mortality was high. Defying tradition and male prerogative, the Child Welfare Commission affirmed the state's responsibility to secure for illegitimate children the "nearest possible approximation to the care, support and education they would be entitled to if born of lawful marriage." Its chief goal was to "provide the illegitimate child with a responsible father"—that is, one who provided economic support—and therefore it drafted new procedures for establishing and enforcing legal paternity. All these proposals are conventional in their assumptions about home and gender, but they broke new ground in 1917 by ascribing innocence to the children of unwed mothers and treating them as the deserving poor.[72]

The contrast with "defectives" could not be starker. While most of the Child Welfare Commission report focused on protecting children, the section on "protecting feeble-minded children" was more concerned with protecting society. "Almost every community in the state furnishes examples of hereditary feeblemindedness," the commission observed, and "cases are not infrequent of mentally subnormal children whose presence in the community is a serious public menace, and for whose own welfare the wise and kindly segregation of the state institution is needed, but whose parents cannot be induced to take the simple steps necessary for admission." Capping off A. C. Rogers's long campaign for compulsory eugenic commitment, the Child Welfare Commission drafted new legislation that combined the superintendent's long-standing goal of forcing reluctant families to institutionalize feebleminded relatives with a bill prepared by the State Association of Probate Judges which simplified procedures related to insanity commitment. The new bill empowered probate judges to commit "Persons Alleged to be Feeble Minded, Inebriate or Insane" to the custody of the State Board of Control (or, in cases of insanity or inebriety, the superintendent of a state hospital) without the consent of parent or kin. The Board of Control, as guardian of the feebleminded, had the power to compel institutionalization. Echoing Rogers, the commission noted that compulsory commitment was especially important for "girls and women of child-bearing age."[73]

Despite its avowed goal of lessening the "number of defectives in coming generations," the Child Welfare Commission took a cautious approach to eugenics legislation. It deemed it unwise to pass any law "so far in advance of public opinion as to be inoperative" and thus focused mainly on marriage, where state authority was already well established. It attempted to prevent "improvident" marriages by requiring a ten-day waiting period to get a marriage license and added venereal disease and tuberculosis to the existing restrictions on the marriage of the feebleminded and insane. Although thirteen US states had eugenic sterilization laws by 1917, Waite's commission simply called for further study.[74]

The careful attention to public opinion paid off. Thirty-five of the forty-three proposed bills were enacted with remarkable swiftness. Although six bills were withdrawn before coming to a vote, nearly all that passed received the unanimous vote of both houses of the legislature. Social worker William Hodson, the commission's secretary, attributed its success to three factors: legislators were uninterested in the subject of child welfare, there was little opposition from business or industry, and no one objected to centralizing power in the State Board of Control. As well, the commission shrewdly insisted that the measures be considered as a package and withdrew the bills facing certain defeat. The bills that failed to pass—the restrictions on marriage, the inheritance rights of illegitimate children, state oversight of private boarding schools, and two child labor laws, including a proposal for regulating the street trades opposed by most newspapers—reveal the limits of progressive reformers' influence and the ongoing resistance to extending state aid to illegitimate children, who were still seen by many as the undeserving poor.[75]

Social workers across the country celebrated the enactment of the Children's Code, which made Minnesota "one of the leading states measured by its children's laws" and launched a "new era" in social welfare. As late as 1930, the federal Children's Bureau praised the vision and courage of the Waite commission, to which "not only Minnesota, but the people of the United States, owe a very real debt of gratitude." The Children's Code confronted the stigma of illegitimacy, modernized adoption procedures, and hastened the shift away from orphanages and institutional care for poor children and toward community services and the chance to live at home. Many destitute mothers and children avoided the poorhouse as a result of the Children's Code, and some of Minnesota's most vulnerable residents—people with intellectual and physical disabilities—gained much-needed protection from abandonment, exploitation, and abusive families. Yet the Children's Code also established new norms for citizen behavior and gave the state unprecedented power to impose certain behavioral and economic standards on the poor. In the name of protecting innocent children, it defined as a "serious public menace" people whose physical appearance, poor earning abilities, or troublesome behavior marked them as feebleminded, thereby legitimizing compulsory institutionalization and the denial of their civil rights.[76]

The death of Superintendent Rogers in 1917 and passage of the Children's Code less than four months later marked a crucial change in how the state of Minnesota would henceforth treat those considered to be feebleminded. The previous decades had witnessed a gradual shift away from fluid nineteenth-century ideas about inherited degeneracy and the interchangeability of the "defective, dependent and delinquent classes" and toward a binary system characterized by growing optimism about the prospects for "normal" dependent and delinquent children and a deeper distrust of so-called defectives. But the Children's Code opened a Pandora's box. The state's new child welfare responsibilities collided with local relief practices and increasing budgetary constraints. Within a few years, as feebleminded commitments exploded in number, the consequences of the new law became clear. The Faribault School grew dangerously overcrowded, and the county child welfare boards were overwhelmed. At about the same time, the newly formed Minnesota Eugenics Society launched an aggressive campaign for an all-encompassing sterilization law. The next chapter examines how the crisis in the child welfare system persuaded once-reluctant state officials to support a eugenic sterilization law.

TWO ROADS TO STERILIZATION

Just eight years after Judge Waite and the Child Welfare Commission dismissed sterilization as "too distasteful to the public," both houses of the state legislature voted overwhelmingly in favor of a eugenic sterilization law.[1] What changed between 1917 and 1925? The resurgence of eugenics activism after a temporary hiatus during World War I is an obvious answer. Equally important, though less analyzed, is the changing nature of the state: the courts' growing child welfare authority, the World War I–era expansion of the state's administrative capacity, and the shift from indoor relief to community-based social welfare services.

This chapter examines eugenics and child welfare as two interlinked roads to sterilization in the aftermath of World War I. The eugenics part of the story is well known. Indiana enacted the first sterilization law in 1907, and within ten years fifteen more states had legalized eugenic sterilization. The legitimacy of eugenic surgery remained in dispute, however, and many of the laws were either struck down by the courts or infrequently used. As a result, the vast majority of operations were performed in one state, California. After the end of the war, mounting anxiety about the influx of immigrants from southern and eastern Europe, the northward migration of African Americans, changing sexual mores, and the wartime deaths of the nation's "fittest" men created a more hospitable climate for eugenics advocacy. In 1922, the Eugenics Committee of the U.S.A. (later the American Eugenics Society) formed to "stem the tide of threatened racial degeneracy," and Harry Laughlin published his massive compendium of sterilization laws, stimulating a new wave of state sterilization statutes that had procedural safeguards that stood up to constitutional challenges. Eugenicists celebrated some momentous policy successes in the 1920s. The Johnson–Reed Immigration Act of 1924 restricted the entrance of "undesirable" immigrants from southern and eastern Europe based on the 1890 census, barring Asians entirely, and Virginia passed the Racial Integrity Act, a harshly punitive antimiscegenation law. By the time the United States Supreme Court upheld Virginia's compulsory sterilization law in *Buck v. Bell* (1927), seventeen states had sterilization laws. Five years later, the number had jumped to thirty.[2]

The new social welfare landscape created by World War I and the Children's Code paved the second, less familiar road toward sterilization. The code gave the State Board of Control new legal power over dependent, neglected, delinquent, and feebleminded children under court-ordered guardianship and created a new administrative apparatus, a state children's bureau and county-level child welfare boards, which took the state board's welfare authority into every corner of the state. As a result of the Children's Code, illegitimate children, unmarried mothers, families dependent on relief, and individuals who were designated feebleminded but lived outside institutions came under state jurisdiction for the first time. Although poorhouses and orphanages continued to operate and even expanded in the interwar period, the main site of social welfare provision shifted away from indoor relief and toward community welfare programs. As social work professionalized after World War I, charity organizations' tradition of friendly visiting evolved into social casework, with its emphasis on individual diagnosis and psychological treatment. By the 1920s, trained social workers used techniques from psychology and medicine to help the "maladjusted"—unmarried mothers, the dependent poor, and even the so-called feebleminded—adjust to community life.[3]

Historians describe World War I as a turning point in the state's increased intervention into ordinary peoples' lives. Nationally, an array of new agencies gave the federal government unprecedented regulatory power over business, agriculture, and labor. The federal Children's Bureau designated 1918 as Children's Year and provided free physical examinations for infants and school-age children, promoted better nutrition, and launched a back-to-school initiative intended to keep children out of the workforce. The Committee on Public Information flooded the country with pro-American propaganda, and the Espionage Act of 1917 made it a crime to make "false statements" promoting disloyalty or the enemy's success. The War Department worked with private organizations to eradicate drinking, venereal disease, and vice. By the end of the war, the state's presence was felt in every aspect of social life.[4]

Politics and policy in Minnesota exemplified these national trends. Less than two weeks after the United States declared war against Germany, the Minnesota legislature approved both the Children's Code and the wartime Minnesota Commission of Public Safety (MCPS), ensuring that the expansion of the state's warfare and welfare systems would be entwined. The MCPS was given sweeping powers to prosecute the war, and while it raised money, increased production, and distributed food, it also banned strikes, required the registration of noncitizens, and suppressed dissent. To expunge disloyalty and eliminate any threat to the state's wartime mobilization of resources, the MCPS suspended the civil liberties of pacifists and German Americans and waged a partisan political campaign during the 1918 election against the Nonpartisan League, a socialist-leaning farmers' organization. The commission also fostered a climate of suspicion and intolerance against people with disabilities and the seemingly undeserving poor who would not (or could not) follow its order to "fight or work." The commission's strong-arm tactics tarnished its credibility and contributed to the rise of the Farmer–Labor Party, but its Women's Auxiliary, which focused mostly on maternalist causes, stayed above the political fray. Operating independently of the main commission on issues that male politicians considered of little concern, the MCPS Women's Auxiliary worked closely with the Red Cross, the federal Children's Bureau, private women's organizations, and the new county child welfare boards to mobilize support for child welfare and warfare work alike. An estimated twenty thousand women contributed to the war effort in Minnesota. They organized children's health programs, got involved with food conservation, policed sexual immorality and alcohol consumption near army camps, and taught English and "American" values to immigrants. The MCPS women's committee had a branch in nearly every county and was a remarkably successful networking and state-building agency. In just two years, it strengthened the personal networks and organizational infrastructure necessary for the smooth operation of Minnesota's eugenics–child welfare system and helped consolidate and modernize an ethnically diverse and politically divided state.[5]

The end of the war in 1918 and subsequent dissolution of the MCPS brought uncertainty for eugenicists and maternalist reformers, but also new opportunities. The postwar expansion of child welfare and the enlarged authority of the Minnesota courts to make feebleminded commitments brought many individuals under state control who would not have been considered feebleminded a decade earlier. Yet the war's impact on eugenics and the "defective, dependent, and delinquent classes" was ambiguous. Three major developments—Prohibition, the fight against venereal disease, and the army intelligence tests—simultaneously intensified and undercut eugenicist concerns about mental degeneration and the menace of the feebleminded. First, the army's efforts to protect recruits from the dangers of drinking and sex put federal power behind the temperance and moral reform measures long supported by maternalists. In 1917, the War Department banned the sale of intoxicating liquors in or near army training camps, and Congress passed the Eighteenth Amendment prohibiting the manufacture, sale, or transportation of alcoholic beverages. The amendment was ratified in 1919 and went into effect in January 1920. During the war, the army also worked with social hygienists and women's groups to educate recruits about venereal disease and force prostitutes and delinquent teens who tested positive for venereal disease into detention hospitals. As a result of these efforts, popular perceptions of female sexuality and vice changed. Although moralists were shocked by sex-mad teenage girls and the number of Minnesotans who casually broke the law to make moonshine and patronize speakeasies and dance halls where liquor was sold, it was clear that such behavior was not limited to the feebleminded. Most "problem girls" were recognized as intellectually normal.[6]

The army intelligence tests also had the contradictory effect of giving ammunition to eugenicists while convincing skeptics that feeblemindedness was not causally related to pauperism and crime. During the war, a distinguished group of psychologists led by Harvard's Robert Yerkes convinced the army to let them test recruits so that enlisted men could be assigned duties appropriate for their level of intelligence. Over two years, psychologists gave alpha tests (for the educated) or beta tests (for the illiterate) to more than 1.7 million recruits. The results demonstrated the stunningly inadequate education of young American soldiers—nearly one-quarter of draftees were illiterate—and, in the minds of eugenicists, a frightening racial disparity in the capacity to learn. According to the testers, 47 percent of white draftees and 89 percent of black draftees had a mental age of twelve or under. To eugenicists, the army test results constituted proof of the exceedingly low mentality of the typical American, fueling fears of the feebleminded menace and the nation's mental decline. To critics, they showed the absurdity of eugenicists' claims. If so many "morons" were serving their country, feeblemindedness was not as menacing as previously thought.[7]

Ultimately, the 1925 passage of Minnesota's sterilization law owed more to the aftereffects of the Children's Code than to the ideas and actions of the state's eugenics lobby. As Randall Hansen and Desmond King have shown, eugenic ideas had the greatest impact when they intersected with the material interests of social workers, superintendents, women's groups, and politicians—as well as, we might add, budget-minded welfare administrators.[8] While eugenics society president Charles Fremont Dight plastered the state with heated expositions about the menace of the unfit, the State Board of Control quietly turned the idea that the feebleminded should not reproduce into a concrete social policy.

Yet Minnesota's example also reveals the importance of fiscal politics and organizational structures. The Children's Code did not simply expand state power over the so-called feebleminded; it also perpetuated the traditions of local welfare responsibility, reliance on the voluntary sector, and keeping costs low by weeding out the undeserving poor. The code made the State Board of Control responsible for child welfare and the feebleminded, in addition to its established duties for managerial oversight of the state institutions, but it also gave considerable authority to local probate courts and welfare boards. Equally important, it established a new legal category, "feeble-minded persons," which was embedded in normative assumptions about illicit sexuality, persistent poverty, and undeservingness. Within a few years, the new child welfare policies of 1917 generated a new politics of sterilization.[9]

The Administrative Consequences of the Children's Code

The Children's Code gave the State Board of Control "general duties for the protection of defective, illegitimate, dependent, neglected and delinquent children" and legal guardianship over children and feebleminded adults committed by a court to its care (or to the custody of an institution under its management). Yet exactly how the board was supposed to carry out these new duties remained uncertain. The law authorized the Board of Control to appoint an executive to administer the act, and it moved quickly to establish a state children's bureau within the Board of Control. William Hodson, who had been the Child Welfare Commission's executive secretary, was named the first director. The main feature of the new law, however, was the county child welfare boards, which were supposed to assist the state board in fulfilling its duties at the local level. Upon a county's request, the State Board of Control would appoint three local residents (at least two of whom had to be women) to serve without compensation alongside two county representatives—the superintendent of schools and another official named by the county—on a five-member child welfare board. The county child welfare board could only be established at the county's request, and all its costs, including salaries, were to be paid out of the general revenue fund of the county. Child welfare responsibilities were thus shared between the Board of Control in St. Paul, county officials, and local, mostly female volunteers.[10]

The law carefully spelled out the state's new child welfare duties. The State Board of Control, as the legal guardian of disadvantaged children, could make any arrangement that "necessity and the best interests of the child" required, with two restrictions: no child who was not adjudged delinquent could be placed in an institution for delinquents, and the board could not authorize the adoption of a delinquent child. The board was required to take action to protect an illegitimate child as soon as it learned that an unmarried woman was pregnant—by initiating legal action to establish paternity, for example—and it was required to cooperate with the juvenile court and with "reputable" public or private child-helping agencies. In practice, this meant that the female volunteers on the county child welfare boards arranged adoptions, provided casework for unmarried mothers, and (upon a county's request) served as probation or truant officers and helped investigate and administer mothers' pensions. And since the Board of Control held legal guardianship over persons adjudged feebleminded in probate court, the county boards also supervised supposedly feebleminded children and adults who were not institutionalized.[11]

The problem was that the working relationship between the county boards and the board in St. Paul was far from smooth. In theory, the county child welfare boards were the "official representatives of their constituents . . . [and] the keeper of the community conscience in doing justice to childhood." The female board members' knowledge of local issues was supposed to enable the boards to address problems quickly, while the presence of elected county officials was supposed to increase the child welfare board's prestige in the community and lead to higher appropriations. It soon became apparent that this would not be the case. A federal investigation published in 1927 concluded that the presence of elected officials on the county child welfare boards had not only failed to lead to higher appropriations but also often made it more difficult for the State Board of Control to "correct local abuses or weaknesses in local administration." State (and federal) officials were frustrated by the untrained county board members, and the county child welfare boards resented the so-called experts in St. Paul. Even Hodson conceded that the state–county power-sharing arrangement could be a "barrier to good results."[12]

Chronic underfunding compounded the problem. The general prosperity of 1920s America did not extend to agriculture, and Minnesota's farm economy foundered in the early 1920s after wartime price supports were removed. The price of wheat dropped from $2.96 to 92 cents per bushel between 1920 and 1922, and economic adversity persisted even after prices improved. The state's legal and administrative authority over child welfare thus expanded at a time when public welfare funding remained inadequate (and, in many counties, nonexistent), and budgetary worries deepened after the antitax crusader Theodore Christianson was elected governor in 1924. A promise from "Tightwad Ted" of deep budget cuts created a bleak outlook for state agencies, and the new programs for child welfare and the feebleminded operated in an increasingly tightfisted fiscal climate. Take the example of mothers' pensions: although the Children's Code had required the state to reimburse counties one-third of the cost of a mothers' pension, no appropriation was ever made, and mothers' allowances remained the county's responsibility. Similarly, because the state's new policy of compulsory commitment for the feebleminded got off the ground in a period of fiscal restraint, it predictably intensified county officials' belief that "defectives" were a social and economic burden.[13]

To make matters even more complicated, child welfare responsibilities were not simply divided between the state and county welfare boards; the courts and the public institutions also had considerable authority. This was especially true when the person was feebleminded. Although the probate court determined feeblemindedness and, if appropriate, committed the feebleminded person to the guardianship of the Board of Control, the Faribault School provided the actual care once the individual was institutionalized. As supervisor of the state board's department for the feebleminded, Mildred Thomson was pulled between the different and often conflicting demands of the institution and the courts. She recalled, "I felt sometimes like a circus performer with a foot on each of two horses that were not always going in parallel directions."[14]

Compulsory commitment brought huge changes to the School for the Feebleminded, changes aggravated by the new superintendent, Guy C. Hanna. As we saw in chapter 1, admission to the Faribault School was voluntary prior to 1917. Even after the Board of Control began to oversee the state institutions, Superintendent Rogers made the decisions about admission and discharge and essentially managed the institution as he saw fit. After 1917, the superintendent's authority was diminished. Henceforth feeblemindedness would be determined by a probate judge, an elected official not required to have any legal or medical training, and the State Board of Control made the decisions about institutional placement. The policy of compulsory commitment thus transformed the Faribault School population and exacerbated the long-standing problem of overcrowding. Probate judges and county child welfare boards used compulsory commitment to rid their communities of troublesome or "defective" individuals —girls with wild tendencies, poor women of childbearing age, and youth from particularly "bad" homes—on the grounds that they were a menace to the community.[15] Under the new policy of compulsory commitment, the Faribault School had to make room for—and actually give preference to—feebleminded persons committed to the state institution as a means of behavior control.

In some respects, these changes were minimal: institutionalization had always been a punishment for "bad" behavior. As we saw in chapter 1, Rogers gave admissions priority to individuals who were considered sexually irresponsible or criminally inclined, especially "immoral" women during their childbearing years. Such admissions priorities continued in the early 1920s. The difference was that the new commitment policy brought an end to voluntary admissions and therefore weakened the influence of the inmate's family. Although voluntary applications were still permitted under the 1917 law, voluntary patients could be detained as if they had been committed under the compulsory law, and a court order was required for discharge. Allegedly feebleminded adults now could be committed to guardianship and institutionalized without the input and even against the wishes of family members, and families who wanted to take their relatives out of the institution needed to go to court. Superintendent Hanna, a staunch eugenicist, decried the voluntary admissions policy that had shaped A. C. Rogers's tenure at Faribault, and it was not long before the Board of Control dropped voluntary admissions altogether. Families could no longer negotiate with state officials over the duration and details of institutional placement, monitor the conditions at Faribault, or easily bring loved ones home.[16]

Still, the power of state eugenics authorities should not be overstated. Minnesota was a large and mostly rural state, and a combination of bad roads, poor train connections, and long winters kept most child welfare authorities in the Twin Cities. As a result, the ties between the State Board of Control and the county child welfare boards in remote counties were tenuous at best. The state children's bureau had just six field representatives, each of whom had a caseload of about one thousand clients in districts covering about fourteen thousand square miles. This meant that, in rural counties especially, the new child welfare laws were implemented largely by local leaders. Few child welfare board members in rural counties had any social work training, and only one-quarter of the boards had any paid staff. Indeed, thirteen of the state's eighty-seven counties did not have a child welfare board at all.[17] Eugenics abuses in Minnesota found fertile ground in local prejudices, uneven child welfare practices, and the incongruities of state power; they cannot be blamed simply on elite experts or a too-powerful state.

Child Welfare in the Counties: Illegitimacy and Feeblemindedness Reconnected

The Child Welfare Commission's divergent portrait of the innocent illegitimate child and defective menace reproduced the traditional distinction between deserving and undeserving poor. At the same time, the commission proposed an administrative structure that placed responsibility for children adjudged illegitimate, dependent, delinquent, and defective within the same agency, casting all of them as undeserving. As a result of the Children's Code, the mostly female volunteers on the county child welfare boards became frontline workers in the state's guardianship program for unmarried mothers and the feebleminded, two new and related responsibilities that soon became the county boards' most time-consuming and expensive tasks. Despite the Child Welfare Commission's efforts to uncouple illegitimacy and feeblemindedness, many child welfare board members believed that illicit sex and mental degeneration were related. This belief was reinforced by administrative structures. In most rural counties, the same child welfare board—indeed, the same individuals—supervised unwed mothers and the feebleminded with the same basic goal: ensuring that their clients and their clients' offspring did not become a public charge.

Recent scholarship has been sharply critical of social work interventions into women's sexual lives. Several historians point out that social workers enhanced their own professional status by characterizing young sexually active women as "problem girls" or "mental defectives" who needed casework and treatment. Professional social workers are sometimes contrasted to evangelical reformers who attempted to redeem fallen sisters through domesticity and prayer, but religious maternity homes in Minnesota played a central role in "state" interventions. For example, the House of the Good Shepherd, a Catholic home for prostitutes and delinquent teenagers in St. Paul, worked closely with law enforcement officials, private charities, and the Board of Control to supervise wayward women and girls committed by the courts for delinquency, dependency, or defectiveness. Some of the women were unmarried mothers, and the House of the Good Shepherd also received Ojibwe girls who were designated delinquent in tribal court and sent to the House from their reservation.[18] Religious and secular organizations joined forces to monitor girls' sexuality, return delinquents to respectability, and "protect" unmarried mothers and children from becoming a public charge.

The shame of illegitimacy shaped the social experience of most unmarried mothers, especially in rural communities, where secrets were hard to keep. The state's new policy of protecting the interests of the illegitimate child directly confronted this issue—and the sexual double standard. The 1917 illegitimacy law established the state's duty to ensure that children born out of wedlock received approximately the same level of care, support, and education as children whose parents were married. Its central feature was the state's responsibility for establishing paternity—that is, getting the child's father to admit paternity and pay for maternity care and child support. Prior to the Children's Code, welfare officials had no involvement with illegitimacy unless the child became a financial burden on the county. Only the mother could file a paternity charge, and the accused father had the right to a trial by jury, which meant that he could call witnesses to testify that they had had sexual relations with the woman around the same time and raise doubts that he was the father. After 1917, county officials or the State Board of Control (as well as the mother) could initiate legal action against the putative father, and the judge could exclude the public from court. The woman no longer had to tell her story before a crowded courtroom in her hometown. These new procedures, while possibly shielding some mothers from public shame, mainly protected the taxpayer by reducing the chance that the child would become dependent on county relief.[19]

Proving paternity was a difficult, time-consuming, and usually unsuccessful task that drained board members' energy and spirits, but it quickly became the primary undertaking of the child welfare boards. A federal researcher estimated in 1927 that illegitimacy work consumed from one-third to one-half of the time of Minnesota's children's bureau and the county welfare boards, far more than the number of cases warranted. Of 4,860 unmarried mothers followed during the two years ending June 30, 1924, paternity was established in just 701 cases. Even when the state did manage to secure a court order for support, it encountered "considerable difficulty" collecting payments. The county had to pick up the slack, a fact that bolstered the belief that unmarried mothers were a burden on the public purse and probably feebleminded. According to one researcher, one-half of illegitimate children known to the state in 1924 had been supported by the public for at least four years, at an annual expenditure of about $500,000. She concluded that it would be more economical to prevent illegitimate births by increasing the budget for the identification and control of the feebleminded.[20]

The Board of Control also tried to prevent illegitimacy and keep welfare costs low by preventing and punishing extramarital sexual misbehavior. Knowing that most people wanted to keep single pregnancies secret, county child welfare board members nosed around schools, hospitals, and local hangouts, kept in touch with the police, and followed up on neighborhood gossip. Sexual intercourse between any man and a single woman was already a misdemeanor, but in 1917 the legislature made fornication that resulted in pregnancy a felony, punishable by up to two years in prison, if the man tried to leave the state to evade a paternity charge. In 1919, punishment for sexual misbehavior was extended to women, with a ninety-day imprisonment or a $100 fine for each party whenever a man and a single woman had sexual intercourse. State officials also used the carnal knowledge law, which criminalized sexual intercourse with a child under the age of eighteen, to prosecute illegitimacy cases involving teenage girls. To the dismay of the federal Children's Bureau, they prosecuted teenage fathers in criminal court as if they were adult offenders. These laws were undoubtedly motivated by economics as well as morality; the 1919 law, for example, increased the likelihood that an accused father would pay child support by making it difficult to thwart paternity proceedings by getting his friends to testify to the woman's promiscuity. But they had a chilling effect on young women's (and men's) heterosexual expression.[21]

Minnesota also tried to protect the illegitimate children of "normal" mothers by enforcing upon them the mother role. Even though the state could take guardianship of an illegitimate child, social workers in the 1920s encouraged normal-seeming mothers and babies to stay together. New maternity hospital regulations, for instance, made it more difficult for pregnant single women to secure an abortion or put a newborn up for adoption, and a highly praised state regulation obliged unmarried mothers in maternity hospitals to keep—and breastfeed—their babies for at least three months. In addition, the Minnesota Supreme Court ruled that an illegitimate child could not be taken away from its mother because of dependency alone. In 1927, the federal Children's Bureau reported that two-thirds of babies born outside marriage in the previous two years remained in their mothers' care. Only if the mother was "mentally defective" would she definitely lose custody of her child.[22]

The divergent treatment of "normal" unwed mothers and those considered feebleminded is starkly portrayed in a 1924 Children's Bureau study by Minnesota social worker Mildred Mudgett. Historians have described Mudgett's report as a "darkly pessimistic" narrative of feeblemindedness spawning illegitimacy. (At one point Mudgett writes that "a mental examination of any girl after she reaches a maternity hospital is like trying to repair the dam after the flood has occurred.") Mudgett does attribute some unplanned pregnancies to feeblemindedness. Yet she also argues that the relationship between mental defect and illegitimacy has been "overstressed" and makes a point of stating that the unmarried mothers in her study were of a "higher mental type" than was generally supposed. Mudgett recommended IQ testing not to prove that most unmarried mothers were feebleminded, but to identify and control the "defective" minority—that is, to separate unmarried mothers who deserved a second chance from the truly undeserving poor.[23]

As Mudgett described Minnesota's unmarried mothers, they were young, overwhelmingly rural, and easily victimized. She blamed their families and communities for failing to protect them. Out of 1,385 illegitimacy cases she studied, 59 percent of the mothers, but just 23 percent of the fathers, were under the age of twenty-one. Nearly one in five was under the age of eighteen. In Mudgett's view, the fact that most of the mothers were young while the fathers were usually mature men proved that Minnesota's innovative illegitimacy law was protecting innocent children, not helping scheming gold diggers advance their claims. Mudgett also stressed what she saw as the damaging effects of a bad home environment: nearly 30 percent came from homes "broken" apart by death or (less frequently) separation or divorce, while 19 percent came from large families with more than six children, where supervision was presumed to be poor. Moreover, most of the girls whose occupations were identified had jobs that brought them into contact with "undesirable" men. One-third did domestic work, and the rest worked in restaurants or factories or were rural schoolteachers. In a few cases, Mudgett reported, illegitimacy occurred because "the whole moral tone of the community [was] low." In one case, "the girls in the factory talk of nothing but sex matters." In another, "all the girls have relations with the boys when they go out." Mudgett concluded that the illegitimacy problem was mainly environmental, caused largely by commercialized recreation, the sexual double standard, and the "rural problem"—poor schools, unqualified teachers, and weak school attendance laws that allowed farm families to keep their daughters out of school. With better educational and professional or vocational opportunities, she maintained, the "most promising" unmarried mothers should be able to keep their children and win back the community's respect.[24]

But what of the least promising mother? When Mudgett thought that the woman's weakness was intrinsic to her person and not her environment, her tone grew harsh. She criticized county leaders for their ignorance of "the subject of reproduction of the unfit" and complained that many feebleminded women had not been committed. Indeed, although Mudgett's report argues for an end to the stigma of illegitimacy, her most vivid cases are bleak illustrations of mental defect, dysfunction, and abuse. For example, she described a nineteen-year-old unwed mother with an IQ of 58 who passed on a syphilitic infection that blinded her child and a twenty-four-year-old "girl" who had three illegitimate children by three different men. The second mother was committed to the state institution for the feebleminded until the pastor of her church convinced the judge to release her on the grounds that she had "learned her lesson." Referring to another case in which a feebleminded woman had sexual relations with so many different men that paternity could not be established but was released from Faribault because of "political pressure," Mudgett declared that the community did not understand "the increased taxation which will result if girls of this grade of mentality are not safeguarded."[25]

Mudgett's grim description was intended to prove two points: there was an urgent need at the county level for professionally trained social workers and judges who could differentiate between capable and incompetent mothers, and there was also a need for more funding for family casework services. Like the Child Welfare Commission, however, she advocated a two-track policy, making the case for better treatment of the most deserving mothers by setting them apart from those she considered undeserving and unfit.

This bifurcated vision shaped state policy toward unmarried mothers, and it increasingly shaped ideas about the feebleminded as well. By the mid-1920s, a growing number of superintendents expressed doubts about their earlier views on the causal connection between feeblemindedness and sex delinquency and reconsidered the need to institutionalize all the unfit. Superintendent Walter Fernald, whose famous 1912 essay "The Burden of Feeble-Mindedness" described the feebleminded as a "parasitic, predatory class, never capable of self-support" and feebleminded women as "almost invariably immoral," recanted his earlier alarmism. He and other experts now believed that at least some of the social problems arising from feeblemindedness were environmental and could be fixed with rehabilitation and training. More and more, experts distinguished between innocent feebleminded people who could live under supervision in the community and *defective delinquents* who would always remain a menace. The philosophy of individualized treatment, touted for "normal" delinquents and dependents before the war, now applied to defectives as well. Each feebleminded person was unique, children's bureau director Hodson observed, so decisions about institutionalization and supervised release had to be based on individual needs. While some people would always require permanent segregation, he believed that most would benefit from institution-based training followed by parole and community supervision.[26]

To make the case for parole, Minnesota officials drew on the familiar language of child welfare reform. Most feebleminded troublemakers were not inherently vicious, the Board of Control explained; they were simply "victims of a poor environment in youth" and usually responded positively to casework and training. Just as children of normal intelligence could be saved by removing them from unfit parents, feebleminded youth could benefit from a change of environment, a period of institutional training, and casework supervision.[27]

The board's emphasis on feebleminded youth was structural—the program for the feebleminded was located in the state children's bureau, after all—but it was also rooted in the traditional belief, promoted by an earlier generation of institution superintendents such as Rogers, that individuals with intellectual disabilities were simply children in mind. Like children, feebleminded people were considered morally irresponsible, lacking in self-control, unable to make competent legal or political decisions, and incapable of raising children or managing their personal affairs. Also like children, most responded to friendly encouragement, discipline, and control. Indeed, one Board of Control memo advising welfare boards on how to handle feebleminded wards could have been written about any modern adolescent. Feebleminded persons must

> not go to dances; must not go out alone with one of the opposite sex; must not 'keep company'; must be in at an early hour; must not associate with persons who would exert a bad influence; must not spend nights away from home or the home where placed; must have some responsible person in any group gathered for pleasure (in going to a picture show for instance, just a group of girls or boys is not sufficient); should not be left alone in the house for any length of time; must have his whereabouts known at all hours and, if not in when expected, the family should investigate.[28]

The fixation on going out reflected the reality that sexual attitudes and recreation were changing. By the 1920s, even small towns witnessed the loosening of sexual mores, and the commercial amusements that had seemed so troubling to maternalists in the 1910s were now common throughout the state. Movies led to "early sophistication" and the relaxation of taboos, blurring the lines between normal and delinquent behavior. Automobiles heightened the threat. Cars figured prominently in sex crimes involving youth, as we saw with the infamous Bragdon case discussed in chapter 1. A study of one hundred inmates at the Sauk Centre Home School for Girls found that cars and dance halls were "contributing causes" of delinquency in nearly every case. "Modern conditions have created a psychology of movement, of impatience, of waste, of futility—a craze for movement, for haste, for change," Board of Control member Blanche La Du explained in a 1925 paper. In a rebuke to eugenicists, she added that young offenders came from every social class and a growing number came from good homes. Drawing on Chicago psychiatrist William Healy's theory that the causes of delinquency were multidimensional and every young person was unique, La Du declared that the best way to handle the "very distressing amount of delinquency among the young people of today" was to treat each delinquent as an individual, not as a type.[29]

La Du's reference to automobiles and movies reflects the continuing importance of maternalists' moral protection campaigns. Indeed, her very appointment to the Board of Control in 1921 was a formal recognition of maternalists' child welfare successes, as well as women's political influence after suffrage. A widowed lawyer and mother of two, La Du had been active in the Woman's Christian Temperance Union and Republican Women's State Committee prior to her appointment; she would later become the first female president of the American Prison Association. La Du maintained a close working relationship with women's groups during her fifteen years on the Board of Control, and in

1924 she engineered an agreement with the Women's Welfare League of Minneapolis to operate a residential clubhouse exclusively for feebleminded women "on parole" from the state institution.[30]

The partnership between the Board of Control and the Women's Welfare League reveals the fluid boundaries between public and private which had long characterized US welfare policy. Founded in 1911 as a maternalist reform club, the league was by the early 1920s an established social service organization that operated a convalescent home and several boarding homes for single women workers. League officers took special pride in their Club House for Girls at Harmon Place, which provided "safe shelter, good food and protection in a home-like, uplifting, atmosphere" to wayward girls refused assistance by other agencies. In 1922, as league secretary Elinor McIntosh reported, nearly half the clubhouse residents were delinquent, one out of six was pregnant, and a few were feebleminded or insane, making the club "more vitally necessary than any other branch of our work." The next year, the league decided that the Harmon Club should "take a few of the higher type of subnormals for a longer period of time . . . as an experiment." By 1924, it was operating exclusively for so-called feebleminded women under state guardianship. For a per capita subsidy of $20 per month, the private agency cared for twenty feebleminded women whom the Board of Control and Faribault superintendent had approved for institutional release. The league helped the women find employment, provided shelter and supervision, and offered them "some pleasure in life, at the same time relieving the state of expense for their care and making room in the school for the more vicious type needing control." The Harmon Club thus combined the maternalist tradition of providing safe housing for wage-earning women with the social work profession's new casework orientation. Given the upsurge in feebleminded referrals that resulted from the compulsory commitment law, a residence for subnormal girls must have seemed a promising field for both fundraising and professional rewards. It certainly cemented the partnership between the private, female-run agency and the State Board of Control.[31]

The different interests of maternalist women's clubs and state welfare institutions shaped the clubhouse program from the beginning. The Women's Welfare League viewed the Harmon Club as similar to its other projects for young female wage earners, but La Du and the Board of Control saw it as a solution to the problem of overcrowding in the Faribault School. They modeled the program on the parole policy pioneered by Superintendent Charles Bernstein of the Rome (New York) Custodial Asylum for the Feeble Minded. In the early 1910s, Bernstein had convinced the New York legislature to let him give inmates who were well behaved and exhibited a good work ethic the chance to work in colonies, or halfway houses, run by the institution. Within a decade, he was operating a dozen colonies for feebleminded men and women who worked in domestic service, factories, or farms. The colonies tested their ability to live a more normal life than was possible in the state institution, and many were eventually discharged. Largely as a result of Bernstein's work, most superintendents in the 1920s no longer believed that all feebleminded people were public menaces who should be institutionalized for life. Instead, they endorsed the "Rome plan" of social adaptation. Although Bernstein's parole program was still in the early stages when A. C. Rogers died in 1917, Massachusetts superintendent Walter Fernald insisted that he was "bubbling up with interest and enthusiasm" about Bernstein's ideas. His successor, Guy Hanna, remained skeptical.[32]

For the Board of Control, a colony for feebleminded girls, such as the one at Harmon Club, was a humanitarian answer to the state's fiscal and welfare needs. Hodson had recognized as early as 1918 that not all the feebleminded could or should be placed in institutions. There were many gradations of feeblemindedness requiring different levels of supervision, and "public opinion will never sanction wholesale confinement in institutions, even of those who are defective." At the same time, he knew that the public expected the state to exercise "proper control" over the feebleminded. State officials believed that, by ensuring that feebleminded parolees were well supervised, a residential clubhouse could dampen popular opposition to institutional release. Yet when Mildred Thomson, the new supervisor of the state program for the feebleminded, visited the Rome asylum in May 1924, she thought that the colonies for women were "very drab—both as regards the houses and the girls themselves," and seemed like an extension of the institution. The houses were cheaply furnished, the women all wore similar institution clothing, and they had to turn over most of their pay to the institution to cover the colony's costs. By contrast, she recalled, the Harmon Club was cheery and bright. The matron was a social worker, not a member of the institution staff, and although residents had to pay board, they could buy their own clothes and keep some of their earnings for themselves.[33]

The Board of Control and Women's Welfare League were optimistic about the clubhouse experiment, and both issued glowing descriptions of the Harmon Club in their annual reports. As usual, the state stressed the project's practical benefits and low cost. "It will never be possible to herd all defectives into institutions," the board wrote in its 1924 biennial report, "and their useful labor under supervision will be an economic gain to the community." The Women's Welfare League, which depended on private donations and elite women's largesse, emphasized the project's similarity to the group's other programs. The Harmon Club brought feebleminded girls out of the institution and "back into social life, under supervision, making them self-supporting and happy," Secretary McIntosh explained. She stressed "how little chance in the world, some of these unfortunate have had," and exhorted the league's privileged membership to provide financial support.[34]

The feebleminded women in McIntosh's reports bore strikingly little resemblance to the ill-kempt degenerates of *Dwellers in the Vale of Siddem* and the mentally defective mothers in Mudgett's illegitimacy study. The "girls" at Harmon Club were not depraved, and they did not have large broods of unattractive children. Instead, they were portrayed like ordinary adolescents: stormy and misbehaving at times, but responsive to maternal authority and interested in domestic pursuits. As the Harmon Club matron declared, feebleminded girls were "just like everyone else, only more so!" Board of Control member Carl Swendsen agreed. Feebleminded women were not the immoral menaces they were made out to be, he insisted, but were "almost normal; in many matters they are normal." They could support themselves and live a "normal life" in the community if they were strictly supervised. "From an economical point of view [parole] is of course a great thing for the state," Swendsen declared, "and just think what it is for the girls!"[35]

Such benign claims about feebleminded girls' similarity to "normal" working-class women obscured the unique vulnerabilities of women labeled feebleminded and the extent to which institutionalization was an ever-present threat. Institutional segregation and community surveillance were two sides of the same policy, and many feebleminded women bounced in and out of the Faribault institution for years. Still, board officials considered community supervision a marked improvement over what they saw as the main alternative, segregation for life in the state institution. Compared to permanent institutionalization, Thomson observed decades later, the clubhouse was a "great advance—a beginning of a gradual change in attitudes."[36]

The appointment of Mildred Thomson as supervisor of Minnesota's Department for the Feeble-minded and Epileptic in 1924 was itself a milestone that reflected the state's growing emphasis on community care: Thomson had no experience with custodial institutions. The youngest child of an Atlanta lawyer, Thomson had graduated from Georgia's Agnes Scott College at a time when few southern women attended university. She worked as a special education teacher after graduation and then earned a master's degree under psychologist Lewis Terman at Stanford University; her thesis concerned the validity of the Stanford–Binet IQ test as the basis for predicting school success. At Stanford, Thomson became friends with another Terman student, Maud Merrill, who had grown up at the Owatonna orphanage, where her father was superintendent, and completed *Dwellers in the Vale of Siddem* after A. C. Rogers died. Thomson applied for a job to work with Minnesota psychologist Frederick Kuhlmann, a former classmate of Terman and director of the state board's research department, but was offered the position of supervisor in the department for the feebleminded of the state children's bureau. She stayed at the job for thirty-five years.[37]

Although Thomson had a master's degree from Stanford, her sex, her department's location in the state children's bureau, and her community (as opposed to institutional) orientation defined her as a social worker and put her on a collision course with Guy C. Hanna, the combative superintendent of the School for the Feebleminded. Hanna was hired in June 1917 to trim a budget the Board of Control felt had grown too high under Rogers. He was uncompromising in his efforts to reduce expenditures and consistent in his portrayal of the feebleminded as a burden to society, noting ominously in his 1922 biennial report that caring for the feebleminded in the Faribault School had cost taxpayers about $10 million since the school was established. At a per capita cost of $265 annually, just seventeen families with four or more children in the institution cost the state about $20,000 per year. Although Hanna did not mention eugenics, the implication was clear.[38]

Hanna and Thomson agreed on the basic eugenics principle that the feebleminded should not reproduce, but they held very different views on social welfare policy and the state. Thomson complained that the superintendent was "negative rather than positive" toward Board of Control policies and showed "no enthusiasm" for community placement. Hanna called an early plan to parole feebleminded women into the town of Faribault under the supervision of the child welfare board a "mistake from every standpoint" which would only cause trouble for him and the board. People with feeble minds would never be able to "hold their own" in society, he insisted, and parole gave the erroneous impression that their mental faculties had improved. Moreover, he added, anyone intelligent enough to function outside the institution should not have been institutionalized in the first place. "The commitment of the feebleminded is for life and it is unthinkable that those released could have their lives regulated until they die, by state authority."[39]

Hanna was forced to soften his position on parole, but the tensions with Thomson did not abate. Writing in her memoirs nearly forty years later, she was still angry that the superintendent refused to meet with her on her first visit to the Faribault School and apparently instructed staff members to keep their distance. "If an atmosphere could actually freeze a person," she recalled, "I would have become frozen in that institution." The woman who had administered Minnesota's eugenic sterilization program for thirty years was appalled by Hanna's lack of affection for his patients, claiming that he prided himself on never having seen an epileptic seizure and cared for the feebleminded "only to the extent of trying to reduce their number and the money spent on them."[40] The disagreements between Hanna and Thomson were rooted in gender, professional orientation, and the conflict between his institutional perspective and her community one, but they were played out on the bodies of institutionalized women and men, an injustice that is painfully clear in their correspondence about who should be released on parole.

Hanna strongly opposed the release of any woman he considered oversexed, even (or perhaps especially) if they were good workers in the institution. He resisted the "considerable effort" Thomson and her staff put into securing the parole of Greta Acker, who had been one of Saidee Devitt's research subjects in 1914 and was now the unmarried mother of her father's child. Despite admitting that Greta was well behaved in the institution, Hanna considered her "coarse and self-willed" and managed to delay her release for nearly three years. Even after Greta was sterilized in August 1926, she remained in the institution for another eleven months. She was only discharged to the Harmon Club the following July, a few months after Hanna resigned as superintendent.[41] The fight over Greta's discharge shows both how casually the lives of vulnerable people were bandied about and how the ill treatment Greta received from the Board of Control could have been even worse if Hanna had gotten his way.

Welfare Officials Debate Sterilization

The gulf between Hanna's hard-core eugenics perspective and the social work orientation of most other Minnesota officials burst into the open in February 1925 at the quarterly conference of the Board of Control. The sterilization bill was then before the legislature, and the conference attendees seemed on edge. First, Frederick Kuhlmann clashed with psychiatrist Smiley Blanton, the director of the Minneapolis Child Guidance Clinic, over Blanton's claim that some youngsters who tested feebleminded were simply maladjusted and could be cured. Then, Hanna read a confrontational paper entitled "The Menace of the Feebleminded," which sparked a tense debate. The paper began with the startling image, clearly intended to provoke, of a "low-grade idiot entirely devoid of intelligence, whose existence is little more than vegetable, whose only sound is a screech, whose appearance is loathsome and repulsive to those unused to such sights." From there, Hanna asserted that mental deviations such as criminality, pauperism, and prostitution had a physical basis and that 90 percent of feeblemindedness was hereditary. Years after other superintendents stepped back from such overheated rhetoric, Hanna pronounced the mentally deficient an "ever-increasing burden on the public . . . the principal cause of all human misery and suffering" and called the feebleminded woman a "greater menace" than the man. He scoffed at efforts to provide charitable aid to defectives and denounced the progressive child welfare policies that the social workers in the audience held dear. Lambasting infant health clinics, the federal child labor amendment, and school attendance laws as a burden on the brightest people and a dangerous expansion of government power, Hanna disparaged social workers who believed that feebleminded men and women could be released into the community. "At least four generations are required to remove the danger of a throwback," he claimed, and no amount of training could make a moron normal. Intelligent people should decide once and for all if they wanted to stop the feebleminded from reproducing or "continue the present fatuous policy of the survival of the unfittest."[42]

The president of the state eugenics society applauded, but Hanna's rambling tirade offended many in the audience. Some were plainly affronted by his attack on the poor and working class. To Hanna's claim that modern machines made the working class redundant, they retorted that many of the world's greatest minds came from the lowest strata. "The Savior of the world was a carpenter," one of them said. Others used Hanna's commentary as a springboard for debating sterilization and parole. Although the Child Welfare Commission had refrained from endorsing eugenic surgery in 1917, the issue regularly came up at Board of Control conferences. By 1920, two prominent officials—board member Carl Swendsen and Arthur Kilbourne, superintendent of the Rochester State Hospital—had gone on record in favor of eugenic sterilization "if properly safeguarded." However, Sauk Centre superintendent Fannie French Morse and Charles Vasaly, Swendsen's Board of Control colleague, remained opposed. Vasaly had been the board's representative on the Child Welfare Commission, and his opposition to sterilization may have been a factor in its rejection. Vasaly assumed—incorrectly, as it turned out—that legislation compelling an individual to undergo surgery that benefited the state but not the patient would be ruled unconstitutional, and he also questioned the efficacy of a policy that prevented procreation but left the "moral menace" intact. If sterilization did not affect the sex drive, he wondered, would it not lead to promiscuity and the spread of venereal disease?[43]

Catholic attendees were particularly vocal in their opposition to sterilization, although the papal condemnation of eugenics was still five years away. Pope Pius XI's 1930 encyclical on Christian marriage barred Catholics from using artificial birth control and stated unequivocally that where no crime had taken place public magistrates had no right to "tamper with the integrity of the body, either for the reasons of eugenics or any other reason." But even before 1930, most Catholics objected to sterilization as a mutilation of the human body and also feared that sterilization would encourage sexual immorality. Although some Catholics embraced the eugenic principle of race betterment and a small minority believed that the state had the right to sterilize the mentally deficient in some cases, most Minnesota Catholics who spoke publicly about sterilization opposed it. A St. Paul priest described surgical sterilization as similar to euthanizing the aged or infirm because they were a burden to their families. Sterilization was both evil and dysgenic, he wrote, and "if we violate the moral law, physical and mental degeneracy will follow." Only God had dominion over life; the state did not have the right to take the lives of "guiltless individuals" as yet unborn.[44]

Most participants at the 1925 conference agreed that the unfit should not reproduce and differed only on sterilization. Only R. M. Phelps, the medical superintendent of the St. Peter State Hospital, spoke out against the very concept of a feebleminded menace. Disputing the alarmist claim that the "whole race was degenerating," Phelps insisted that the apparent increase in mental deficiency could be explained by new modes of classification. "We are studying down into the minor grades of feeblemindedness, which we never touched years ago," he reminded the audience, and heredity was a predisposition, not a "definite result." Many so-called defectives were "good, respectable citizens," and "we all fall short of perfection more or less."[45]

Phelps was virtually alone in his dissent, and the storm over Hanna's argumentative presentation masked an emerging consensus. By 1925, most members of Minnesota's welfare establishment agreed with eugenics hardliners that the economic and social burden of feeblemindedness was staggering, and something had to be done. Although the arguments for and against sterilization had changed very little since 1917, the legal and administrative context in Minnesota was drastically different. The enlarged authority of the courts to make commitments had strained the resources of the School for the Feebleminded and the State Board of Control, and the county child welfare boards were overwhelmed. Carl Swendsen observed despondently that even the occasional placement seemed "very insignificant" given the magnitude of the problem.[46]

Blanche La Du, concluding the rancorous discussion of Hanna's paper, emphasized the need to "get away from this philosophy of despair" and look at the problem of feeblemindedness from the "standpoint of prevention." A sterilization bill with proper procedural safeguards promised to do just that. Although Phelps remained unconvinced, two influential sterilization skeptics were no longer involved with the Board of Control, and this smoothed the way for its support for sterilization legislation. Fannie Morse had left Minnesota for a career in the East, and Charles Vasaly, now the superintendent of the St. Cloud Reformatory, was no longer a board member.[47] Equally important, the board's successful partnership with the Women's Welfare League provided the infrastructure needed to supervise and control feebleminded women living outside the institution. As the board's sterilization bill was making its way through the state legislature, however, the MES launched a spirited campaign for a mass sterilization law.

The Minnesota Eugenics Society and the Battle with the Board of Control

Eugenics had deep roots in welfare circles, yet Minnesota's eugenics movement is often assumed to have begun in the early 1920s, when physician Charles Fremont Dight founded the MES. In late 1922, Dight organized a gathering of Minneapolis activists, including former child welfare commissioner Catheryne

Cooke Gilman, to establish a society that would spread "knowledge of the laws of heredity and the principles of eugenics, for the social good that might result."[48] University of Minnesota zoologist Henry Nachtrieb had been a member of the eugenics committee A. C. Rogers organized in 1913, but all the other attendees came to eugenics through their involvement in left-wing and feminist circles. Catheryne Gilman had worked with the Women's Welfare League on the Bragdon sex crime case and was the executive secretary of the Women's Cooperative Alliance, an organization devoted to preventing sex delinquency. Her husband, Robbins Gilman, was the head resident of the North East Neighborhood House. Victoria McAlmon, a charter member of the Minneapolis Federation of Teachers, was the first president of the Minnesota Women's Trade Union League and would later be a Farmer–Labor Party candidate for Congress. Dight was a former city alderman with a long history of activism in Minneapolis socialist and temperance politics. When the MES was formally launched in January 1923, Dight became its president, and nearly ninety Minnesotans were listed as members of a statewide eugenics advisory council.[49]

Despite the broad support for eugenics, the MES was essentially a one-man show. Dight had a medical degree from the University of Michigan and taught in two Minnesota medical schools in the early 1900s, but he was an eccentric. He lived for a time in a tree house and had a part-time job as medical director for the Minister's Life and Casualty Union, which left plenty of time for activism. Dight had been an alderman in Minneapolis from 1914 until 1918, but he left municipal politics and the Socialist Party over its handling of the Russian Revolution and took up the cause of eugenics. Dight was the public face of eugenics in Minnesota. During his decade-long campaign for race betterment and mass sterilization, he published more than three hundred pamphlets, radio talks, and letters to the editor.[50]

Dight came to the eugenics crusade relatively late, so perhaps it is unsurprising that his numerous popular pamphlets mostly restated the ideas and arguments of his predecessors. Like Nachtrieb and an earlier generation of natural scientists, Dight used agricultural metaphors to advance his contention that "there should be at least as much importance attached to the production of human thoroughbreds as there is to the breeding of good hogs and dogs." Like University of Minnesota anthropologist Albert Jenks, a member of the MES advisory council who studied "primitive" Filipinos and Native Americans, Dight maintained that there was a hierarchy of races and worried about the potentially dysgenic impact that immigration from Mexico and southern and eastern Europe would have on the United States. Finally, like Gilman and her fellow maternalists, Dight emphasized the importance of sex education. He urged Minnesotans to abandon their "silly prudery" and make sure their marriages were eugenically sound.[51]

Yet Dight disdained the welfare-oriented eugenics that the Board of Control and most Minnesota reformers espoused. Although he regularly approached women's clubs to talk about eugenics, he had harsh words for maternalists (like Gilman) who tried to prevent sex delinquency by focusing on what he saw as superficial things like "poolrooms, dance places, moving picture shows . . . and parental negligence," and he criticized a psychopathic clinic that aimed to "prevent waywardness and unfitness" through psychiatric treatment but did nothing to improve the human stock. The damage caused by bad heredity could not be undone by "any amount of medical, surgical or hospital care, prayers, tears or repentance," he sneered; a wise state must employ eugenic measures to improve its population just like a "good farmer does his stock."[52]

Dight's contemptuous critique of maternalist reformers was obviously gendered, but it also reflected his socialist politics, which associated moral reform with the bourgeoisie. Yet although Dight considered himself a champion of industrial democracy, he never championed positive eugenics policies, such as family allowances, which could have provided an economic benefit to most working people. Instead, he focused on negative eugenics. He used the army intelligence tests to prove that the nation's mentality was low—and declining—and claimed repeatedly that there were more patients in Minnesota's insane asylums than there were students at the state university. The growing numbers of feebleminded, insane, epileptic, diseased, criminally inclined, and avaricious Americans constituted a "peril to this nation," he declared, for a "good house cannot be built with rotten lumber."[53]

Like other eugenicists, Dight identified two main sources of mental degeneracy. The first, found in isolated regions where a "grossly degenerate stock" of poor whites never "mingled their blood" with better people, reflected the continuing influence of the eugenics family studies, as well as Minnesota's rough rural economy. The second, which was perhaps more timely given the American eugenics movement's support for immigration restriction in the early 1920s, was the influx of mentally inferior foreign laborers with large families. The importation of African slaves and the influx of undesirable European immigrants were "the two great errors committed by this republic—both of them for private profit making," he charged, reflecting national eugenics concerns more than Minnesota politics. "The worship of the dollar will finally damn any nation."[54]

Despite Dight's brazen words and personal acquaintance with the Minneapolis elite, his impassioned eugenics campaign was in many ways a failure. He failed to get his 1922 pamphlet "Human Thoroughbreds, Why Not?" distributed nationally (one publisher called the booklet "distinctively offensive to certain classes of readers") or even circulated to Minneapolis schoolteachers. Two years later, he failed to get a "fitter families" contest at the Minnesota State Fair. Dight had more success with his sterilization crusade, and in his 1935 history of

Minnesota eugenics he claimed credit for generating the "sentiment favorable to the adoption of eugenics measures." Yet despite his proficiency at networking, propagandizing, and self-promotion, there is no evidence that Dight's role in Minnesota's sterilization drive was decisive.[55]

Dight wanted Minnesota to enact eugenics legislation based on Harry Laughlin's Model Sterilization Law, but instead the state legislature enacted a narrower bill that the Board of Control had authored. Laughlin's model bill, which provided the framework for the 1924 Virginia law upheld by the United States Supreme Court, proposed an office of state eugenicist with sweeping powers to collect the personal and family histories of anyone in the state who was deemed socially inadequate. The state eugenicist would present his assessment of an individual's social inadequacy in court, and the court would issue a sterilization order if judged necessary. Although Laughlin's bill established due process procedures for notification, judicial hearings, and appeals, the targeted population —"potential parents of socially inadequate offspring," both in institutions and in the population at large—was exceedingly broad. A "socially inadequate person," according to Laughlin, was one who "failed chronically in comparison with normal persons" to be a useful member of society. The "socially inadequate classes" included the feebleminded, insane, epileptic, inebriate, criminalistic, diseased, blind, deaf, deformed, and dependent (the last group specifically included "orphans, n'er-do-wells, the homeless, tramps, and paupers"). This broad definition clearly had much in common with the concept of the defective, dependent, and delinquent classes, but Laughlin preferred "socially inadequate" to the older "scrap-basket title" because he thought that it allowed for a more precise enumeration of the subclasses needing restraint. Significantly, his bill did not restrict sterilization to patients who were *themselves* socially inadequate, but targeted anyone who might have an inadequate descendant. In Laughlin's (and Dight's) view, there was no chance that a child from the socially inadequate classes could become the deserving poor.[56]

Laughlin's model law was not used in Minnesota. Whereas Dight wanted to sterilize everyone who was "obviously unfit," Minnesota law limited sterilization to "feeble-minded and insane persons" already under state guardianship, and only after careful investigation, consultation with three experts (the superintendent of the School for the Feebleminded, a "reputable" physician, and a psychologist), and the written consent of the patient's spouse or nearest kin. In cases of insanity, the person also had to be a patient in a state hospital for the insane for six consecutive months and give his or her personal consent. (Feebleminded persons, having been declared legally incompetent, could not provide their own consent.) Although the Board of Control, as legal guardian of the feebleminded, could consent to sterilization if no relative could be located and the "duly appointed guardian" of an insane patient could consent on the patient's behalf, the legal requirement for consent to sterilization made the Minnesota law highly unusual. Several states ultimately enacted a voluntary as well as compulsory sterilization law, but Minnesota was one of only two US states with an exclusively "voluntary" eugenic sterilization law.[57]

Dight objected that Minnesota's sterilization statute was too restrictive, but most of the state welfare establishment disagreed. Although Dight convinced a small but prominent group of men, including Dr. George Eitel, founder of the private Eitel Hospital in Minneapolis, to support a more sweeping law, even strong supporters of sterilization, such as Frederick Kuhlmann, opposed his mass sterilization plans. Kuhlmann told Dight privately that it was wrong to operate on people "simply because they are defective." Surgical sterilization, he said, should be a last resort.[58] Most legislators saw sterilization as a child welfare measure. The bill was introduced by the House Public Welfare Committee along with bills supporting the child labor amendment to the US Constitution and legitimizing children born out of wedlock if the parents subsequently married. Two of Minnesota's first female legislators, Mabeth Hurd Paige and Hannah Kempfer, gave it their support. Dight was disappointed with the bill's restrictions, but he saw it as an "entering edge for more advanced legislation" and worked hard for its passage. The sterilization law passed with little debate, 86–37 in the Minnesota House of Representatives and 40–4 in the state senate. Governor Theodore Christianson signed it into law on April 8, 1925, and it went into effect the following January.[59]

Dight's persistent lobbying did not lead to the passage of his preferred bill, but his association with Dr. George G. Eitel, an officer of the MES and the surgeon who performed the sterilizations, was rewarded with an invitation to observe the first group of operations performed at the Faribault School's hospital on January 8, 1926. As Dight looked on, Eitel and two assistants performed bilateral tubectomies on five women between the ages of nineteen and twenty-four, as well as a hysterectomy on a forty-year-old woman. The next day, Dight went with Eitel and two other MES officers to meet with Governor Christianson and the Board of Control to try to convince them to widen the law. Appealing to the traditional concern that legalizing sterilization would promote vice and promiscuity, Dight claimed that "some if not all" of the first six sterilized women actually wanted the operation because they were prostitutes. Unless the law was applied more broadly, he warned, the public would surely conclude that the law was promoting prostitution and repeal it. Dight also tried to convince the board to expedite the sterilization process by collecting signed consent-to-surgery forms at the initial commitment hearing in probate court. The Board of Control was unmoved.[60]

Over the next months and years, Dight continued to fight for a broader sterilization law. In March 1926, he called on "Miss Florence Thompson" (Mildred Thomson), who told him that sterilizing every feebleminded person in Minnesota was unnecessary and would generate opposition "which should not be aroused." Dight refused to give up. Thomson recalled that every time Dight visited the board's office, he "entered into a long discussion" about the need to prevent feeblemindedness. She found him so annoying that "it got to the point where if I saw him soon enough, I was out another door and so 'not in' when he arrived." Dight's relationship with Blanche La Du, the only woman on the Board of Control, was even worse. He was furious that she rebuffed the eugenics society's offer to collect signatures on consent forms, saying that it would result in too many people to sterilize and that the legislature had not placed the administration of the sterilization program in the eugenics society's hands. Dight also took exception to the board's practice of selecting candidates for sterilization from a list of names the Faribault superintendent prepared and to its requirement that all sterilization operations be performed at the hospital of the Faribault School. He observed, correctly, that the board primarily used the sterilization law to make room for new patients at Faribault and prioritized the sterilization of sexually delinquent wards. These policies limited the law's effectiveness as a eugenics measure, he complained.[61]

The board was unyielding, but the ever-determined Dight submitted new sterilization bills to the state legislature in 1927, 1929, 1931, 1933, and 1935. The existing law was inadequate, he stated repeatedly, because it applied only to wards of the Board of Control and because written consent was required "before even a blank idiot . . . can be sterilized." He prepared a number of bills, all of which were killed in committee, he believed, by the "adverse acts and indifference" of the Board of Control.[62] Dight's dispute with the Board of Control derived partly from the mismatch between his abstract eugenics philosophy and the board's practical public welfare perspective. Although the two sides agreed that the state should be able to limit some people's reproductive rights, Dight believed that mass sterilization was a necessity while the Board of Control stressed the importance of individual casework. La Du told Dight that the decision to render someone infertile was too serious to make without a personal connection and that supervision following sterilization was essential. Sterilization should not be performed only for the benefit of the state, she said; the patients themselves should derive "some actual benefit" (such as being released from the institution). Their differences soon became personal. Dight accused La Du of prejudicing legislators by calling his bill dangerous and threatening to resign if it was passed into law. At the end of one particularly heated phone conversation, she complained about spending her Sundays arguing with him and hung up.[63]

Dight's highly publicized sterilization drive also rankled nonelite activists. Maude Baumann Arney, a schoolteacher, farm wife, and mother of six, wrote angrily that "so-called race betterment" would be unnecessary if social conditions were improved. "The people are up in arms against a good many recent 'welfare' methods in regard to children," she warned, and no one has a "God-given right to torture or maim another." Another letter attacked sterilization as an unchristian, uncivilized, and un-American attempt to suppress the working class. Dight's files contain surprisingly few references to religious opposition to sterilization. He did complain, after one of his bills died in committee, that legislators with "little or no scientific knowledge, decide scientific matters—especially where religious prejudices enter into the question," yet he never engaged with Catholic arguments against sterilization and showed little reaction to the 1930 papal encyclical, which banned birth control and sterilization. Although resistance from Catholics was certainly a factor in Minnesota's rejection of Dight's sweeping sterilization proposals, his rage remained focused on the Board of Control.[64]

Eventually, Dight's obsession with the Board of Control alienated even his staunchest supporters. His allies were furious when in 1930 he appended their names, signed to a letter they thought was simply endorsing a new sterilization bill, to a twelve-page attack on the Board of Control and sent it to every member of the state legislature. "Increase of the Unfit a Social Menace" accused the board of "autocratic and unnecessary interference in eugenic legislation" and caring only about increasing its appropriations, even though welfare spending only encouraged the unfit to reproduce. The Board of Control, Dight insisted, failed to serve "the best eugenic interests of the state."[65]

Dight continued his frenzied sterilization campaign into the mid-1930s, but by then most Minnesotans were preoccupied with the economic and political turmoil of the Depression and the New Deal. Some of the original members of the eugenics society passed away or retired (Dight himself died in 1938), but others simply drifted away. Yet if Dight was frustrated by the indifference to his eugenic sterilization crusade in Minnesota, he was buoyant about developments abroad. In the summer of 1933, he published a letter to the editor in the *Minneapolis Journal* praising Hitler's "scientific plans" to stamp out mental inferiority. He sent a copy of the letter to the führer, along with a note expressing his hope that Germany's success would "advance the eugenics movement in other nations as well," and received a thank-you card and form letter inviting him to a conference in response.[66] If Dight's brief correspondence with Hitler seems, at first glance, to confirm the affinity between eugenics in Minnesota and Nazi race hygiene, a closer examination of his sterilization crusade shows that the loudness of a political campaign is not necessarily an indication of its effectiveness. Although the mean-spirited rhetoric of eugenicists like Dight leaps off the page, Minnesota's road to sterilization was equally paved by welfare administrators who rejected the eugenics society's intemperate rhetoric.

As the example of Minnesota shows, state sterilization policies emerged from a wide variety of worldviews and political agendas. In the years after 1917, when the Children's Code dramatically expanded the state's child welfare responsibilities, a broad alliance of child welfare reformers, institution superintendents, doctors, social workers, politicians, ordinary people, and eugenicists endorsed sterilization (and its alternative, institutionalization) as the best way to protect poor young women from pregnancy, defend their communities from the burden of the feebleminded, and manage the "defective, dependent and delinquent classes" at little public cost. The next chapters focus on the routine operation of Minnesota's eugenic sterilization program during its most active years, when the gap between eugenic discourse and bureaucratic imperative was especially marked.

WHO WAS FEEBLEMINDED?

With the passage of Minnesota's eugenic sterilization law in April 1925, the Board of Control faced a difficult question: who should be sterilized? This question was at the heart of the board's dispute with the eugenics society, and it shaped the day-to-day deliberations of the probate judges, child welfare board members, institution superintendents, and psychologists who implemented different facets of the state's eugenics program. Under Minnesota law, eugenic sterilization was restricted to feebleminded or insane persons under state guardianship, and the law further required that the insane person had to be an inmate of a state mental hospital for six consecutive months and provide written consent prior to the surgery. Because of these stringent guidelines, the vast majority of people sterilized in Minnesota were categorized as feebleminded.

Who was likely to be designated feebleminded, and on what grounds? Historians often describe feeblemindedness as a "catchall term" for a variety of conditions and perceived social inadequacies, rooted in crude scientific theories about heredity and the innate superiority of the elite. "Feebleminded," most writers agree, was an astonishingly broad description that social workers, progressive reformers, psychologists, doctors, and other elites used to castigate immigrants, blacks, poor whites, tramps, prostitutes, criminals, and teenage girls overly interested in sex—in short, anyone who "offended the [eugenicists'] middle-class sensibilities."[1] This casual definition, while not inaccurate, is more a criticism than an explanation, for it cannot explain why only a small proportion of the "feebleminded" people listed above were actually brought into court, forcibly institutionalized, and sterilized. Although the sterilization approval process differed from state to state, it always involved several steps: the initiating action or arrest, adjudication in court, commitment to the state institution, and the authorization of surgery. This meant, in practice, that the feebleminded designation was inseparable from the implementation of policy. This chapter examines the initial commitment process in Minnesota, with particular attention to why some individuals—but not others—were designated feebleminded and institutionalized. The next chapter focuses on the different but related considerations that went into the authorization of sterilization surgery.

At the turn of the century, experts used the word *feebleminded* in both specific and general ways: it was a precise term for the highest level of functioning within a mental deficiency diagnosis, and a generic term for every type of mental defect. Yet whether they used the term in the specific or generic sense, even eugenics practitioners recognized that feeblemindedness was a social construct. In their influential 1918 textbook *Applied Eugenics*, Paul Popenoe and Roswell Hill Johnson described feeblemindedness as a "condition in which mental development is retarded or incomplete" and then added, "It is a relative term, since an individual who would be feeble-minded in one society might be normal or even bright in another." Unlike a medical disease, which one either had or did not have, there were many gradations of feeblemindedness, and a person who seemed intellectually normal in a small peasant village might appear feebleminded in a large urban environment.[2]

Discussions of how to identify feeblemindedness usually centered on poverty and class. In 1911, Henry Goddard, the Vineland Training School psychologist who coined the term *moron*, defined feeblemindedness broadly, as a mental defect existing from birth or a young age which left the individual "incapable of performing his duties as a member of society in the position of life to which he was born." The most widely accepted definition came from England's Royal College of Physicians, which characterized a feebleminded person as one who could earn a living under good conditions, but who lacked the capacity to compete "on equal terms" with normal people or manage one's affairs "with ordinary prudence." Both of these definitions were fundamentally economic. They reflected superintendents' public welfare orientation, as well as the widespread belief that the feebleminded were a burden to society because they lived "more or less at public expense." In addition, as many scholars have pointed out, the broad definition of feeblemindedness fused all sorts of dependencies, delinquencies, diseases, and disabilities into one diagnostic label. At a time when mass migration, urban growth, labor turbulence, and westward expansion challenged race and gender hierarchies, feeblemindedness provided a language for the expression of social anxieties. The vagueness of the term meant that there was "no limit to its misappropriation and resulting abuse."[3] The feebleminded person was the embodiment of the undeserving poor.

Most scholars writing about feeblemindedness have analyzed it as a cultural discourse and (pseudo)scientific diagnosis. But feeblemindedness was also a legal and administrative category by which persons deemed to be incompetent for citizenship were made to surrender their political and civil rights in exchange for the state's "protection." Just as recent legal scholars have argued that race is at least partly constructed by the law, so too was feeblemindedness. The law did not simply codify a preexisting scientific or social category; as with race, it actually created the category of feeblemindedness, using science and common sense to fix the boundaries of normality and define a subordinate identity. A person committed to state guardianship as feebleminded in Minnesota could not vote, own property, manage his or her financial affairs, or marry without the state's permission. Feebleminded wards of the state had no legal right to control their own bodies. The State Board of Control, as the legal guardian of the feebleminded, made the decisions about institutionalization or (after the passage of the Minnesota sterilization law in 1925) sterilization. Since the feebleminded ward could not legally consent to a medical procedure, the Board of Control had the power to consent to sterilization on her behalf.[4]

It would be easy to see the 1917 enactment of a eugenic commitment law and the resulting increase in feebleminded commitments as the unambiguous triumph of eugenics expertise. As is always the case with public policy and the law, however, a closer examination shows a more complicated story. Until an individual was actually placed under guardianship, surprisingly little authority rested in the hands of the doctors, psychologists, or social workers employed by the state. Any family member or "reputable citizen" living in the same county as the alleged defective could initiate the commitment proceedings, and a probate judge—an elected official not required to have any medical or legal training—decided whether the petition had merit and should proceed. The probate judge could appoint a board of examiners, consisting of himself and two licensed physicians appointed by him, to determine whether the person under investigation was really feebleminded, and the Board of Control could send someone "skilled in mental diagnosis" to examine the alleged defective and attend the commitment hearing. However, the state-appointed expert had only an advisory role. If the individual was "obviously feeble-minded," the judge could dispense with the board of examiners and, with the consent of the county attorney, make the commitment decision on his own.[5]

Experts complained bitterly about their negligible role in the commitment process. Psychologist Frederick Kuhlmann, the director of research at the Faribault School (and, after 1921, the Board of Control), objected that the law placed inordinate power in the hands of the probate judge, a nonprofessional. Most judges, he complained, lacked not only the expertise to recognize a feebleminded person but also the courage to commit someone over the objections of relatives and friends, especially in an election year. Kuhlmann was also frustrated that the law made medical doctors full-fledged members of the board of examiners but gave psychologists with expertise in mental testing only an advisory role. It was the "delusion of the layman that a physician must be skilled in mental diagnosis because he is a physician," he protested. Feeblemindedness was not a disease, and the physician's opinion should be irrelevant.[6]

Kuhlmann's objections may have been motivated by professional self-interest, but he certainly posed an important question: who was feebleminded, and who got to decide? The definition of a "feebleminded person" in the 1917 statute was vague: "any person, minor or adult, other than an insane person, who is so mentally defective as to be incapable of managing himself and his affairs, and to require supervision, control and care for his own or the public welfare." The Minnesota statute did not include the standard references to competing "on equal terms" with normal people or managing one's affairs with "ordinary prudence," but it gave probate judges wide latitude in making commitment decisions that could result in a person being institutionalized for life. Most judges considered various factors when making a feebleminded diagnosis, but few were familiar with the professional literature on mental deficiency, and they mainly encountered people already in trouble with welfare agencies or the law. Even judges prepared to follow the experts' advice faced a confounding array of theories about the taxonomy of feeblemindedness and, in many cases, had to sort out conflicting testimony from local doctors, ministers, school officials, police officers, and neighbors. As a result, while some judges depended on intelligence test results and family pedigree charts when assessing mental abnormality, others paid more attention to delinquent behavior or economic dependency, or looked for physical stigmata such as an "ugly" appearance or racialized features. Still other judges, especially those from rural areas, rejected any "scientific" explanation for aberrant behavior and viewed feebleminded commitment through a moral or religious lens. All of this illustrates the profound uncertainty in how judges with the authority to commit individuals to guardianship interpreted the law.[7]

Whether or not they were familiar with eugenic science, Minnesota judges were acutely aware of the administrative usefulness of the *feebleminded* category. For that reason, delinquency and dependency remained the standard criteria for a mental deficiency designation. Most women committed to guardianship and eventually sterilized in Minnesota were either sex delinquents—often, unmarried mothers of children they could not support—or slightly older married women with a number of children on public assistance. The men generally exhibited antisocial behavior that made them seem like a threat to the innocent child. As we shall see, specific decisions about who was feebleminded did not only flow from the class bias, racial prejudice, and professional self-interest of the elite; they were also shaped by local fiscal and administrative considerations and the everyday interactions between county officials, the families of the so-called feebleminded, and the allegedly feebleminded individuals themselves.

Determining Feeblemindedness in Rogers's Day

Expert ideas about the nature and causes of feeblemindedness changed surprisingly little between the turn of the century and World War II. Despite the growing reliance on the Binet intelligence test and, in the interwar years, greater use of psychiatric terminology, Minnesota's eugenics–welfare program remained static, rooted in Faribault superintendent A. C. Rogers's turn-of-the-century ideas about the menace of hereditary feeblemindedness.[8]

To be sure, administrative procedures and the legal status of the feebleminded in Minnesota changed dramatically after the enactment of the compulsory commitment law in 1917. Previously, the power of diagnosis rested with the superintendent of the School for the Feebleminded, a doctor who diagnosed mental deficiency through a time-consuming and highly subjective medical examination. Rogers and other superintendents recognized that the physical and mental capabilities of people considered to have intellectual disabilities varied widely, and they often commented on the need for a scientific classification system. Yet despite the absence of standardized criteria for a mental deficiency diagnosis, most were confident about their diagnostic skills. As historian Leila Zenderland points out, most superintendents believed that, "after years of experience treating feeblemindedness, they simply knew it when they saw it."[9]

Probate judges also relied on intuition when deciding who was feebleminded. Although most considered a range of factors, including economic status, social behavior, family background, school or work record, and IQ, they usually looked first for the physical stigmata of mental deficiency—a disabled, disfigured, or "ugly" appearance. Indeed, as Susan Schweik has shown in her study of municipal anti-begging ordinances, a major reason that public institutions for the feebleminded expanded so dramatically in the late nineteenth century is that they removed physically disabled beggars—the lowest of the undeserving poor—from the public eye. Pennsylvania superintendent Martin Barr, to use one example, had described feeblemindedness as a mental or moral defect "usually associated with certain physical stigmata of degeneration." While certain types of intellectual disability, such as Down syndrome, had easily identifiable visual characteristics, Barr and other superintendents and judges also looked for other visual markers, such as a drooling mouth or undirected gaze, when diagnosing "low-grade" idiots and imbeciles. Long-standing assumptions about racial degeneration also persisted in terms such as "Mongolian idiocy" and in the visual association of racialized features, such as dark skin and thick lips, or the prominent cheekbones and deep-set eyes supposed to be characteristic of American Indians, with subnormal intelligence and innate criminality. At the same time, as Frederick Kuhlmann explained in numerous speeches, physical traits were a highly inaccurate gauge of mental acuity. Many "high-grade" feebleminded women were healthy and normal in appearance, even beautiful. The difficulty of recognizing mental deficiency in "moron girls" made them, like the figure of the attractive mulatto who passes for white, exceedingly dangerous to unsuspecting men (and the taxpayers who might have to support their illegitimate children). In Kuhlmann's view, this visual uncertainty proved the need for psychological expertise.[10]

Inappropriate behavior or comportment was another highly subjective indication of feeblemindedness. Disturbing behaviors, such as violent outbursts, public masturbation, rocking or head banging, and playing with fire, were considered obvious signs of mental deficiency, but so too were more ambiguous behaviors, such as truancy, vagrancy, petty theft, sexual transgressions, and difficulties learning to read. Many "high-grade" feebleminded were diagnosed at the beginning of the school years or—of even more relevance for sterilization—at the onset of puberty. The problem, psychologists admitted, was that many of the behavioral signs of feeblemindedness showed up in the "normal" population too.[11]

The most widely accepted sign of feeblemindedness was another attribute rooted in the three Ds and shared by many "normal" Minnesotans: the inability to achieve success in life and be self-supporting. A. C. Rogers and his coauthor Maud Merrill adopted this fundamentally economic test in *Dwellers in the Vale of Siddem*. Quoting Britain's Royal College of Physicians, they defined a feebleminded person as "one who is capable of earning a living under favorable circumstances, but is incapable, from mental defect existing from birth or from an early age, (a) of competing on equal terms with his normal fellows; or (b) of managing himself and his affairs with ordinary prudence." The reference to "ordinary prudence" reveals the moral stigma of chronic poverty. As Merrill and Rogers explained, a few feebleminded families in southern Minnesota "left a trail of criminals, paupers, and degenerates, who will patronize our county jails, poor houses and houses of prostitution for several generations."[12] In a remote rural economy where most people were poor, the high-grade feebleminded were indistinguishable from the undeserving poor.

The belief that feeblemindedness was inherited led to a fourth sign of feeblemindedness: a family history of social inadequacy. Henry Goddard observed, and most other superintendents agreed, that the "vast majority of feeble-minded persons are so because a parent or grandparent was feebleminded." To A. C. Rogers, the rediscovery of Mendel's laws of inheritance in the early twentieth century constituted proof that feeblemindedness was a genetic trait, and the eugenics pedigree studies conducted by Charles Davenport's ERO provided a promising means of confirming the feeblemindedness of borderline cases who might otherwise escape detection and his institution's control. It was "self-evident," he wrote in a funding letter to the Board of Control, that the "most important foundation" for predicting the appearance of feeblemindedness was an "accurate knowledge of the family history of those families in which two or more defectives are found." Even if a definitive medical diagnosis was impossible, a family history of feeblemindedness could justify classifying a person as feebleminded, rather than normal, so that he or she could be institutionalized on eugenic grounds.[13]

Family history moved to the forefront of feebleminded diagnosis in the 1910s, when the ERO's famous fieldwork project gave scientific legitimacy to this diagnostic measure. Even after field-workers Saidee Devitt and Marie Curial began their investigations of the families of Faribault School patients in 1911–1912, however, not every Minnesota welfare administrator welcomed the approach. At the quarterly meeting of the Board of Control, the superintendent of the St. Peter State Hospital for the Insane, Harry Ashton Tomlinson, disputed the idea that feeblemindedness and insanity ran inexorably through families and emphasized the circular bias implicit in the field-workers' family investigations. First, he pointed out that many normal individuals came from feebleminded families, since "the mistakes of Nature tend to rectify themselves." Second, he argued that eugenics field research was methodologically flawed. Since the field-workers believed that individuals with a feebleminded relative were themselves feebleminded, they naturally assumed that the families they were investigating were defective. "In other words," Tomlinson stated acerbically, "If you hunt a Jukes family, you will find a Jukes family."[14]

Rogers conceded that "we naturally, all of us, have unconsciously a little prejudice, and we are very likely to interpret things in a way favorable to what we are looking for." But his cautious words rang hollow given the premature conclusions he drew from the field-workers' early research. Indeed, Rogers presented his first report on Devitt's findings in 1912, when she had been at work for less than nine months. With only partial information collected on 99 families, Rogers announced confidently that only 17.8 percent of the inmates' relatives were definitely normal, and preliminary data confirmed that feeblemindedness was hereditary. Over the next four years, Rogers took his message about inherited feeblemindedness to welfare officials, juvenile court judges, charity workers, clergy, and women's clubs. Hereditary mental deficiency caused most dependency and delinquency, he always told them, and containing it was the key to preventive child welfare work.[15]

Rogers became ill with pernicious anemia and died before he finished analyzing Devitt's and Curial's fieldwork data, but their unpublished notes and narratives reveal much about the process by which some of Minnesota's rural poor were marked as feebleminded and unfit. Each report centered on the alleged hereditary pathologies of one family, beginning with the proband (the institutionalized person whose genetic history was under investigation). It then listed the informants, gave a short overview of the patient's home and general health, and cataloged what each informant had to say about each member of a set of relatives—the patient's siblings, the patient's father's (and mother's) siblings, the patient's grandparents, and so on, as far back as they could go. Repetitive and inward looking, the reports described in mind-numbing detail the dilapidated homes, supposedly unattractive children, and depressed personalities of the rural poor, while downplaying any possible social or environmental explanation for the patient's alleged deficiencies.[16]

Davenport instructed the ERO field-workers to gather data, not analyze it, but Devitt and Curial turned their research notes into sensationalist narratives of pauperism and degeneracy in the Root River Valley. In "Timber Rats," Devitt vividly recounted her hellish descent "down & down" to the foot of the ravine, and then along a rocky road where the walls of the gully rose so high there seemed like no other way to get out. Eventually, she and her driver came to a little log shanty where a number of children were playing in the yard. The youngsters ran into the house when they saw the visitors. A pig ran out from under the doorstep. The house was small and filthy, and there was a little garden, but no crops. Devitt wondered how the family survived. She was told they were "timber rats" who endured the harsh Minnesota winter by cutting wood and trapping foxes and raccoons. As Devitt's narrative shows, the field-workers who ventured into rural Minnesota felt themselves in an alien and depraved environment and translated their prejudices into their field notes, proving that "if you hunt a Jukes family, you will find a Jukes family." The effect was to prejudge those who later would find themselves in front of a probate judge.[17]

Rogers, like most eugenicists, was intensely worried about the feebleminded marrying their own relatives. He instructed Devitt to investigate the subject of cousin marriage (loosely defined), and she tracked down a farmer who was married to his niece. She diagnosed Henrik Olsen as a borderline case. He was, she wrote, a "very lazy and shiftless" old man who never did a "decent day's work in his life." His wife was "very slovenly in her appearance & neglects her home." Since she could not read or write, Devitt identified her as a moron. She described the couple's cramped one-room dugout as "one of the worst places for humans to live in that can be imagined." Six adults and three children crammed into a small dark room with a low ceiling, which was crowded with broken furniture and the rags they used for beds.[18]

To the modern reader, "Timber Rats" is a distressing depiction of rural isolation and poverty. The gloomy one-room cabin that Devitt interpreted as evidence of feeblemindedness was uncommon by the 1910s, but similar houses had dotted the landscape in the nineteenth century. Devitt, however, viewed the dugout as proof of its occupants' low morals, disreputable characters, and feeble minds. Her report, submitted to the ERO after Rogers died in 1917, showed no sympathy for the desperately poor families who struggled to farm the rocky soil during a short growing season and no concern for the children she said were thinly dressed in winter, "never had enough to eat and were abused terribly." Devitt pointedly rejected the suggestion that being "brought up in poverty in a secluded ravine" might have contributed to their lack of economic success. "It is true environment counts," she conceded, but biology mattered more.[19]

The child welfare movement was in full swing when Devitt was writing her reports, but her submissions to the ERO contained no reference to those reformers' ideas. Minnesotans were engaged in heated battles over prohibition, women's suffrage, farm conditions, and child labor, and maternalists were working to bring innocent dependent and delinquent youngsters into the deserving poor. Devitt, however, discussed dependency, delinquency, and drunkenness only in relation to hereditary defect. For example, her thirty-page report on Mary Schmidt, the oldest of five children in a German farm family, scarcely mentioned the fact that the seventeen-year-old girl had only two years of schooling (counting her year in the School for the Feebleminded as a year of school). Instead, it began with the observation that Mary had spasms at age two, did not talk until she was four, and left the Faribault School prematurely. The Schmidts considered their daughter capable of "considerable rough outdoor work," but not very useful inside the home, so the teen spent her days working in the fields with her alcoholic father. An environmentally oriented reformer might have seen Mary's story as demonstrating the need for child health care or compulsory schooling, but in her report Devitt never doubted that the girl's feeblemindedness was inherited and incurable. After all, the girl's father was a moron, and her mother, "a woman of no force or energy, [was] somewhat slow and dull." Devitt admitted that Mrs. Schmidt was "about up to the average of her class in mental make-up," but was uneducated and thus "never had a chance to grow mentally." As a youngster, she worked on a farm, and after getting married, she cared for her invalid mother-in-law and "endure[d] much hardship." Although Devitt acknowledged Mary and her mother's heavy workload and lack of schooling, she still concluded that Mary's feeblemindedness was inborn and incurable.[20]

Field-workers' refusal to recognize any role for the environment was particularly cruel in cases of family violence and sexual abuse. The write-up on twenty-year-old Susie Herman, an unwed mother who died of pneumonia just three months after giving birth, is a poignant example. Devitt began her 1914 report on the Herman family with a summary of what she considered the salient facts: Susie Herman was "feeble-minded and a sex offender." She was pregnant on admission to the Faribault School and later gave birth to an illegitimate child. All but two of Susie's eight siblings were feebleminded. According to Devitt, the low mentality of her siblings explained why, although Susie attained the sixth grade, her mental age was only eight.[21]

Susie's female relatives and neighbors, however, accentuated a different set of facts to explain her mental status. They said the girl's stepmother treated her shamefully, beat her head with a stick, and was "dreadfully cruel." Susie used to be a "bright little girl," her uncle's wife recalled; "I think Susie's defect is due to her step-mother's ill treatment." Another woman reported that Susie was "criminally intimate with at least a dozen of the young fellows about here," but she "never knew any other life." Her stepmother and father were brutal: they locked Susie in a room and stuffed clothes in her mouth so she could not cry out while her brother sexually assaulted her. Devitt recorded these shocking stories, but gave more space (and thus more credibility) to the views of the county attorney, who stated only that Susie "could not get on" with her stepmother. He thought that Susie's refusal to work for a respectable farm family was proof that she was "mentally weak" and "irresponsible." Devitt's report showed no consideration for Susie or the trauma she endured.[22]

In report after report, the flat inventory-like catalog of family failings obscured the conflicting viewpoints of relatives, neighbors, and public officials, and the opinions of officials carried the most weight. Consider Devitt's 1914 report on eleven-year-old Greta Acker, the incest survivor whose release from the institution Superintendent Hanna so vigorously opposed. Devitt described Greta, the daughter of German immigrants, as a strong, healthy child who had only a few days of schooling before she went to Faribault. Although two informants called Greta's parents unkind and abusive, the report gave more credence to the views of the Humane Society officer, who said he could not verify the neighbors' claims that the girl was beaten and mistreated. The Ackers seemed respectable because they lived in a good neighborhood and kept their house fairly clean and neat, so Devitt summarized Greta's home treatment as "probably kind but neglectful." She portrayed Greta's troubled family life and lack of schooling as the symptoms, not the cause, of her handicap.[23]

Devitt's reports are powerful evidence of eugenicists' disparaging assessment of poor "white trash," but that alone does not explain a feebleminded diagnosis. Why were some destitute rural people, but not others, labeled feebleminded and sent to Faribault? Local dynamics may provide a clue. The field-workers relied heavily on interviews with county commissioners, sheriffs, teachers, physicians, relatives, and neighbors, and their eugenics reports may have reflected local resentments and frustrations as much as their own preconceptions. All of the families under investigation already had someone in the School for the Feebleminded, and many had other relatives on relief or in trouble with the law as well. To the local officials who had to deal with these families on an everyday basis, and perhaps even to some of their better-off relatives, people from these families may have seemed innately defective, the undeserving poor. Despite their designation as scientific researchers, Devitt and Curial were not very different from the charity workers, parole agents, and police who intruded into working-class family life on a regular basis. It is too simple to see the feebleminded label only as something eugenicist outsiders imposed on the rural poor.

The concordance between charity work and eugenics research is revealed in Devitt's correspondence about an allegedly feebleminded single mother, the sole support of her family, who was fighting the Associated Charities' efforts to send her father to a mental hospital and remove her bright five-year-old daughter from their home. Devitt told Rogers that after several "friendly visits" to the family, she could see that the woman loved her daughter deeply and would be brokenhearted if charity workers took the little girl away. She confided that she almost wished that the little girl were feebleminded so the mother and daughter could go to the Faribault School together. Yet Devitt did not mention the little girl's heredity, which could be a eugenic justification for placing her in Faribault, nor did she question the need to remove her from the home.[24] In this case, eugenicist ideas about inherited degeneracy were secondary to the social work objective of rescuing an innocent normal child from a supposedly bad home environment. For social workers and eugenicists alike, the state had a moral responsibility to protect innocent children—and the wider society—from their feebleminded parents who were the undeserving poor.

The Power of IQ

By 1910, most superintendents acknowledged the subjective nature of the criteria for diagnosing feeblemindedness and emphasized the need for a more reliable and scientific means of assessment. Rogers believed he had found this standardized assessment tool in the Binet intelligence test, which measured an individual's reasoning and problem-solving skills ("mental age") in comparison to average children of the same age. He was one of the first superintendents to recognize the usefulness of the test. In 1910, when the American Association for the Study of the Feeble-Minded endorsed the Binet test as the "most reliable method at present" for determining the mental status of feebleminded children, Rogers was enthusiastic. "Who is there that does not have a mental picture always in view, of the activities and capacities of normal children at different ages?" he wrote in a *Journal of Psycho-Asthenics* editorial; "What more natural or rational than to compare the mind, backward in development, with a normal one?" The association also adopted a new method of categorizing the feebleminded. Under the new classification system, there were three classes of feebleminded: *idiots* had a mental age of about two years old and an IQ under 25; *imbeciles* had an IQ of 26–50 and a mental age of up to seven years old; and *morons* had an IQ of 51–70 and a mental age of about twelve.[25]

Eugenicists used intelligence testing to identify, classify, and control feebleminded people who could pass as normal, but it was originally designed for a different purpose: to spot schoolchildren who could benefit from special education. French psychologist Alfred Binet developed the tests because he wanted a more precise measurement of children's innate intellectual abilities in order to distinguish those who had permanent disabilities from those who were merely underperforming in school. Struck by the similarities in the intellectual level of "normal" young children and older people of below-average intelligence, he developed the concept of "mental age." This triggered a major shift in experts' understanding of intellectual disability from weak-mindedness to developmental delay. In bringing the Binet test to America, Goddard helped redefine mental deficiency as a deficit in "intelligence"—a problem of psychology rather than medicine—and narrow its measurement to a test score.[26]

IQ testing enabled experts to identify as feebleminded people who had no physical stigmata and, to the casual observer, seemed more uneducated than defective. This led to a spectacular increase in the number of people labeled feebleminded. In 1890, when Rogers first declared that feeblemindedness was a greater problem than previously thought, he estimated that as many as one in five hundred Americans was feebleminded. By 1915, Frederick Kuhlmann maintained that one in two hundred was a conservative estimate. Many experts drew a causal connection between low IQ and economic deprivation, criminal recidivism, and moral lapse. As proof that feeblemindedness and criminality were linked, Kuhlmann pointed out that 25–35 percent of reformatory inmates tested feebleminded, but Goddard estimated that as many as 50 percent of criminals, prostitutes, and almshouse paupers had feeble minds. Some overzealous corrections officials went so far as to claim that 70–100 percent of prisoners were feebleminded, a finding Kuhlmann dismissed as "extreme to the point of absurdity."[27]

As these figures suggest, at a national level the impact of intelligence testing was momentous. "More than any other factor," writes historian Mark Haller, the faith in IQ test results "led to the crusade against the menace of the feebleminded." Mass testing took root in prisons and functioned as a weeding mechanism in reform schools and juvenile courts, but it was Goddard's testing of immigrants at Ellis Island and the IQ tests given to World War I army recruits that shaped the national political conversation about race, intelligence, and citizenship. At a time when about one-third of Americans and an astonishing 70 percent of Minnesotans either were foreign-born or had a foreign-born parent, Goddard's early finding that feeblemindedness was present in about 40 percent of immigrants arriving at Ellis Island—and 80 percent of Russians, Jews, Italians, and Hungarians—garnered attention. A few years later, Goddard and another former G. Stanley Hall student, Lewis Terman, joined the team of psychologists who prepared the intelligence tests for army recruits. The disturbing results, which found that nearly half of recruits—and, by implication, the American population—were feebleminded, both reinforced and undermined the eugenics belief that subnormal intelligence was the root cause of most social problems. Critics of the army tests pointed out that the vast majority of "feebleminded" recruits were respectable, self-supporting, and able to manage their own affairs. This realization did not lead to the rejection of mental testing, however, but to a shift in usage: after the war, IQ testing was used not only to diagnose feeblemindedness in criminals and paupers but also to rank and classify schoolchildren. As Michael Rembis has observed, the army tests led experts to differentiate between the "good" feebleminded person, who could be self-supporting if in a wholesome environment, and the "bad" feebleminded person, who was a hopeless case and would always remain the undeserving poor.[28]

In Minnesota, the effects of intelligence testing were more ambiguous. Although Minnesota was home to one of the nation's most prominent test developers, Frederick Kuhlmann, his obsessively narrow focus on IQ testing limited his practical influence on state policy. Kuhlmann had earned his PhD at Clark University, where he was a classmate of Lewis Terman, the Stanford University psychologist who taught Mildred Thomson, but he spent most of his career working for the state of Minnesota, first as director of research at Faribault and then at the Board of Control. Thomson wrote her MA thesis on IQ testing, but she found Kuhlmann a difficult colleague who was "more concerned with his tests than with pleasantries" and had little to do with the children's bureau staff. Whereas Kuhlmann believed that a mental test alone provided all the information needed for a feebleminded diagnosis, Thomson preferred what she considered Terman's wider-ranging approach, which also considered social and familial information. In her view, Kuhlmann was "so dogmatic and tense about his convictions that he cut himself off from the give and take of discussion with groups with whom it might have been fruitful."[29]

Still, Thomson regularly used intelligence tests when a court or county child welfare board wanted to determine whether a person should be committed as feebleminded. If the individual's IQ was below 70, Thomson told the state conference of social workers, the need for guardianship and possibly institutionalization was plain. If the IQ was between 70 and 75, social workers should take both intelligence and environment into account. If the IQ was over 75, Thomson advised, guardianship should be imposed only if there was "extreme failure in adaptation" or if the family was unable to "make plans" (that is, if the family was destitute or "defective" and incapable of controlling the ward). This rigid classification system guided Minnesota policy for decades. "I.Q. tests possess a special magic," a critic observed bitterly in 1965; probate judges still relied to an "astonishing degree" on the rigid formulations for determining intellectual disability which state welfare officials had developed forty years earlier.[30]

Intelligence testing was not a routine part of the adjudication of feeblemindedness in 1920s Minnesota, despite the experts' faith in IQ. The relatively limited role of mental testing was due not only to a shortage of trained examiners who could administer IQ tests outside of cities but also to statutory requirements, which made an elected judge the person responsible for determining feeblemindedness. Sometimes judges ordered IQ tests, but sometimes they did not. The statute authorized the judge to obtain "expert" assistance from two licensed physicians and permitted the Board of Control to send someone "skilled in mental diagnosis" to advise them, and it also stipulated that the county would bear most of the cost. Although the state paid for the examiner it appointed, the county paid all the fees and transportation costs of the physicians on the examining board, as well as of the person who made the arrest and transported the alleged defective to court and each witness who testified. For budgetary reasons, then, the judge had an incentive to dispense with the board of examiners, and experts skilled in mental diagnosis did not usually attend commitment proceedings in remote rural counties. Moreover, even when IQ tests were ordered, they were often administered by poorly trained testers in settings that were far from ideal, such as in "a crowded room, in a home with a child often pounding on the door, in the yard or in the car." Unsurprisingly, the admissions registers of the Faribault School were inconsistent in their recording of IQ.[31]

Early critics of the Binet tests, and countless scholars since, have pointed out that IQ tests measured schooling more than native intelligence, reflected considerable class and cultural bias, and reinforced the hurtful assumption that many of the poor and uneducated were unintelligent and unfit to be parents. Yet scholars' entirely reasonable emphasis on test bias has obscured another important truth: some Minnesota women may have escaped eugenic segregation and sterilization because of their high IQs. One such woman was Agnes Ogden, an Irish American "sex delinquent" from a socially problematic family. Agnes's parents divorced when she was young, and she spent her childhood living a nomadic life with her father until he was killed while robbing a bank. She moved in with her mother after her father died, but she soon got into trouble over alcohol, race mixing, and sex. When Agnes was fourteen, the police raided the house of a black man looking for moonshine, found Agnes in bed with a (different) man, and took her off to jail. Agnes insisted that she was not having sex that time, but the authorities did not believe her because she admitted that she began having intercourse when she was twelve. Still, the officials viewed her sympathetically. Although they complained that Agnes used coarse language and was evasive and crafty during questioning, they described her as a "neglected child, thin, and ill kept," who never had a proper home. They attributed Agnes's delinquencies to her poor associates and bad environment, not her family heredity, for there was no question of feeblemindedness: she had an IQ of 119. Agnes was committed to the Minnesota Home School for Girls at Sauk Centre and discharged six years later at the age of twenty.[32]

A high IQ also saved Vera Hardy, who was committed to Sauk Centre at the age of sixteen for theft, truancy, and sex with a carnival man. Vera's family was a textbook example of social inadequacy; the county sheriff described her home as the worst he had ever seen. Vera's father was a hard-drinking brute who viciously beat his wife and children. Her mother was a pathetic woman who "raised a large family, endured poverty, and wretchedness all her life . . . [and] hasn't the character to even attempt a change." Social workers considered Vera the only person in her family to be of average intelligence, and she had an IQ of 118. Her accomplishments were indeed impressive. Although she left home at the age of twelve, Vera managed to stay in school until the eighth grade while supporting herself and giving money to her siblings. Her social worker admitted that Vera deserved "an immense amount of credit for what she has done," even as she wondered aloud whether the girl's delinquencies were due to the "normal conflicts of adolescence" or the shortcomings of her family inheritance. What is important is that the social worker's musings mattered little. Vera's family may have exemplified the "socially inadequate" stock featured in eugenics narratives, but she herself did not fit the statutory definition of a feebleminded person in Minnesota, for she was clearly capable of managing her own affairs. Vera's brother, mother, and at least one other sibling spent time in the Faribault School for the Feebleminded, and at least one of her sisters was sterilized, but she married and had children (and, not surprisingly, moved far out of state). In Virginia, Vera might have been sterilized as the "probable potential parent of socially inadequate offspring." Instead, she managed to avoid eugenic institutionalization and sterilization because of her ingenuity, high IQ, and luck. The county child welfare board and probate judge recognized that Vera was capable of managing her own affairs and committed her to state guardianship as a delinquent, not a defective. Would the outcome have been different with another judge? Minnesota law gave the probate judge, in Kuhlmann's words, "full power to determine any case as he alone wishes," so there is no way to be sure. As Vera's case illustrates, the IQ test helped some individuals avoid eugenic commitment, even as it put away many others. The only certainty was the capriciousness of the commitment process.[33]

Adjudicating Feeblemindedness: Sex Delinquency and the Practice of Commitment

Kuhlmann never stopped trying to convince social workers and judges of the need for intelligence testing, but he was well aware that most of them were more concerned with practical economic and social assessments. In a 1927 speech, he advised social workers that judicial commitment should be guided by two main questions: was the individual feebleminded, and (since the state could not supervise every feebleminded person) was guardianship required? The first question was "strictly psychological," and Kuhlmann believed that it was easily answered by an intelligence test. The second question was sociological and concerned the alleged defective's home environment, ability to earn a living, and behavior. (Kuhlmann noted that the judge also had to ensure that the commitment process followed the law and did not violate the rights of the alleged defective, but he had little to say about legal procedures.)[34]

Kuhlmann's emphasis on "sociological" considerations reflected both the language of the Minnesota statute, which did not mention IQ, and the new child welfare responsibilities of the courts. Traditionally, probate courts handled matters of probate and the administration of estates, but progressive legal reformers had expanded their jurisdiction. After 1917, probate judges in Minnesota had the power to commit dependent, neglected, delinquent, and illegitimate children, and "defectives" of all ages, to state guardianship. Moreover, as we saw in chapter 1, probate courts in rural areas functioned as the juvenile court, managing delinquents and administering mother's pensions. Probate judges thus worked closely with school officials, welfare agents, and police officers to evaluate the deservingness of mother's pension applicants and the rehabilitative potential of poor kids in trouble with the law. It is hardly surprising, then, that mental deficiency commitments pivoted on customary notions of delinquency and dependency. The three Ds were not only conceptually connected, but the administrative apparatus was the same.

In practice, Kuhlmann considered numerous factors beyond IQ when determining feeblemindedness. In a 1920 speech telling probate judges how they could recognize "obvious feeble-mindedness" and so avoid appointing a board of examiners, he advised evaluating the alleged defective's physical appearance and ability to do the "ordinary things of everyday life" and listening to the opinions of relatives and neighbors. A pleasing appearance and the neighbors' opposition to feebleminded commitment were "no proof of normality," Kuhlmann warned, but if everyone agreed that an individual was "a little odd, peculiar, and so on, but not so bad as to be called feeble-minded," that person would almost certainly test in the imbecile or moron class. Despite his complete faith in the IQ test's objectivity, Kuhlmann's own notes and speeches were rife with clichés about the immoral and inappropriate behavior of people he considered feebleminded. He thought that the majority of prostitutes and unwed mothers were feebleminded and told probate judges that defectives' predisposition to delinquency was a "well-established fact." Even in the era of the IQ test, Kuhlmann's writings show that physical appearance, nonstandard or sexually transgressive behavior, and the social test of self-support remained powerful indicators in testing for feeblemindedness.[35]

Eugenicists had long believed that high-grade feebleminded women were hyperfertile, and fear that these "prolific breeders of defectives" would add to the tax burden clearly shaped the everyday implementation of the state's commitment policy. Many of those committed and eventually sterilized in Minnesota were young, unmarried, sexually active women in their early twenties who either had or might have had illegitimate children they could not support. In Hennepin County (Minneapolis), for example, more than half of the 120 "high-grade" feebleminded committed to state guardianship in 1927 had been "grossly delinquent," while another 20 percent had been charged with incorrigibility.[36] Sometimes unmarried mothers were brought under guardianship simply because they had a child outside of marriage and were financially insolvent. Eugenic considerations were a crucial factor in these commitments, but a narrow focus on eugenic goals can obscure the equally important, but decidedly more mundane, fiscal and administrative aims of the state program. Nearly everyone designated feebleminded and committed to state guardianship in the interwar period was poor. Most were dependent on some kind of public aid. Compulsory commitment to state guardianship was the first step toward institutionalization, which transferred partial financial responsibility to the state and provided financial relief to local communities that might otherwise have to support the dependent individual and family indefinitely. In addition, since guardianship of dependent and delinquent children normally ended when the person turned eighteen, a mental deficiency designation enabled state officials to exercise long-term control.

Promiscuity and prostitution had long been associated with mental deficiency, but the sexual transgressions of adolescent girls took on new meaning in the 1920s, as mass culture, automobiles, and Prohibition-era lawbreaking blurred the line between respectable and deviant feminine behavior. As an older generation of welfare officials and reformers struggled to adjust to the new morality, the courts gained new power to intervene into ordinary people's private lives. Sauk Centre superintendent Fannie French Morse had been a vigorous opponent of the routine IQ testing of sex delinquents, but after she left Minnesota in the early 1920s, the Board of Control regularly approved mental tests for Sauk Centre girls, transferred those with low IQs to Faribault, and had them sterilized. One such girl was Edna Collins, who allegedly ran about the streets at night, used bad language, and had sex with three different men. Kuhlmann described Edna as dirty and vicious and claimed that she taught immoral acts to other children. He set her IQ at 68. Another allegedly feebleminded sex delinquent, Lillian Green, went to dances, used vile language, smoked, read confession magazines continually, and never attended church. She was committed to Sauk Centre at the age of sixteen for "excessive indulgence" with middle-aged men.[37] As both of these cases illustrate, young women's forays outside the norms of accepted sexual practices became a measure for identifying them as feebleminded.

Some historians have portrayed feeblemindedness as a spurious charge leveled against young women, like Edna and Lillian, who refused to conform to the suffocating constraints of Victorian sexual morality. Yet a closer look at the case histories complicates the narrative highlighting these women's sexual rebelliousness and agency. Although some women designated feebleminded may have been resisting the norms of a repressive society, many others were victims of rape, incest, or domestic violence, or came from troubled families unable or unwilling to support their adolescent daughters during economic hard times. Edna Collins's father, for instance, had deserted his family, and Edna began acting out sexually after a fifty-year-old man related to her mother by marriage paid her to have sex in the back of his car (this man was later accused of violating five girls under the age of ten). Lillian Green's hard-drinking father committed suicide when she was fourteen, and social workers considered her mother, who was disabled from polio, to be "very incompetent." Lillian herself was said to be very "hard boiled" and mean. From the age of fourteen, she had regular sexual relations with a number of old and middle-aged men, earning between fifty cents and a dollar each time. (The wife of one of these men initiated the petition that led to her commitment.) As Lillian did not get along well at Sauk Centre, she was committed as feebleminded and transferred to Faribault, where she was sterilized in 1938, two months before her twenty-first birthday. Reflecting on Lillian's case a few years later, Thomson described her as "a girl who needs a family." She was sterilized instead.[38]

At times, the feebleminded label grew out of parents' concerns about their daughters' sexual reputations or was the result of a cruel sexual double standard. For example, Rachel Kopf's parents worried that she was promiscuous and always wanted to go out. She fought with them constantly, but they were unable to restrain her, as she was "lazy and impudent and just 'boy crazy.'" Rachel's caseworker described the Kopfs as respectable, but overly strict, and noted that they once punished her for running away by chaining her to the bed for three days. When she was fourteen, Rachel ran away and rode the rails with a "moron" boy until she was arrested and sent to jail. Rachel was committed on a sex delinquency charge to the Home School for Girls, but her difficulty adjusting to the Sauk Centre routine, combined with her low score on an IQ test, led to her transfer to the Faribault School and eventually to her sterilization. Sarah Berger's experience was somewhat different. She was a young child walking with her cousin when several boys "jumped out from the bushes by the road and pulled them over into the woods and did bad things to them." Everyone received punishment that time, but when Sarah, at age twelve, reported that one of the boys bothered her again, she alone was summoned to court and designated a delinquent. Sarah protested that the boys should have been sent away instead of her, but she spent nearly eight years at Sauk Centre and another six years at Faribault. Finally, at the age of twenty-six, Sarah was sterilized and released.[39] The abstract idea of childhood innocence did not apply to young sexually molested girls.

The psychological trauma of sexual abuse, institutionalization, and loss trapped some women in a tragic vicious circle. Feebleminded women and girls were especially vulnerable to sexual abuse, and sexual abuse made some women and girls feebleminded. For example, Mabel, "an attractive Indian girl" and one of the few nonwhite women mentioned in the state records, was treated as "'common property' in the community" and tormented by men who "not only made vile remarks to her but did things they would never do to a white girl." She was committed as feebleminded at the age of fourteen. Dora was also sexually victimized as a young girl. "Pretty, but sweet and more docile" than most feebleminded girls, she had spent her entire childhood in an orphanage. The things that happened to her in the orphanage would "make your hair stand on end," Mildred Thomson recalled, but Dora had little education, no experience of community living, and an IQ of 72, so she was committed to the Faribault School. Sterilized and released after several years, Dora soon returned to Faribault with a case of gonorrhea. "She was a girl for whom psychiatry could have done much if at that time the feebleminded had been considered capable of responding to treatment," Thomson reflected years later. "Without doubt it would have shown her to be both brighter than indicated by the tests and capable of making a good adjustment. She needed a personal tie of some sort." Instead, she got caught in the state's eugenics program.[40]

Like Dora, many women committed to state guardianship had venereal disease. Although most experts had tempered their views on the menace of the feebleminded by the mid-1920s and no longer viewed all feebleminded women as degenerates who spread venereal disease (as Massachusetts superintendent Walter Fernald claimed in 1912), a venereal disease diagnosis remained a leading cause of a feebleminded designation. Working-class girls who tested positive for gonorrhea were assumed to be hypersexual and probably feebleminded. Even maternalist reformers who campaigned against the double standard and male sexual license generally accepted the conventional medical view that teenage girls with venereal disease either acquired it innocently, from unsanitary objects like toilet seats, or were diseased because of their aberrant sexual desire. Incest and child sexual abuse were invisible. Even when incest was prosecuted and the offender jailed, experts generally viewed the ensuing depression, anxiety, and dissociative or sexualized behaviors as symptoms of the girl's inherited deficiency. Social workers thought that feebleminded women were too dense to be disturbed by sexual abuse and expressed little concern about victims' psychological state. For example, a 1926 study that stressed the possibilities of rehabilitation for "normal" sex delinquents described a fifteen-year-old feebleminded girl who had "immoral relations" with the neighborhood boys as a hopeless case. The girl did not understand the "seriousness" of her sexual behavior, the author explained, because she had been having intercourse with her father since she was eleven years old. Similarly, Faribault superintendent J. M. Murdoch expressed impatience with the fragile mental state of Lucille Johnson, a nineteen-year-old who had two illegitimate children after her mother died as a result of sexual intercourse with her father and brother. (Her father served time in the state prison for incest.) Superintendent Murdoch described Lucille as "quiet, well-mannered, and responds to kind treatment," and he recognized that her "delinquencies seem to have been beyond her control, and she has none of the tendencies towards prostitution." Still, he thought she worried too much about her surviving child. Although one of her babies died at one week old and she lost the other to adoption after she went to Faribault, Murdoch attributed Lucille's "delinquencies" to her intellectual disability. He never considered the possibility that her anxieties—and even her feeblemindedness—might stem from the trauma of incest and the loss of her children.[41]

The tangled interplay of social, behavioral, and physiological factors in a feebleminded diagnosis is apparent in the Faribault School's admissions register. Few judicial commitment records survive, but the intake records of four women admitted in July 1924 (and eventually sterilized) show how poor health, disability, family troubles, and dire poverty intersected with sexual misconduct to create troubled personalities and feebleminded diagnoses. Eighteen-year-old Kate, a farmer's daughter, suffered from polio, heart trouble, and a stubborn disposition; she also had sexual intercourse with her neighbor and a brother. Sixteen-year-old Prudence had venereal disease and an "incorrigible" disposition, the result of sexual relations with her uncle and several other men. Twenty-nine-year-old Alice, the daughter of German immigrants (her father was deceased), had "slow speech." Another twenty-nine-year-old, Lucy, came from a Swedish immigrant farm family. Her father was disabled from rheumatism, and her brother had spent a year in a state hospital for the insane, but the onset of Lucy's problems allegedly began when she contracted diphtheria at the age of twelve. Despite her sixth-grade education, Lucy was "immoral" and suffered from venereal disease.[42]

The range of factors leading to feebleminded commitment reflected, at least in part, the increasing regulation of young women's lives. By the 1920s, working-class teens had considerable contact with social workers, truant officers, nurses, and psychologists who had the authority to intervene into their family lives and try to fix their bad behavior. Sometimes the girl's own parents invited officials to intervene. Yet no single authority exercised full control, and as a result, the reasoning behind most feebleminded commitments was opaque.

Judicial commitment was particularly unpredictable when the allegedly feebleminded girl was Ojibwe. In the interwar years, many Ojibwe teens, like their nonindigenous counterparts, went to the movies, stayed out at night, engaged in sexual relationships, and became pregnant out of wedlock. These young women had to contend with white stereotypes of Indians as drunk, defective, and disorderly; in addition, some were given IQ tests that found them to be feebleminded. Still, a finding of feeblemindedness did not necessarily lead to commitment in probate court or institutionalization at Faribault. Some judges were reluctant to commit Ojibwe girls to state guardianship as feebleminded on jurisdictional grounds, since most tribal members were wards of the federal government. However, years of intermarriage, allotment, and land loss could make the certification of individuals' Indian status exceedingly complex, and other judges did not hesitate to use their power to commit. For indigenous and nonindigenous delinquents alike, there was no discernible pattern to judicial decisions about commitment.[43]

Even Mildred Thomson, the chief administrator of the state program for the feebleminded, was puzzled by the seemingly arbitrary disposition of cases. Why, she asked, were some sexually delinquent girls committed as feebleminded and transferred to Faribault to be institutionalized indefinitely or sterilized, while others with similar backgrounds, behaviors, and IQs were charged only with delinquency and discharged when they turned eighteen? In 1934, Thomson obtained New Deal funds for a study she hoped would explain the inconsistencies. Taking a group of women with similar ages, IQs, behaviors, and dates of placement, she divided their cases into three different types: those committed only as delinquent and sent to Sauk Centre, those committed only as feebleminded and sent to Faribault, and those under guardianship as delinquent and feebleminded who had been in both institutions. After spending hours mulling over the data, Thomson decided that nothing helpful stood out and (to the historian's dismay) threw out the data. There was "apparently some basis for choice—although it perhaps was established unconsciously," she wrote in her memoirs.[44] In the end, the arbitrariness and unpredictability of the feebleminded designation were the only things Minnesota's poor young "sex delinquents" could count on.

Fixing Poor Mothers: Dependency, Mother Blame, and Child Welfare

Next to having sex out of wedlock, being a "bad" mother or the daughter of a supposedly bad mother was the principal cause of feebleminded commitment, institutionalization, and sterilization. The belief that feebleminded mothers bred feebleminded children was deeply held, and it functioned, in some ways, as a feminine version of the biblical saying that the sins of the fathers were visited on the sons. Maternal behavior and the home environment were also central to popular theories of degeneration, which held that poverty, sexual immorality, and intemperance could damage the germ plasm and be passed on to their offspring. "Bad" mothers also loom large in the classic works of eugenics, from the nineteenth-century "Margaret, Mother of Criminals," a progenitor of the family that Richard Dugdale famously called the Jukes, to the nameless tavern girl who headed the supposedly defective family line in Henry Goddard's 1912 book *The Kallikak Family.* As philosopher Licia Carlson points out, Goddard's study of the Kallikaks exemplifies the good mother / bad mother dichotomy because the same man produced both the good and bad family lines. Martin Kallikak's marriage to a virtuous Quaker woman produced 496 upstanding citizens, whereas an earlier liaison with an unnamed feebleminded tavern girl yielded generations of mental defectives, prostitutes, criminals, and paupers; the only difference was the mother. Even in the 1920s, feebleminded women were symbols of promiscuity and careless procreation and "prolific breeders of defectives." Any feebleminded woman who chose to procreate was by definition a bad mother.[45]

Mothers were held responsible for their children's deficiencies regardless of whether the mechanism for the transmission was considered hereditary or environmental. Perhaps because the Minnesota children's bureau administered its eugenic commitment law, state officials expressed greater concern about the harm caused by neglectful mothering and inadequate homes than about the transmission of genetic defects. Although feeblemindedness was thought to correlate with poverty, messy housekeeping, sexual immorality, and child neglect, in the end it was the failure to meet the standards of middle-class domesticity that marked the feebleminded mother as undeserving and unfit. For example, the brief case reports on four Faribault residents who had feebleminded mothers and were considered for sterilization in 1933 made no mention of other "defective" relatives or the eugenicist concept of family pedigree. Instead, they were written in social work language, using the motif of the undeserving poor. As evidence for the feeblemindedness of two of the mothers, the histories noted that one had an illegitimate child and the other was receiving county aid. Regarding the other two women, who were sisters, the report said only that the family had "no delinquent tendencies . . . just extreme poverty and mental backwardness."[46]

The feebleminded mothers and potential mothers portrayed in the records of state agencies bear little resemblance to the degenerate women in the *"The Jukes," The Kallikak Family*, or *Dwellers in the Vale of Siddem*. Rather, they reflect the image of the dangerous mother which pervaded the social work and child guidance literature of the interwar period. Prior to World War I, psychologists attributed juvenile misbehavior to a range of causes, including heredity, ignorance, and a bad environment, and progressive reformers utilized the rhetoric of good motherhood to demand child welfare measures such as mother's pensions. They portrayed dependent and delinquent youngsters as innocent children who needed mother love and good homes. By the 1920s, however, psychologists saw mother love as a "dangerous instrument" and flawed mothering as the explanation for virtually all behavioral problems. Middle-class housewives were criticized for overprotecting their children, and working-class mothers were accused of neglecting their children by going out to work.[47]

The harshest condemnation was reserved for allegedly feebleminded mothers, who were unfit by definition. Both too much aggression and too little initiative were evidence of feeblemindedness in women; in addition, they were indications of psychological dominance or child neglect, signs of a "bad" mother. In

1934, a Hennepin County social worker reviewed forty-one open cases of the child welfare board's feebleminded files and found that 90 percent of children with a feebleminded parent were neglected. The fact that the welfare board only saw problem cases did not stop this social worker from concluding that there was a "strong relationship between feeble-mindedness and neglect of children." As University of Minnesota psychologist Florence Goodenough stated emphatically, "No feebleminded person shall be entrusted with the rearing of children."[48]

Despite the gender-neutral language, the parents discussed in these reports were invariably the mothers. Every mother who kept a dirty house, "neglected" her children by partying or going to work, or had kids who got in trouble faced the possibility of a feebleminded designation, and every woman labeled feebleminded was cast as an incompetent mother and risked losing custody of her children. In parenting as in sex, women faced a punishing double standard.

The unfairness of state policy toward mothers is discernible in the differential treatment of wives and husbands when both were feebleminded wards of the state. Consider the case of Elizabeth Bergmann, a farmer's wife and mother of two who was committed to state guardianship at the age of twenty-four. Although Elizabeth and her husband were both determined to be feebleminded, she alone was sent to the Faribault School to be sterilized and educated in "habits of cleanliness and good housekeeping." Elizabeth was discharged from Faribault to her husband's family, but she did not get along with them and felt mistreated, so she soon left for the Twin Cities, taking one of her children with her. Three years later, Elizabeth was unemployed, homeless, and unable to support herself or her child and had to return to Faribault. After two more years in the institution, she was so desperate to get out that she agreed to return to her husband. Was Elizabeth's feeblemindedness related to her unhappy marriage? Like many poor Depression-era women, Elizabeth did not have a job or family to fall back on, and as a result, she had few options. Social policies that put all the responsibility for housekeeping and childcare on women but denied employment and mothers' pensions to women like Elizabeth only made matters worse.[49]

If Elizabeth was too defiant and stubborn to be a good mother, most feebleminded mothers were considered too passive and dull. Listlessness, often regarded today as an indication of fatigue or depression, was a common justification for feebleminded commitment and institutionalization in the 1920s and 1930s. Pearl Morgan, for example, had five children, a hard-drinking husband, and very poor health, but social workers described her unsympathetically as dull, listless, and lacking in initiative. Mary Peterson, a thirty-six-year-old mother of ten, was "dull and rather slovenly." Although she did not use alcohol or drugs, she was a poor housekeeper and had been a weak student twenty years earlier, so the Faribault medical staff reasoned that she was mentally deficient and incurable. As usual, they recommended sterilization for Mary, but not for her husband, who was also a feebleminded ward.[50]

Listlessness and rebelliousness were both considered symptoms of feeblemindedness in women. They were also, in the thinking of 1920s psychiatrists, indications of a pathological or rejecting mother who posed a danger to her child. That is why, in spite of a general policy of family preservation and programs like mothers' pensions which enabled most poor children to live at home, social workers often removed the children of feebleminded mothers. As an officer of the Children's Protective Society explained, "Mental defectives have undiminished powers of procreation, but often have not the power to support children and generally have little or no ability either to guide or to discipline them. Often the children of a feebleminded mother by the time they are 10 years old have more intelligence than their mother and consequently dominate her."[51] By expressing special concern for the normal children of feebleminded parents, social workers revealed both their narrow view of proper maternal behavior and their social welfare (as opposed to strictly eugenic) orientation.

The damage a feebleminded mother could inflict on a normal child was hammered home in the case of Martin X, an illegitimate and allegedly neglected child of a feebleminded woman whose case was "fairly typical." The fifth of seven children, Martin had no respect for his mother because he was smarter than she was—and knew it. School officials considered him neglected; he was dirty, often absent, and uninterested in his studies. A visiting nurse said Martin's mother was "simply impossible" and worried what would become of the boy if he continued to live with "this woman in this environment." In the spring of 1933, when Martin was ten, the nurse's fears came true. Martin joined a gang, looted automobiles, broke windows, and stole from his mother. When a social worker advised Martin's mother to hide her money, the boy sneered, "I am smarter than her, she can't hide her money where I can't find it." The social worker concluded that the boy's delinquency was "a natural result of his mother's inadequacy."[52]

Martin's case was written up to demonstrate that social workers were powerless to prevent Martin's delinquency. As a feebleminded ward of the state, Martin's mother bore no legal responsibility for her son's care. It was only after Martin tangled with the law and became a "delinquent" that the county welfare board was able to remove him temporarily from his mother's custody. For the social worker who wrote up the case, the system had failed Martin. If social workers were to "protect the child handicapped by being born to mentally deficient parents," they needed more power to intervene. Of course, the state already did have the power to institutionalize a feebleminded mother to prevent her from reproducing, but the reality of tight budgets, overcrowding at Faribault, and community opposition meant that this approach was not always possible; it was much simpler to remove the child from the home. Orphanages, rescue homes, and American Indian boarding schools had a long history in the United States, and even judges who would never institutionalize a noncriminal adult did not hesitate to remove the children. Despite the scholarly emphasis on sterilization, the eugenics campaign to prevent the feebleminded "from becoming responsible for the care and rearing of children" also supported a policy of child removal.[53] Child removal was more common than sterilization because it was less controversial, but it, too, was traumatic. At a time when child welfare policies encouraged deserving poor mothers to rear their own children, the feebleminded mother who lost custody of both her child and herself was truly the lowest of the low.

Feeblemindedness in Men: Delinquency and the Institutional Career

The manifestations of feeblemindedness and thus the reasons for commitment were deeply gendered. As we have seen, the vast majority of women committed to guardianship and eventually sterilized were sexually delinquent or economically dependent "bad" mothers or potentially bad mothers, and, in most cases, the county child welfare board initiated the petition to commit them. In contrast, the police filed most of the petitions to commit teenage or adult feebleminded men, and they were far more likely than women to be accused of a crime. For both men and women, the reasons for commitment varied. Some men committed to guardianship were school truants or juvenile delinquents transferred to Faribault from the Red Wing Training School for Boys. Others were committed to Faribault with their mothers and grew up there. Still others were committed as adults after a sexual offense or a vagrancy charge. Male and female "defectives" were both portrayed as a threat to the innocent child, but the nature of the threat was quite different.

During the economic crisis of the 1930s, joblessness, transiency, and dependency on relief led to a crisis of masculinity. Tens of thousands of "loafers" and unattached men roamed the countryside, freed from the discipline of job and family, and male defective delinquents replaced fertile feebleminded women as the chief object of state officials' institution-management concerns and societal fears. Historian Margot Canaday demonstrates that New Deal social workers attempted to distinguish the Depression's new transients, "normal" needy strangers whose rootlessness came from the economic collapse, from habitual tramps and vicious perverts, whose wanderlust and degeneracy were supposedly inborn. The former were deserving of work relief or transient services, while the latter remained the undeserving poor. Minnesota's policy of sterilization and parole had reassured state officials and the public that feebleminded women could live in the community without jeopardizing public safety, as long as they did not have children, but the Depression had intensified concerns about feebleminded men. Compulsory commitment provided a means of controlling hard-to-manage men.[54]

Most of the feebleminded men who show up in the Faribault School superintendent's correspondence regularly exhibited illegal and antisocial behavior, such as heavy drinking, thievery, vandalism, sexual offenses, and family violence. Troubled men from desperately poor families, they often spent a good portion of their lives in and out of the state institutions. Ryan McDonald, for example, was committed to the Red Wing Training School for truancy at the age of ten, and by the time he was adjudged feebleminded in his twenties, he had been implicated in a variety of charges, from carrying dangerous weapons to selling moonshine to forcing his wife into prostitution. Peter Knowles was "considered a menace in the community and excluded from school because of his attention to girls." He was first committed to Red Wing as a delinquent, but he was sent to the School for the Feebleminded when he was twelve. He ran away several times until he was discharged while an escapee five years after his initial admission. Peter lived at home without incident until 1937, when his family fell on hard times and, because no one would hire Peter, the whole family went on relief. He was readmitted to Faribault at the age of twenty-one, sterilized, and released, but after only six weeks he was returned to the institution because he had attempted to strangle his father. Richard Meyer also had a troubled childhood. His parents were divorced, his brother was feebleminded, and he could not "get" his lessons. Richard was committed to Red Wing for drinking, stealing, and running away from home, and then transferred to Faribault a year later. Sterilized and released so he could work on his family's farm, Richard was returned to Faribault because his mother and sister were so frightened by his heavy drinking and aggressive behavior that they pleaded for the state to readmit him.[55] While probate judges and child welfare boards used the eugenic commitment of women to ease counties' relief responsibilities, the same law could be used to incarcerate men who exhibited aggressive behavior, including domestic violence, but had served out their jail sentences or committed no actual crime.

For men and women alike, sexual misconduct was a leading cause of feebleminded commitment and institutionalization. At one point in the mid-1930s, 60 percent of the fifty-eight inmates in the men's locked building at Faribault had committed some kind of sexual offense. Twenty-five were guilty of "sexual delinquencies," a term that included indecent assault, child molestation, incest, and rape. Eleven exhibited sexual "perversions," eight had venereal disease, and twenty-nine suffered from "emotional instability" (they were impulsive, attacked other people, and could not concentrate). In addition, the superintendent explained, sixteen of the men were excessive drinkers, twenty-five were thieves, and thirteen were psychotic. Nearly 40 percent were repeat offenders, and more than two-thirds had previously escaped.[56]

Several scholars have observed that eugenics laws targeted gay men. In Minnesota, however, there is little evidence that men were committed to guardianship as feebleminded when homosexuality was their *only* offense. Edward Wood, for example, was described as a sex pervert "in love with a woman's life," but he had also been arrested for auto theft, was visibly disabled (with a "crippled" arm and leg), and allegedly attempted illicit relations with his sister. Jim Beattie was first committed to Red Wing as a teenager for theft and indecent sexual behavior with older men, but he also drank heavily, stole a car, fathered an illegitimate child, and appears to have had several psychotic episodes. Although sterilized as part of a plan for release, he did not stay outside the institution for long and spent much of his life in state institutions.[57]

The disturbing stories of two men who were arrested for sex offenses and later alleged to be feebleminded reveal the unstable line between "normal" and "abnormal" sexual behavior, the emotive power of perceived threats to women and children, and the smug assertions of the experts who insisted on mental deficiency diagnoses. The first case involved Brian Murphy, a nineteen-year-old farmhand who had spent four years in the state reformatory for attempted rape when a psychiatric evaluation prepared for his parole hearing claimed that the young man was feebleminded and thus more dangerous than he seemed. The psychiatrist said that Brian's poor school report and record of truancy, along with the fact that he had a sister at Faribault, pointed toward a mental deficiency diagnosis, but the conclusive proof that Brian was feebleminded was his behavior on the night of the crime. At about eight o'clock in the evening, when the village streets were still full of people, the young man started to follow a girl he had never met before. He showed her his sexual organs and pulled up her dress to see hers, but he did not follow through with the assault. The subsequent trial revealed that Brian had exposed himself to two other women but never attempted to do more. The psychiatrist, reviewing the case four years later, expressed doubts about the original charge because the teen's behavior on the night in question was so peculiar: he exposed himself on a crowded street but did not attempt intercourse. "Mentally he is a moron and his reasoning and judgment are not particularly good," the psychiatrist explained; his penchant for exhibitionism over rape was proof that Brian's abnormality was incurable. Since the young man was almost certain to reoffend, the doctor recommended that Brian be committed to guardianship and sent to the School for the Feebleminded. The evidence suggests, however, that the psychiatrist's recommendation was not heeded and Brian was not committed.[58]

We know more about the disturbing case of a World War I veteran named Herman Fechner because he challenged his feebleminded designation all the way to the state supreme court. Fechner's tragic story illustrates the terrible vulnerability of men deemed both sexually abnormal and mentally slow. Nearly forty-five years old and never married, Herman Fechner was an unemployed janitor who lived with his parents when a Rice County probate judge determined him to be feebleminded. With his parents' support, Fechner appealed his commitment, and the district court reversed the order of the probate court, ruling that Herman was not so feebleminded as to justify permanent guardianship. The state then filed a second commitment petition with some new information. Based on this new filing, the probate judge committed Fechner a second time, and this time the district court upheld the order. Fechner appealed to the Minnesota Supreme Court, which sustained the lower court's decision in 1934.[59]

The chief of police brought the initial petition for Herman's commitment, citing that he "talks to himself, curses, swears, strikes the barn with his fists, I.Q. is low, urinates in public, [and] has attempted crime against nature." According to the police chief and his neighbors, Herman was seldom seen but often heard. The man next door testified that Herman had loud spells of "swearing and cursing and, well, rapping around the barn and making a lot of noise." His wife, the mother of two girls aged five and seven, complained that Herman's screaming and pounding "made me nervous." Police chief Albert Hanson, who called on the Fechners after the neighbors made a complaint in the summer of 1933, agreed. "He saw me coming," the officer explained, "and he started to curse in the kitchen and told me he didn't want to see me, he didn't want to have anything to do with me at all, for me to get out of there, that I had caused him enough trouble now, and called me awful names, and so on, and told me to get out." Frustrated, the chief issued a warning: if Herman did not stop his ravings, "we would have to do something about it." He filed a commitment petition shortly thereafter.[60]

The trouble to which Fechner alluded was the police chief's role in his arrest the previous year for attempted sexual assault. According to court documents, the incident took place in the wee hours of the morning in June 1932, when a twenty-three-year-old gas station attendant treated Fechner to a bottle of Prohibition-era near beer. The young man testified that he talked with Fechner for half an hour and let him unbutton his pants, but when he realized what Fechner intended, he hit him on the nose with his gun. At that point (the young man continued), another man appeared on the scene and fired two shots at Fechner, who then fled. Fechner was arrested for attempted sexual assault. The police obtained a signed confession, which the police chief had written. Without consulting a lawyer, Herman admitted that he attempted to have oral sex with the gas station attendant and that on another occasion he had had sex with another man. At the criminal trial, three doctors and a psychologist testified that Fechner was feebleminded. If he had had a higher IQ, Fechner might have gone to jail. Instead, he was institutionalized for the rest of his life. His ordeal had just begun.[61]

The transcript of Fechner's hearing is a powerful demonstration of how the criminalization of homosexuality, combined with narrow definitions of intelligence and normality, affected ordinary people. Fechner had the support of his parents, the tenants of buildings where he worked as a janitor, and some of his neighbors, but the gas station attendant, police chief, several other neighbors, and a psychologist all testified that he was feebleminded. His lawyer did his best to prove his client's harmlessness by pressing the gas station attendant to explain the circumstances of the alleged assault. Why was he at the station so late? How long had he known Herman? Why did he offer Herman a drink and then let the older man unbutton his trousers? When did he realize that somebody else was there?

Q. And so you kind of coaxed him along, did you?
A. No, I didn't coax him along.
Q. Well, when he said "Come on," you didn't say, "No, I won't do it," or something like that.
A. Well, I just thought I would see what to hell he would do. . . .
Q. And you are sure you didn't encourage him in any way?
A. No, I didn't.
Q. But you didn't tell him no, or tell him to go out of there and stop that, did you?
A. No.

Fechner's case concerned his alleged feeblemindedness and not his sexual predilections, however, and the court's main concern was his (lack of) mental agility. Herman scored between 55 and 62 on several IQ tests. His lawyer objected that at least one result should be discarded because the assessment had been conducted in an intimidating setting (the judge's private office) and Herman had had a toothache. The psychologist, however, insisted that the location of an IQ test was irrelevant and dismissed the seven-point gain in his scores as the result of Fechner's growing familiarity with the test.

As part of the court proceedings, the state's attorney posed a series of questions to Fechner in order to demonstrate his lack of intelligence. Fechner fared badly. For instance, he could not name the word opposite of *war*, could not say how a ship was like an automobile, could not count backward from twenty, and claimed that he had held nine different jobs over a period of forty-seven years—even though he was not yet forty-seven years old. Finally, after a long period of humiliating questioning, Fechner lost his temper. To the psychologist, the outburst proved that Fechner was feebleminded: he lacked self-control. To his attorney, however, Fechner's outburst showed that his client was normal. What ordinary man would put up with such badgering? Fechner had answered most of the questions correctly, had an honorable discharge from the army, had a good record at most of his jobs, had the support of his parents and some neighbors, and did not look abnormal or ugly. All of this, said his attorney, demonstrated that Fechner was sufficiently intelligent to manage his own affairs. He did not require permanent supervision, for he did not cause any harm.[62]

Unfortunately for Fechner, the statutory definition of feeblemindedness was expansive, and the belief that mental defectives (and homosexuals) posed a danger to innocent children ran deep. The real issue before the court was not Fechner's past or present conduct, but his future behavior. The psychologist insisted that feeblemindedness was a serious birth defect with no hope of a cure. Although it was difficult to recognize feeblemindedness in the absence of physical stigmata, he admitted, lifelong supervision was definitely required. Fechner's behavior disturbed little children, and his two arrests (one for public drunkenness in 1931 and one for the alleged gas station assault) proved that he lacked normal self-control. As time passed, the psychologist warned, Herman's elderly mother would find him increasingly difficult to manage. He was almost certain to wind up on poor relief or in jail.[63]

The Minnesota Supreme Court concurred. There was factual evidence to support both sides, but the jurisprudence that would have protected Herman Fechner in a criminal trial did not apply to civil commitment proceedings. For instance, the state was not required to prove its case beyond a reasonable doubt; the only question was whether there was sufficient evidence of feeblemindedness to sustain the finding of the lower court. The court also dismissed Fechner's procedural objection to the state bringing a second petition for commitment after the first one was denied; since Fechner was not charged with a criminal offense, double jeopardy did not apply. All of this illustrates the very different rules that governed civil commitment proceedings and the difficulties that individuals like Fechner confronted when attempting to escape the grasp of state guardianship.[64]

Herman Fechner spent the rest of his life in an institution. He was confined first at Faribault, but then in 1939 he was transferred to the St. Peter State Hospital, where he was eventually put in the ward for the dangerously insane. Yet he and his family continued to fight for a discharge. Fechner's second court challenge reached the Minnesota Supreme Court in 1941, but the court ruled against him again. Fechner remained at St. Peter until his death in 1946. He was just fifty-eight years old.[65]

Fechner's legal battle was unusual, and the court rulings against him show why. It was almost impossible for an allegedly feebleminded man to contest his commitment in court, especially if he was termed a sex offender who might endanger an innocent child. It is no wonder that most men (and women) committed to Faribault resisted eugenic incarceration by fleeing. In the 1920s and 1930s, officials watched helplessly as a steady stream of inmates ran away, the vast majority of them men. For example, fifty-eight men and eighteen women escaped from Faribault in the biennial period ending in June 1930. In 1934, the year of the first *Fechner* decision, the Faribault School superintendent admitted in his biennial report that sixty-eight men and fourteen women had escaped.[66]

The runaway problem worsened during the Depression, as high unemployment, rising relief costs, and public concerns about transients led to a substantial increase in feebleminded commitments. By the late 1930s, the most secure building at Faribault, the Main Boys' Annex, was full to capacity with adult men with criminal records, many of whom had served time in the state prison or reformatory. Some of these men had spent time at Faribault as youngsters, but others were committed as feebleminded in jail and transferred to Faribault because "they were considered unfit to return to society upon completing their sentences." Conditions in the annex were abysmal. Inmates could not go outside the building without close supervision, and the only activities they could participate in were shoemaking and basketry, which held little interest, so they generally remained behind bars, bored and restless, except when they went to exercise in the annex's tiny yard. Many of the inmates came to Faribault from tightly locked prisons, and the fact that the Main Boys' Annex had only a high wire fence was an invitation to flee. At one point in the mid-1930s, nearly 70 percent of inmates had tried to escape. The annex was a tinderbox of hopelessness and rage.[67]

In the late 1930s, Faribault superintendent Edward J. Engberg warned state officials that the annex had become a "place of imprisonment" for feebleminded men who were chronic lawbreakers interested only in getting transferred or planning their escape. On October 1, 1938, his fears came true. Eleven men escaped. They had convinced two unsuspecting "lower-grade" boys to take two hacksaw blades from the kit of a worker and sawed through the steel bars on a porch. Although all but two of the men were caught within two months, the incident bolstered the calls for a secure separate facility for male defective delinquents. As Engberg explained, the ease of escape not only was a problem for the institution but also endangered the families and communities to which the men returned. A separate institution for defective delinquents would enable the School for the Feebleminded to return to its mission of training and care for innocent feebleminded wards "not possessing persistent and serious anti-social tendencies."[68]

The problems at the Main Boys' Annex strengthened officials' deepening conviction that there was a distinction between the "good" and "bad" feebleminded. The eugenic attitudes that prevailed in Rogers's day—that every feebleminded person was a potential pauper or criminal—had long been supplanted by efforts to differentiate between the undeserving "defective delinquent" and the fundamentally innocent, feebleminded "child." Walter Fernald, the Massachusetts superintendent whose mean-spirited 1909 paper "The Imbecile with

Criminal Instincts" had disparaged institutionalized persons as "criminals who have actually committed no crime," wrote a decade later that there were "both bad feeble-minded and good feeble-minded, that not all the feeble-minded are criminalists and socialists and immoral and anti-social. . . . We have really slandered the feeble-minded." Yet despite Fernald's own evolution, his 1909 paper was cited well into the 1940s as proof of the inherent viciousness of a small number of defective delinquents whose presence in a regular school for the feebleminded was the "equivalent of wolves loose in a flock of sheep."[69]

While institution officials struggled behind the scenes to control disruptive inmates, a highly publicized sex crimes panic gave new life to the idea of a feebleminded menace and the supposed need for new laws. In 1939, the Minnesota legislature extended the compulsory commitment provisions of 1917 to "persons having a psychopathic personality," and in 1945, a new Annex for Defective Delinquents (ADD) opened within the St. Cloud Reformatory. In contrast to Faribault, where volatile offenders had nothing to do, defective delinquents in the prison annex could exercise and play ball in a secure area from which it was nearly impossible to escape. A glowing article in the *Minneapolis Star Journal* reported that the men were much better off than they had been at Faribault and their families spared much anguish in the knowledge that they could not escape, revealing both the continuing antipathy toward "defectives" and the terrible bleakness of life at Faribault.[70]

A total of 291 men designated "defective delinquent" and accused of offenses ranging from major felonies to the generic "difficult to manage" passed through the ADD's doors by the time it closed in 1963. Thomson's office initially assumed that these men would remain incarcerated for life, partly because the county welfare boards supposed to supervise them bitterly opposed their release, but prison officials with experience in releasing once-dangerous offenders at the end of prison sentences insisted on parole. For some of these men, sterilization was the price of freedom from the state institution. Most annex inmates remained incarcerated, however. Committed to guardianship in probate court, they remained in the St. Cloud Reformatory indefinitely, effectively part of the general prison population despite not having had a criminal trial. These men were viewed as monstrous, menacing, and a threat to the innocent child. They generated little sympathy, and many spent the rest of their lives in an institution.[71]

Officials' anxieties about female sex delinquents in the 1920s and defective delinquent men in the late 1930s reveal both the centrality of gender norms to a feebleminded classification and the ways that gender shaped the basic structure of Minnesota's eugenics program. While male troublemakers at Faribault were locked up more tightly, unruly female inmates were sterilized and released. Gender was also central to the taxonomy of feeblemindedness which eugenicists developed in the early twentieth century, as poor women considered sexually "delinquent" and economically dependent (that is, dependent on relief rather than on their husbands and fathers) were deemed prolific breeders of defectives and probably feebleminded. As many critics have pointed out, the idea of feeblemindedness was so broad that it could apply to any poor or uneducated person who failed to live up to the middle-class white respectable ideal.

Feeblemindedness was not just a sorting system or a slur, however; it was also a legal and administrative category, and specific decisions about who was feebleminded were more arbitrary than is often assumed. Eugenics-inspired doctors, psychologists, and social workers delineated the supposed characteristics of the feebleminded at conferences and in written texts, but in Minnesota after 1917 individual determinations of feeblemindedness actually rested with a local probate judge. These probate judges took a range of issues into account, but in general their judgments about who was feebleminded had less to do with abstract eugenic theories about human heredity than with practical economic and social concerns. In everyday practice, the question of who was feebleminded was inseparable from local welfare costs, fiscal politics, and the enduring distinction between deserving and undeserving poor.

The next two chapters examine the routine operation of Minnesota's sterilization program and explore how sterilization became the price of freedom from the state institution. As we shall see, Minnesota's sterilization program was not simply a means of reducing the reproduction of the unfit or punishing sexual transgressors, nor was it simply a means of institution population control. Ironically, it was also a routine welfare practice that some social workers imagined could "fix" the worthiest feebleminded women and transform them into the deserving poor.

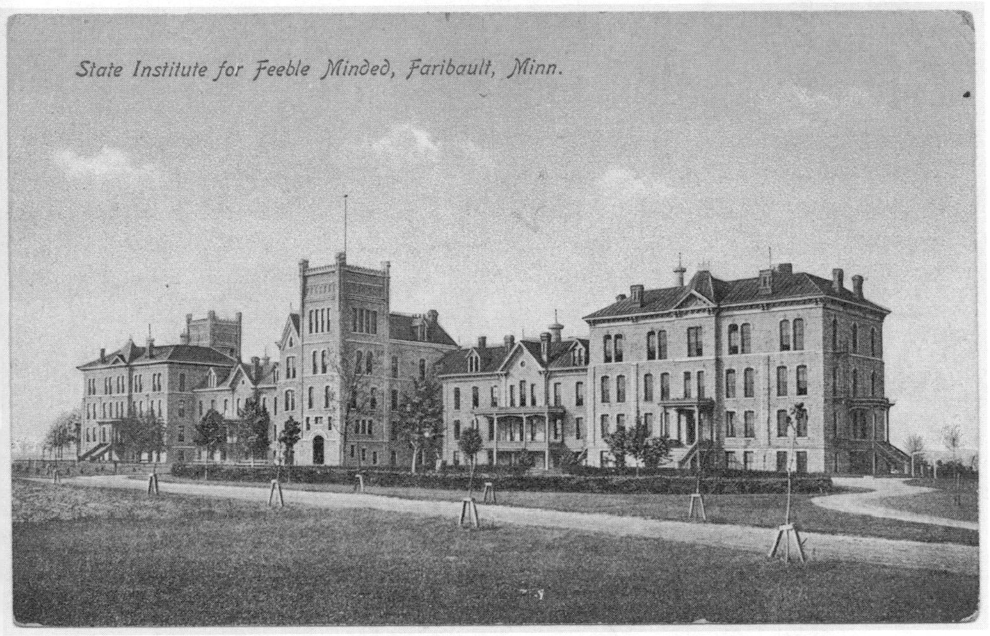

Most sterilizations performed under the 1925 eugenic sterilization law took place at the Minnesota School for the Feebleminded in Faribault, shown here in a 1905 postcard. The school's modern buildings, inviting green lawn, and pastoral landscape portray the school as a point of pride in the local community, a far cry from its reputation in later years. Faribault's population peaked at 3,355 residents in 1955, and the institution closed in 1998. It is now the Faribault Correctional Facility, a medium-security prison. Reprinted with permission of the Minnesota Historical Society.

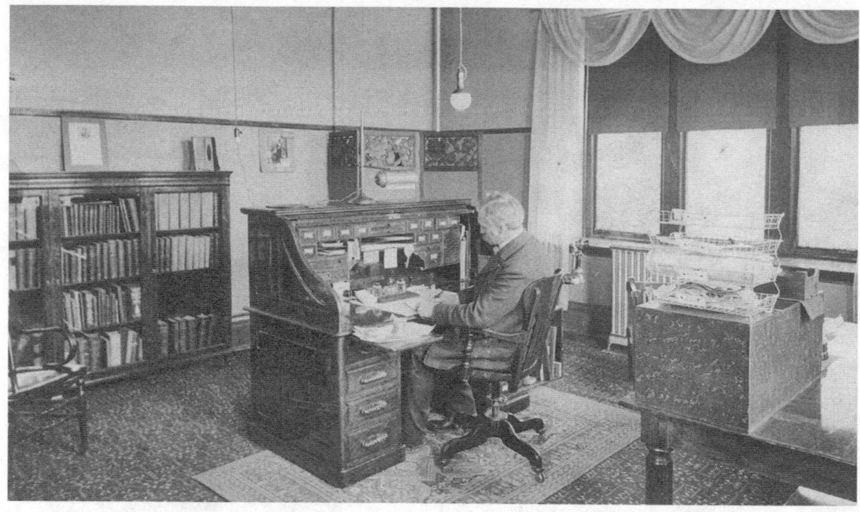

Dr. Arthur C. Rogers in his office at the School for the Feebleminded at Faribault, where he was superintendent from 1885 to 1917. A man of science and letters, Rogers was editor of the *Journal of Psycho-Asthenics*, a leading journal for the study of the feebleminded, and one of the nation's most influential superintendents. Although he died in 1917, Rogers's turn-of-the-century ideas about eugenics and the feebleminded menace shaped Minnesota policy into the 1940s. Reprinted with permission of the Minnesota Historical Society.

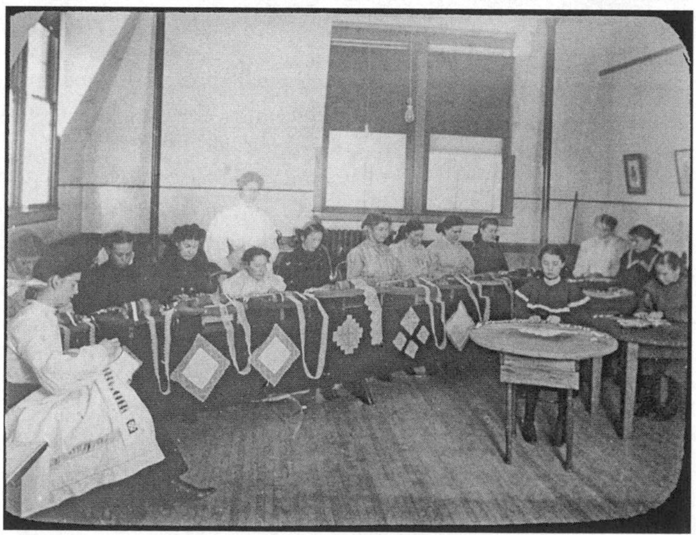

This undated photograph taken by A. C. Rogers was one of a series of slides depicting the skills taught at the Faribault School. Pupils were separated by sex and ability. The "high-grade" men learned carpentry and brush making, while women engaged in sewing and other feminine pursuits. Lace making, seen here, was an especially popular activity. Reprinted with permission of the Minnesota Historical Society.

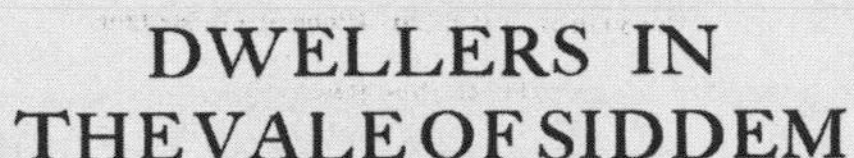

DWELLERS IN THE VALE OF SIDDEM

A True Story of the Social Aspect of Feeble-Mindedness

BY

A. C. ROGERS

Late Superintendent of the Minnesota School for Feeble-Minded, and Colony for Epileptics

AND

MAUD A. MERRILL

Research Assistant in the Department of Research of the Minnesota School for Feeble-Minded and Colony for Epileptics

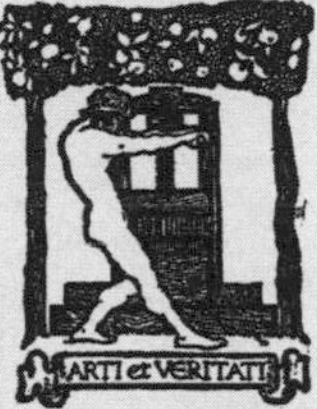

BOSTON
RICHARD G. BADGER
THE GORHAM PRESS

Beginning in 1911, the Eugenic Record Office sponsored two field-workers who traveled throughout southern Minnesota collecting information about hereditary feeblemindedness in the families of Faribault inmates. The resulting volume, *Dwellers in the Vale of Siddem* (1919), completed after Rogers's death by his young assistant Maud A. Merrill, was typical of the eugenics family study genre. Merrill later became a distinguished psychologist at Stanford University, well known for her work with Lewis Terman on the Stanford–Binet intelligence scale. *Dwellers* is rarely included in her list of publications. Reprinted with permission of the Minnesota Historical Society.

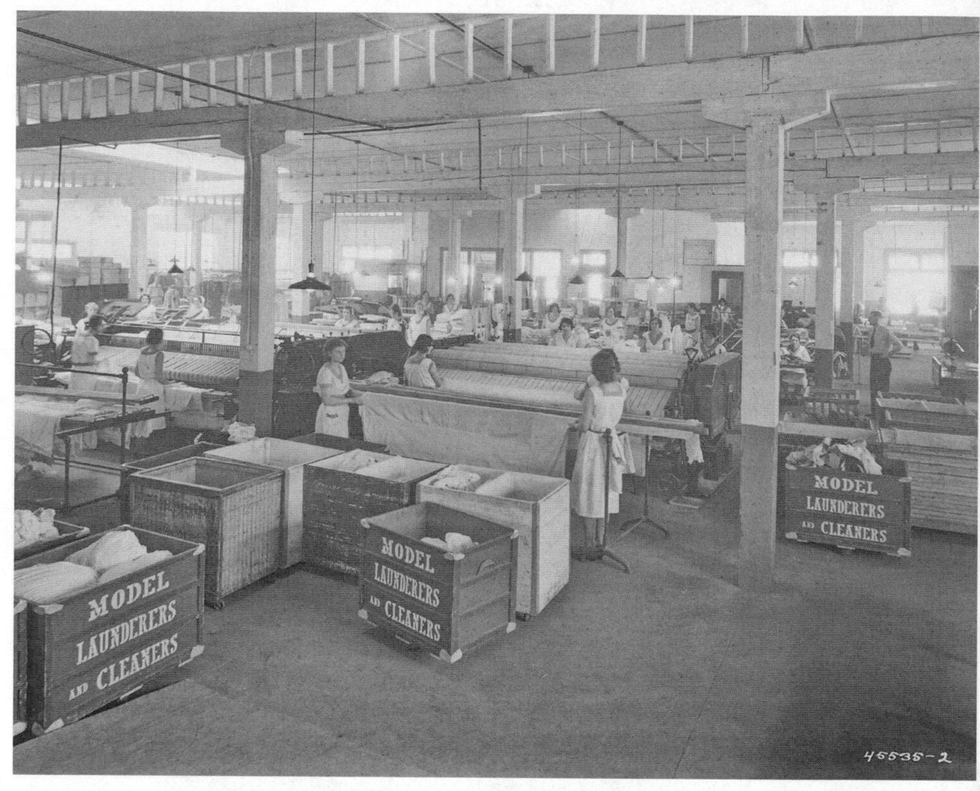

Women sterilized and released from the School for the Feebleminded found work in low-wage jobs, such as this Minneapolis laundry. Interior, Model Launderers and Cleaners, Minneapolis, ca. 1930. Reprinted with permission of the Minnesota Historical Society.

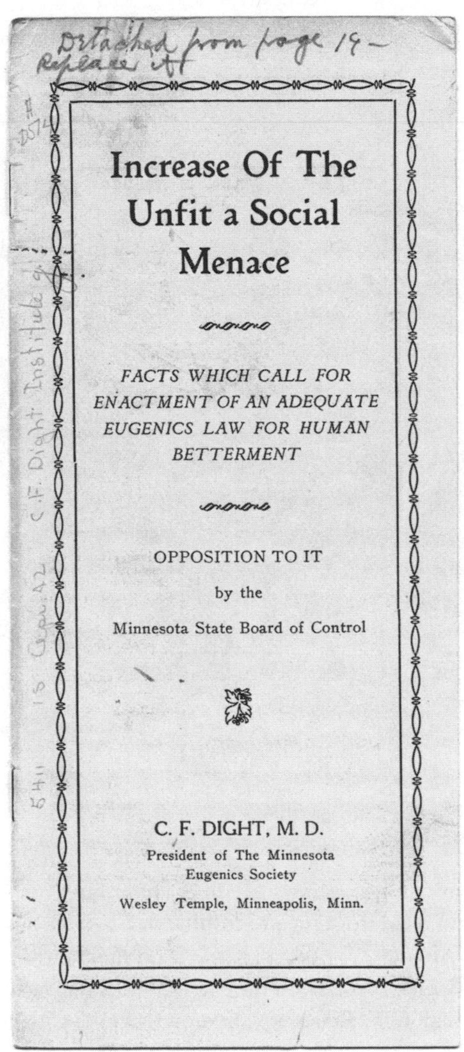

Increase Of The Unfit a Social Menace

FACTS WHICH CALL FOR ENACTMENT OF AN ADEQUATE EUGENICS LAW FOR HUMAN BETTERMENT

OPPOSITION TO IT

by the

Minnesota State Board of Control

C. F. DIGHT, M. D.

President of The Minnesota Eugenics Society

Wesley Temple, Minneapolis, Minn.

Minnesota Eugenics Society president Charles Fremont Dight waged a vigorous campaign to extend Minnesota's voluntary sterilization law to provide for the compulsory sterilization of all the unfit, a plan he believed was thwarted by the State Board of Control. In 1930, Dight distributed this pamphlet to every member of the state legislature. Reprinted with permission of the Minnesota Historical Society.

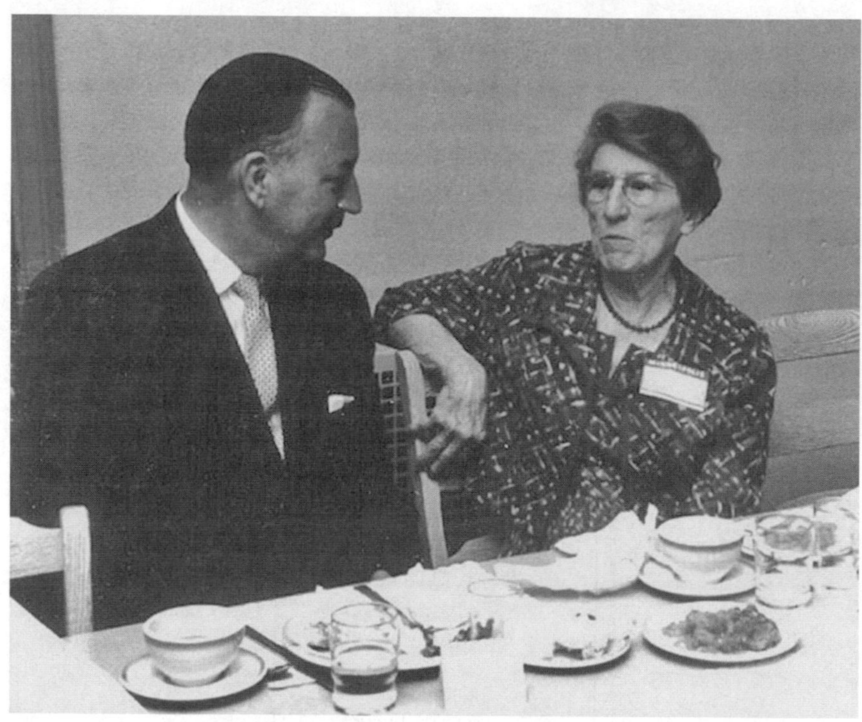

This photograph from the 1950s shows Mildred Thomson, supervisor of Minnesota's Bureau for the Feebleminded from 1924 to 1959, with Governor Elmer L. Andersen. As lead administrator of Minnesota's eugenic sterilization program, Thomson was the person most responsible for its "success." In the postwar years, she facilitated the formation of the National Association for Retarded Children (later ARC), winning praise for her enlightened outlook. Reprinted with permission of the Minnesota Governor's Council for Developmental Disabilities.

A MAJOR MINNESOTA PROBLEM – Institutions for Retarded

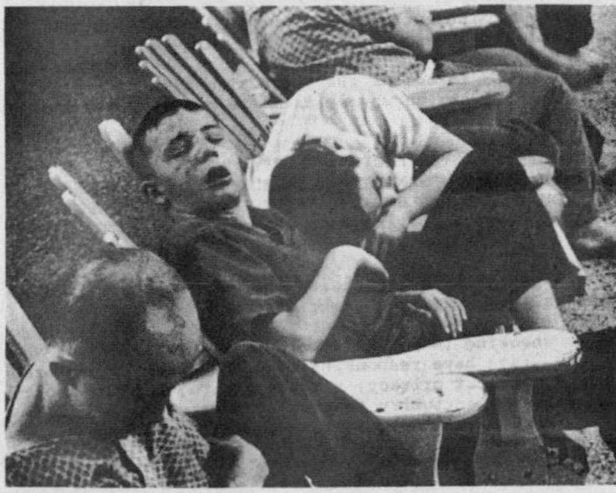

Lack of adequate staff to provide proper care and programs results in scenes like these --- young boys with nothing to do lolling in chairs, the unhappy figure of a girl in soiled clothing sitting on a bare floor.

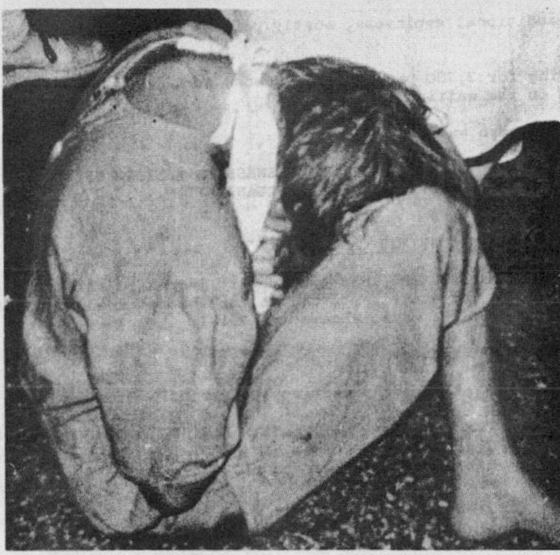

In this 1964 flyer, the Minnesota Association for Retarded Children (MARC) used shocking images to raise public awareness about the inadequate level of care at Faribault. Special education and community programs increased opportunities for people with mild intellectual disabilities outside the institution. Most who remained institutionalized had severe disabilities and complex medical needs. MARC sponsored bus tours to the institutions and lobbied the legislature to address the funding crisis and increase the number of staff. Reprinted with permission of the Minnesota Historical Society.

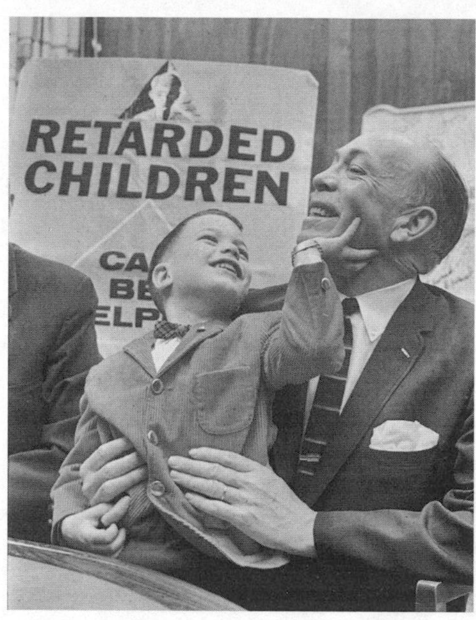

This *Minneapolis Tribune* photograph shows five-year-old Dickie Bach, the National Association for Retarded Children poster boy for 1965, with Governor Karl Rolvaag. NARC used images of innocent children like Dickie to challenge eugenicist portrayals of the "mentally retarded" as genetically inferior, low-class, and menacing. They wanted to show that mental retardation also affected respectable families that were innocent and deserving of aid. *Source*: *Minneapolis Tribune*, May 6, 1965. Reprinted with permission of the Minnesota Historical Society.

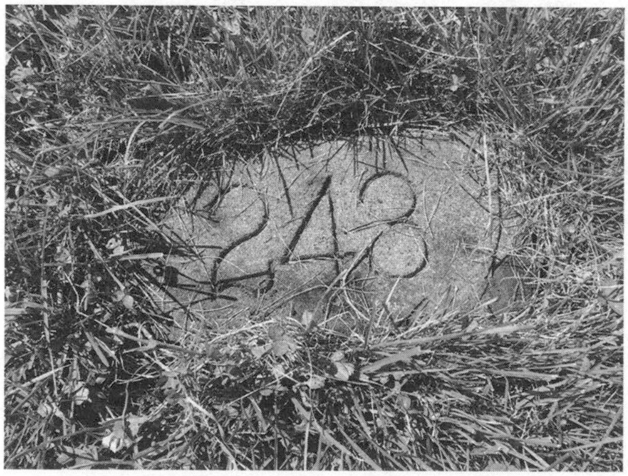

In 1994, the disability rights group Remembering with Dignity launched a public awareness campaign to honor the people who lived and died at Faribault and other state institutions. Approximately thirteen thousand Minnesotans were buried in anonymous numbered graves, such as the Faribault grave shown here, between 1866 and 1997. As of 2016, Remembering with Dignity had placed proper gravestones on the majority of unmarked graves. It also secured an official state apology in 2010.

THE PRICE OF FREEDOM

Minnesota's sterilization program was well under way when the United States Supreme Court, by a vote of 8–1, issued its precedent-setting decision, *Buck v. Bell* (1927). By the time Virginia's Carrie Buck underwent surgery in October 1927, 120 Minnesotans had been sterilized. Most historians agree that the *Buck* case launched a "new era in eugenics" because it established the constitutionality of compulsory sterilization and added legitimacy to eugenics ideas.[1] Yet when Carrie Buck's story is examined from a social welfare perspective, it is the continuities and, sadly, the ordinariness of her story that stand out. Carrie was not the first poor, allegedly feebleminded woman to undergo sterilization, and her experiences of poverty, sexual assault, illegitimacy, forced institutionalization, lost child custody, and nonconsensual medical intervention were replicated across the country, before as well as after *Buck v. Bell.* Although historians have focused on the surgeon's knife, sterilization was just one aspect of a protracted and often callous crusade to "fix" the poor.

Many scholars have pointed out that while eugenics theories led to the development of state sterilization laws, the actual administration of those laws was often more socially oriented than specifically eugenic. Others posit that eugenicists shrewdly shifted their arguments to make their ideas more palatable —talking more about welfare, for example—but their eugenic intentions remained unchanged.[2] In fact, pragmatic social and economic concerns were fundamental to sterilization decisions from the beginning. While Justice Oliver Wendell Holmes's disturbing statement that "three generations of imbeciles are enough" has captured the most attention, a lesser-known phrase from *Buck v. Bell* is equally revealing: "many defective persons . . . if incapable of procreating, might be discharged with safety and become self-supporting with benefit to themselves and to society."[3] The goal of reducing the cost of the "defective, dependent, and delinquent classes" shaped the adjudication of feeblemindedness in Minnesota probate courts and was equally important to sterilization. In the context of America's decentralized and locally funded public welfare system, it was never possible to separate "eugenics" from welfare concerns.

In Minnesota, as in other states, the decision to sterilize was usually part of a plan to parole the person from the state institution. This meant that prosaic considerations about employability and housing were often as relevant to sterilization authorizations as abstract ideas about hereditary fitness. As we saw in chapter 2, by the 1920s most superintendents and social workers had moved away from the harsh rhetoric emphasizing the menace of the feebleminded. They argued instead that most people with intellectual disabilities, like children, were capable of adjusting to community placement if (also like children) they remained under supervision and did not have their own children. The United States Supreme Court made the connection between sterilization and parole explicit when it ruled in *Buck v. Bell* that Virginia's sterilization law did not violate the equal protection clause of the Constitution insofar as "the operations enable those who otherwise must be kept confined to be returned to the world, and thus open the asylum to others." As James W. Trent Jr. points out, sterilization had an institutional as well as a medical function; it was a routine technique to manage the population flow in and out of the state institutions.[4] The Minnesota case shows that the policy of sterilization and parole was also part of a larger welfare-policy shift away from poorhouses and toward community services and surveillance.

Minnesota's example also underscores the importance of individual administrators and institutional structures in shaping sterilization practice. As we saw in the previous chapter, the process of committing an allegedly feebleminded person to state guardianship in Minnesota was highly decentralized, and the identification of what constituted feeblemindedness varied from court to court. In contrast, sterilization was an administrative decision made in St. Paul. Under Minnesota law, the power to authorize sterilization rested with the Board of Control, which rendered its decision after careful investigation; consultation with the superintendent of the School for the Feebleminded or hospital for the insane, a reputable physician, and a psychologist; and obtaining the written consent of kin.[5] In practice, however, administrative responsibility rested with one person: Mildred Thomson, the supervisor of the Minnesota Department for the Feebleminded and Epileptic and de facto guardian of the state's feebleminded wards.

Thomson was involved in the sterilization process from beginning to end, and the program's "success" owed much to her tenacious resolve. She helped county child welfare boards file the initial commitment petitions, advised probate judges on the adjudication of mental deficiency, and worked with successive superintendents of the Minnesota School for the Feebleminded to arrange for admissions and discharges from the institution. Thomson scheduled IQ tests and medical exams, convinced families to consent to sterilization, and ensured that plans for community supervision after sterilization were in place. In the late 1920s, she personally supervised feebleminded wards who lived in the Twin Cities clubhouses but were legal residents (that is, the financial responsibility) of other counties. Later, when public objections to the state sterilization program were mounting, she attempted to quell disquiet by personally interviewing candidates for sterilization. Thomson's vast correspondence with three successive Faribault superintendents, Guy C. Hanna, J. M. Murdoch, and Edward J. Engberg, and her 1963 memoir, *Prologue: A Minnesota Story of Mental Retardation*, provide rich evidence of how sterilization functioned within the welfare system put in place by the 1917 Children's Code. In her papers, the bureaucratic pressures, fiscal considerations, and professional rivalries that drove sterilization decisions during the first decade of legal sterilization are exposed.[6]

Sterilization was not simply a welfare measure; it was also a medical practice through which the power of the state was written onto the bodies of the vulnerable. The Faribault School's medical record of the first thousand sterilization cases bears witness to how a policy often described in abstractions caused untold physical and emotional harm. From January 1926 to April 1937, Faribault staff recorded the name, birth date, and IQ of each sterilization patient, along with medical information about the nature of the operation(s) and administrative details about residency, consent, and discharge. Together, Thomson's writings and the Faribault sterilization ledger reveal that four surprisingly mundane but deeply gendered factors were paramount in decisions about sterilization: the physical ability to withstand surgery, the mental ability to live in the community without breaking the law or becoming a public charge, the existence of an acceptable plan for community supervision and control, and the willingness of relatives to provide legal consent to the operation. This chapter describes each of these factors, but we begin with a brief discussion placing Minnesota's sterilization program in national context.

Minnesota Sterilization Practice in National Context

MES president Charles Dight was the loudest proponent of eugenic sterilization in Minnesota, but the authors and administrators of the state's 1925 sterilization law clearly saw it as a child welfare measure; this is why they gave the job of administering it to the Board of Control. The board was a logical choice: it oversaw the management of all the state institutions and acted as legal guardian of dependent, delinquent, and defective children living in the community. In addition, its close working relationship with private-sector charities, women's organizations such as the Women's Welfare League, and the mostly volunteer members of the county child welfare boards simultaneously facilitated the supervision of discharged inmates and reduced the likelihood of public opposition to their release.

Most studies of state sterilization laws focus on the exceptional cases: Indiana enacted the nation's first sterilization law, California sterilized the largest numbers, Virginia took the Carrie Buck case to the Supreme Court, and North Carolina continued its aggressive sterilization program after other states had

TABLE 4.1
Sterilizations performed at the Minnesota School for the Feebleminded, 1916–1945

Year	Female	Male	Total	Year	Female	Male	Total
1916	1	0	1	1935	112	28	140
1919	1	0	1	1936	59	21	80
1921	1	0	1	1937	145	43	188
1926	51	2	53	1938	111	40	151
1927	86	4	90	1939	99	37	136
1928	50	7	57	1940	82	34	116
1929	62	6	68	1941	86	42	128
1930	52	8	60	1942	68	27	95
1931	67	8	75	1943	23	19	42
1932	72	7	79	1944	18	15	33
1933	87	6	93	1945	6	5	11
1934	123	21	144	Total	1,462	380	1,842

Source: E. J. Engberg to Carl Swanson, June 22, 1946, Faribault State School and Hospital, Superintendent Correspondence, Minnesota Historical Society.

stopped. In contrast, Minnesota's history helps us understand the operation of an "ordinary" sterilization program. The surgical program at Faribault, where the vast majority of sterilizations in Minnesota were performed, peaked in the 1930s and declined after World War II, and women constituted the majority of patients (see table 4.1). An analysis of Minnesota's welfare orientation and focus on feebleminded women suggests ways to think about postwar sterilization programs, in which poor women of color on welfare—many of them labeled mentally retarded—were the group most vulnerable to sterilization. It also suggests the need for more research into the processes by which individuals initially came to be institutionalized, for institutionalization was always the first step toward eugenic sterilization.

The varied language and numerous revisions to sterilization laws make a comparison with other states difficult. Minnesota's sterilization law was different from those of most states because it did not refer to heredity or "socially inadequate offspring" or use the word *menace*. It was similar in its focus on the feebleminded and insane. In 1940, every single state sterilization law applied to the feebleminded, and all but two applied to the insane. Yet although twenty states sterilized epileptics, Minnesota did not. Nor did Minnesota sterilize habitual criminals (ten states) or sex perverts and moral degenerates (seven states). Ultimately, however, the most distinctive feature of Minnesota's eugenic sterilization law was that it was "voluntary," meaning that the state was required to obtain the legal consent of the guardian or next of kin—and, in the case of insanity, the patient herself—prior to surgery. Only one other state, Vermont, had an exclusively voluntary sterilization law.[7]

It is significant that most state laws did not make eugenic considerations the

TABLE 4.2
Recorded sterilizations per 100,000 in states with active sterilization programs

	1920–1929		1930–1939		1940–1949		1950–1959	
State	Female	Male	Female	Male	Female	Male	Female	Male
California	95.95	90.11	114.86	105.98	63.81	65.16	6.93	2.22
Delaware	n/a	n/a	134.4	99.22	77.4	72.6	21.81	19.58
Georgia	n/a	n/a	n/a	n/a	38.72	6.08	52.97	29.33
Indiana	0.07	0.13	23.43	22.05	29.53	30.73	12.17	10.6
Kansas	25.96	39.78	70.89	94.21	39.91	48.71	0.78	1.57
Michigan	n/a	n/a	50.16	16.22	24.35	11.55	12.54	4.17
Minnesota	n/a	n/a	80.94	23.17	21.36	10.66	6.68	0.81
Mississippi	n/a	n/a	34.22	14.11	7.44	0.74	4.7	0.37
New Hampshire	n/a	n/a	113.75	25.63	47.67	20.95	25.61	12.23
North Carolina	n/a	n/a	40.01	10.51	63.72	16.83	110.75	25.47
North Dakota	2.87	2.0	97.13	38.62	69.77	36.17	33.66	30.22
Oregon	81.34	41.27	95.92	50.84	41.76	29.54	31.78	17.07
South Dakota	n/a	n/a	92.81	47.7	42.22	27.16	9.82	2.05
Virginia	n/a	n/a	194.5	105.07	94.08	52.79	48.32	29.58
Washington	n/a	n/a	50.95	16.63	8.46	3.85	n/a	n/a
Wisconsin	15.46	1.39	45.56	7.41	24.88	11.5	4.11	2.01

Sources: Sterilization data for 1920 are from Harry H. Laughlin, *Eugenical Sterilization in the United States* (Chicago: Psychopathic Laboratory of the Municipal Court of Chicago, 1922). All other sterilization data are from Sterilization Statistics, Association for Voluntary Sterilization Records, Social Welfare History Archives, University of Minnesota Libraries. Statistics on female and male populations for each state are from "Table 17: Age by Color and Sex for the State: 1890 to 1960," in vol. 1, chap. 3 of the 1960 US Census.

only basis for sterilization. Of the twenty-nine state laws in effect in 1940, all but eight included improvement in the condition of the patient as a basis for sterilization. It is possible that this statutory justification made women particularly vulnerable to sterilization in the 1930s. While men constituted 57 percent of sterilizations performed through 1920, table 4.2 shows that the majority of states sterilized women in greater proportion than men. Sterilizations clearly shifted south over time, but otherwise the data defy easy explanation. A deeper understanding of the national impact of eugenic sterilization laws requires more state-level studies.[8]

Minnesota, in its decision to empower the Board of Control to authorize sterilizations, was different from most states, where an institution superintendent initiated sterilization proceedings, and this administrative arrangement likely shaped the sterilization program in two ways. First, the fact that the sterilization program operated out of the department for the feebleminded in the state children's bureau is probably one reason that feebleminded women accounted for the vast majority of sterilizations. An astonishing 87 percent of the first thousand patients sterilized at Faribault were women, even though men and women were committed to the Minnesota School for the Feebleminded in roughly equal numbers. The Faribault School reported in 1928 that women constituted just 49 percent of Faribault inmates, but a stunning 89 percent of those "discharged as unimproved." Minnesota officials consistently used the sterilization law to ensure that women released from the School for the Feebleminded would not bear any children who might become a public charge. Even though the percentage of female sterilizations dropped slightly in the late 1930s and 1940s (owing in part to a wartime shortage of surgical staff), table 4.1 shows that women still accounted for nearly 80 percent of all sterilizations performed at Faribault through 1945. Women between the ages of eighteen and forty were the most likely to be sterilized, although exceptions were made at the upper age limit for married women still having children and for young teens who were "well developed physically and conditions indicate this might be wise for social reasons." The median age was twenty-four.[9]

Second, like the child welfare system itself, sterilization affected people in almost every part of the state. Eighty of Minnesota's eighty-seven counties sent residents to Faribault for sterilization (see fig. 4.1). The three largest cities, Minneapolis, St. Paul, and Duluth, were overrepresented in the sterilization register, likely because cities were magnets for poor people in search of work, adventure, and, in the case of pregnant single women, obscurity. Yet large numbers of individuals from rural Minnesota faced sterilization too. The vast majority of counties had only a few sterilization cases (nearly 90% of Minnesota counties had fewer than ten residents sterilized over the ten-year period), but seven nonurban counties, including Rice County, where the School for the Feebleminded was located, and nearby Goodhue County, sent between ten and fourteen individuals for sterilization. Winona and Crow Wing counties sent between fifteen and nineteen. Sparsely populated Marshall County in the northwest sent six women to be sterilized. Only seven counties, all with populations under fifteen thousand, had no recorded sterilizations, and six of the seven were located near the state border. As these figures suggest, sterilization was a statewide policy that functioned as a vital part of Minnesota's child welfare structure. Perhaps even more than preventing the propagation of the feebleminded and insane, the sterilization program established the boundaries for "normal" feminine behavior in every corner of the state.[10]

Withstanding Surgery: Sterilization as Medical Practice

Sterilization is often discussed alongside euthanasia, human medical experimentation, and other Nazi-like plans to "purify" the race, so it may seem surprising that the state's first consideration when authorizing sterilization was the patient's ability to survive surgery. Such concern for the patient's physical survival was no trivial matter, given the fragile physical condition of many institutionalized

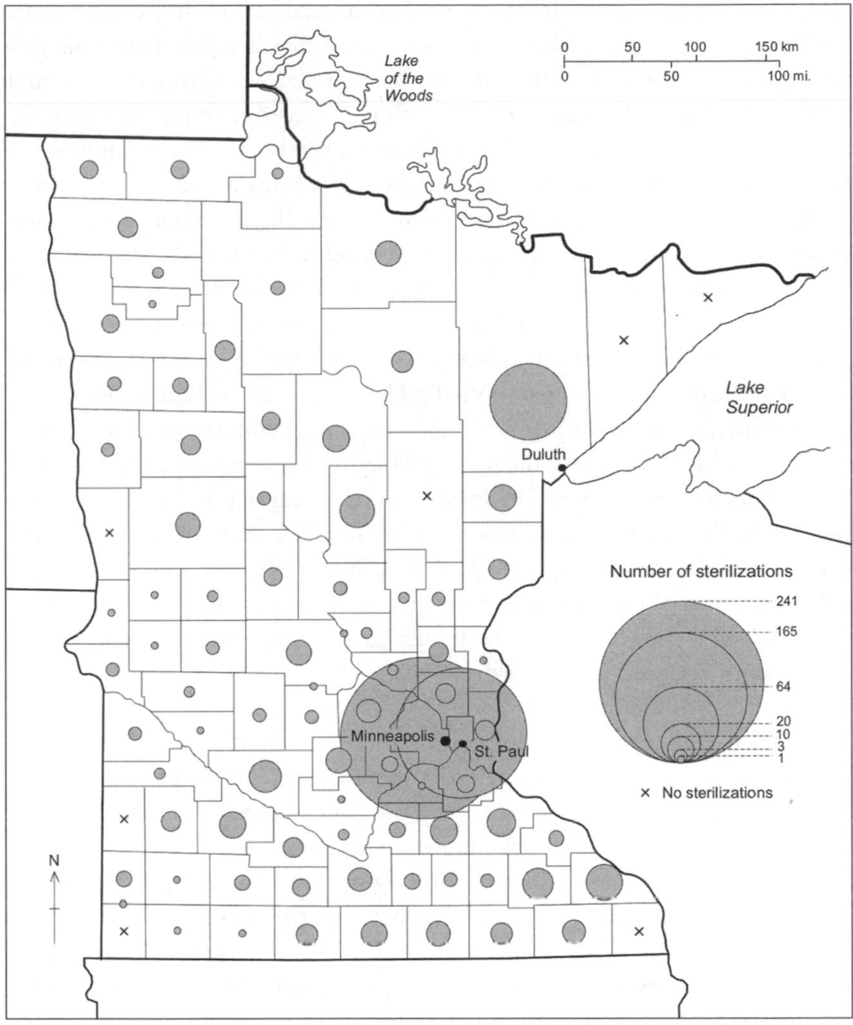

Figure 4.1. County of residence of persons sterilized at the Minnesota School for the Feeble-minded, 1916–1937.

persons. A substantial number of Faribault residents had physical ailments or disabilities. Contagious diseases such as measles and influenza swept the institution with depressing regularity, physical restraints and punishments were all too common, and accidents stemming from broken-down kitchen equipment and plumbing fixtures took a heavy toll on patients' health. Many individuals were already physically unwell when admitted to Faribault—that was often why they came to the attention of the welfare boards in the first place—but even for patients whose health improved after institutionalization, the School for the Feebleminded could be a hazardous place. State officials justified the policy of sterilization and release by telling themselves that feebleminded patients would be happier and healthier outside the institution, if they were "protected" from the stresses of having children. Despite their disregard for the reproductive and bodily integrity of institutionalized persons, they did not see themselves as doing harm.

Medical experimentation on institutionalized bodies has a long history, and sterilization was only one of the many nonconsensual tests and treatments imposed on residents at Faribault. On admission to the institution, poor people with almost no experience of medical care were given a complete physical examination, and by the time a patient was rolled into the operating room, she would have experienced numerous medical interventions, including blood tests, vaccinations, dental checkups, and, in the case of pregnant women whose babies were born at Faribault, medically managed births. While a number of these procedures benefited the patient, the institution's medical staff believed that sterilization benefited patients too. As we saw in chapter 1, A. C. Rogers and other medical superintendents experimented with hysterectomies, oophorectomies, and castration as a cure for masturbation and other supposed sexual abnormalities long before enactment of eugenic sterilization laws. Indeed, the first three sterilizations recorded in the Faribault medical register took place before the passage of the Minnesota law.[11]

Men also endured medical experimentation and sterilization, if they came from the "defective, dependent and delinquent classes." At the end of the nineteenth century, some of America's most prominent physicians advocated the castration of black rapists and child molesters, and the superintendent of a Kansas asylum castrated at least forty-four young institutionalized men for chronic masturbation. Castration blurred the line between therapeutic treatment, punishment, and eugenics, and it was too extreme and too risky to become routine. But the development of vasectomy, a much less drastic operation, opened the way for wholesale eugenic sterilization.[12]

The first and most effective advocate of eugenic vasectomy was Dr. Harry C. Sharp, a physician at the Indiana State Reformatory. Sharp first performed vasectomies on prisoners who suffered from "excessive masturbation" and determined that the operations, performed without anesthesia, had excellent therapeutic results: the prisoner-patients stopped masturbating, felt stronger, slept more soundly, and did better in school, but they did not lose their "normal" sexual desire. Sharp quickly realized vasectomy's eugenic value, and in 1907 he and the reformatory's superintendent, W. H. Whittaker, convinced the Indiana legislature to pass the nation's first compulsory sterilization law. Henceforth, confirmed criminals, idiots, rapists, and imbeciles in the state's institutions could be sterilized on the recommendation of a committee of experts. (The state supreme court struck down Sharp's law in 1921, but a new law, designed to meet the court's due process objections, was passed a few years later.) Sharp was inspired by his success in Indiana and launched an energetic campaign to promote similar laws across the country. His 1908 paper "The Sterilization of Degenerates" appeared in the quarterly proceedings of the Minnesota State Board of Control and prompted much discussion. By 1930, twenty-four states had sterilization laws, and at least 5,134 men and 5,743 women had been sterilized.[13]

When Sharp began his campaign for eugenic vasectomies, female sexual surgeries such as salpingectomies, tubectomies, and oophorectomies were well-accepted treatments for gynecological disorders. Yet unlike vasectomy, which was a relatively simple outpatient procedure, female sterilization was major abdominal surgery that carried considerable risk and therefore required an up-to-date hospital and several weeks of postoperative care. In the early years of the Faribault sterilization program, Dr. George G. Eitel, the highly respected founder of the private Eitel Hospital in Minneapolis and an active member of the MES, performed almost all of the operations. When he died in 1928, his nephew George D. Eitel took over as principal surgeon. For nearly two decades, the doctors Eitel and their associates spent one day each month at the Faribault School hospital performing tubectomies, vasectomies, appendectomies, and an assortment of related surgeries. They performed six to ten operations at a time, with the assistance of the institution's medical staff and their own students, and worked for a nominal fee. According to medical historian Neal Holtan, the surgical team was capable and the operations were as safe as in the community.[14]

Still, surgery carried risks. Although recovery was usually uneventful, there were a number of failures and complications. At least ten women got pregnant in the early years of the program. "It was a great shock," Mildred Thomson recalled of the first pregnancy, which occurred in the program's first year; "A woman who already had a large family bore twins!" Three of the ten women who got pregnant were sterilized a second time, but in 1933 Dr. George D. Eitel modified the surgical technique his uncle had devised, and no more post-sterilization pregnancies were reported. Even so, Thomson recalled with amusement, a woman sterilized in the early years of the program married many years afterward, and "to everyone's consternation there was a child later!"[15]

At least four patients were pregnant at the time of the operation. Of the three discharged to their families after the operation, only one—twenty-four-year-old Susan Hartmann—had her baby's birth recorded; she gave birth to a baby boy seven months after the operation. The other fetuses probably died in utero or were aborted. Sadly, one of the pregnant patients died. Gretchen Fischer was about seven months pregnant and died of a "paralytic illness" about a week after a bilateral tubectomy. The baby's birth was not recorded, and it is likely that the fetus was already dead.[16]

Gretchen was one of seven women whose deaths Faribault staff recorded in the sterilization register. Two deaths were almost certainly due to postoperative complications. In addition to Gretchen, a twenty-two-year-old woman died of postoperative pneumonia four days after her surgery. Five of the deaths occurred many months after the surgery and may have been unrelated. A sixteen-year-old with Down syndrome died of an unidentified cause six months after her operation. Four women died more than a year after their sterilizations, three of them from tuberculosis. That these patients' deaths were recorded in the sterilization register long after their operations reveals both the hospital staff's sense of responsibility for their patients' health after discharge and the long arm of the state's surveillance and control.[17]

These cases underscore the gendered nature of Minnesota's eugenics program and the intense medicalization of women's bodies. That nearly nine hundred of Minnesota's first thousand sterilization patients were women suggests that although *eugenic* sterilization legislation began with vasectomies in Indiana, the history of involuntary female sterilization is inseparable from the professionalization of obstetrics and gynecology. As is well known, gynecology's emergence as a medical specialty rested on surgeries performed on women, sometimes without their consent. J. Marion Sims, the so-called father of gynecology, developed a surgical cure for vesicovaginal fistula by operating on enslaved women. His contemporary Robert Battey, also exhibiting a cavalier attitude toward young women's bodies, pioneered the surgical removal of healthy ovaries as a treatment for a variety of nervous diseases, a technique he developed by operating on private patients. In the early twentieth century, many ordinary people concurred with medical specialists' belief that women's reproductive organs were inherently pathological and various medical conditions could be cured by removing them. Although such attitudes were always highly contested, by the 1920s an increasingly well-organized medical profession, combined with the maternalist campaign to improve infant and maternal health, had strengthened physicians' institutional and cultural power. At Faribault and other state institutions, these ideas reached an extreme. The doctors and nurses who accompanied the doctors Eitel to Faribault had the opportunity to practice their surgical skills on women whose "feeblemindedness" made them the ideal submissive patient, replicating an earlier age when doctors operated on enslaved women unable to consent.[18]

Perhaps unsurprisingly, a sizable number of Faribault sterilization patients—almost all of them women—had multiple operations. Although the surgery was initiated for eugenic reasons, nearly one-quarter of the first thousand patients had more than one operation, and twenty-three patients had three procedures or more. Most second and third procedures took place at the same time as the sterilization. While some seem to have been therapeutic in purpose—eleven patients had cysts on their ovaries or fallopian tubes, and ten had adhesions—others had no medical justification recorded. This is particularly true for appendectomy, the second most common operation listed in the sterilization register (after tubectomy). Doctors at Faribault performed more appendectomies than vasectomies, and the operation grew more common over time. Although appendectomies accounted for less than 10 percent of all operations listed in the sterilization register between 1927 and 1932, they increased steadily over the next few years. In 1937, appendectomies accounted for 27 percent of all recorded operations. Furthermore, the number of appendectomies increased as the reported diagnoses of appendicitis declined. Fifty-eight percent of recorded appendectomies took place between 1935 and 1937, when there was not a single recorded diagnosis of appendicitis. The surge in preventive appendectomies reflected national trends, and at Faribault they seem to have been a regular accompaniment to tubectomies as the sterilization program accelerated. It is telling that nearly three-quarters of appendectomies recorded in the sterilization register were performed on women under thirty years old, and not a single man was subjected to the same procedure.[19]

Why did Minnesota officials perform relatively few vasectomies and not one appendectomy on a man? The obvious answers are that appendectomy and tubectomy (unlike vasectomy) were both abdominal surgery, women's bodies had long been subjected to medical treatment, and the sterilization program operated out of the state children's bureau. However, popular and medical concepts of masculinity also played a role. Well into the 1920s, vasectomy was associated with castration and mutilation, and families and practitioners alike feared that sterilization could impair a man's sexual performance and manliness. There were no similar fears about gynecological surgeries. In addition, young women's sexuality and reproduction already faced parental and societal controls. Thus, many families who cheerfully agreed to the sterilization of a wife or a daughter hesitated when the patient was a man—unless they believed that the operation was therapeutic and could bring about a cure. The earliest vasectomies performed under the 1925 sterilization law may have been considered at least partly therapeutic. The first vasectomy listed in the sterilization register was performed on a "high grade case mentally, but a confirmed criminal" charged with assaulting his six-year-old daughter. The fact that the man was discharged to his wife about a year after the operation suggests that sterilization may have been intended to cure. The second vasectomy, performed at the same time as a herniotomy on a fifteen-year-old boy, was also probably therapeutic. That both men were discharged after the operation suggests that the Board of Control viewed sterilization as a condition of release for men and women alike.[20]

The dynamics of Minnesota's sterilization program foreshadowed national trends. As mentioned earlier, men constituted a slight majority of those sterilized until the 1920s, but feebleminded women always constituted the overwhelming majority of sterilization patients in Minnesota. Minnesota's unwavering focus on the feebleminded was also consistent with some—but not all—state programs. In 1937, the pro-sterilization Human Betterment Foundation reported that just 25 percent of sterilizations in Minnesota were performed on the insane, compared to 60 percent in Virginia and nearly 67 percent in California. Yet Virginia and California were not typical, and states like Michigan and Indiana shared Minnesota's focus on the feebleminded, reminding us that there is no single sterilization story in the United States. The differences were not due to a difference in attitude, for the most ardent proponents of eugenic sterilization in Minnesota as elsewhere strongly supported sterilizing the insane. As the superintendent of the Rochester State Hospital declared in 1925, "The most important thing in the prevention of insanity is the non-production of the insane."[21]

Incomplete records and the absence of an eager administrator like Mildred Thomson are more likely explanations for the relatively few sterilizations among Minnesota's insane. Although Thomson worked closely with child welfare boards to identify feebleminded prospects for sterilization, she did not have any authority over the non-feebleminded insane. Sterilizations performed on mental patients at the Fergus Falls, Rochester, and St. Peter hospitals were not recorded in the Faribault sterilization register (or any other central location), and they may have been undercounted. The Rochester State Hospital had the most complete reporting, and it appears that the majority of sterilizations performed on mental patients took place there, with most of the surgeries performed by Mayo Clinic staff. The superintendent's biennial reports declared fourteen tubectomies and nine vasectomies (as well as eight hysterectomies) between 1926 and 1928, although the Board of Control expressly authorized only four tubectomies and two vasectomies, presumably for mental patients who were also feebleminded wards. By 1944, the Rochester State Hospital had sterilized 109 female and 96 male patients, more than half of the 392 sterilizations performed on the insane which Minnesota reported overall (table 4.3).[22]

The relatively small proportion of eugenic sterilizations performed on the mentally ill was probably an artifact of the law: unlike the so-called feebleminded, mentally ill Minnesotans had to be an inmate of a state hospital for the insane for six months and give their personal consent to the operation prior to sterilization; consent of kin alone was not enough. The six-month hospital stay and a stipulation that the insane person had to be sterilized by a "competent surgeon" were amendments to the original bill, and it is revealing that these provisos were not extended to the feebleminded.[23]

Eugenics provided an abstract justification for sterilizing the insane, but Minnesota's sterilization law did not refer to the prevention of hereditary defects, and sterilization operations may have been performed as much for therapeutic or administrative reasons as for eugenic ones. As the historian Joel Braslow ar-

TABLE 4.3
Sterilizations performed at the Rochester State Hospital, 1928–1946

Biennial year ending June 30	Female	Male	Total
1928	14	9	23
1930	12	7	19
1932	25	16	41
1934	23	12	35
1936	12	38	50
1938	12	10	22
1940	9	4	13
1942	2	0	2
1944	0	0	0
1946	0	0	0
Total	109	96	205

Source: Rochester State Hospital (Minn.), Annual and Biennial Reports, Minnesota Historical Society.

gues in his study of psychiatric treatment in California state hospitals, many institution doctors saw sterilization "not as an instrument of the state to prevent the procreation of the insane but as a therapeutic intervention to alleviate individual suffering." Although they used eugenics rhetoric when justifying sterilization to administrators, these psychiatrists viewed sterilization as a surgical cure for the physical and psychological strains of pregnancy and child-rearing and as a treatment for nervousness in men. The evidence suggests that Minnesota psychiatrists saw sterilization the same way.[24]

For the Board of Control, however, sterilization was primarily an administrative means of reducing hospital overcrowding. Always concerned with the population flow in and out of state institutions, the board considered a policy of sterilization and release to be beneficial both to the individual, who got to leave the institution, and to the taxpayer. In light of the board's concern with overcrowding and psychiatrists' interest in therapeutic treatment, it is intriguing that the number of sterilizations dropped at the Rochester State Hospital just as the number of lobotomies increased. Twelve sterilizations and three lobotomies were performed between 1938 and 1940, but in the 1944 biennial report four years later, the hospital reported 58 prefrontal lobotomies and no sterilizations in the previous two years. Intriguingly, the superintendent now described lobotomies in much the same terms as sterilization two decades earlier: as a surgical intervention that would allow patients who would be otherwise doomed to permanent institutionalization to live in the community and lead "normal lives as useful members of society."[25] For the insane and feebleminded alike, sterilization had multiple motivations beyond the eugenic aim of preventing the reproduction of the unfit. It was a medical treatment for mental disturbances until "better" therapies became available, and it was an administrative tool for institution management. Above all, sterilization was a surgical fix for the economic and behavioral problems of the poor.

After Sterilization: Out of the Institution and into the Community, and Sometimes Back Again

Once a patient was determined fit for surgery, the Board of Control (that is, the supervisor of the program for the feebleminded, Mildred Thomson) had to make plans for discharge. This was not always a simple task. While many families welcomed their loved ones home after sterilization, some sterilization patients did not want to go home, and still others had no home to return to. A significant minority of Faribault inmates were in the institution because they were thought to be a community problem, and local officials, their neighbors, and sometimes even their own families did not want them back. In addition, the board had to contend with the intangible fears of those who worried that releasing "morons" into the community after sterilization would be a license to promiscuity and cause an increase in vice, venereal disease, and crime. Thomson's job was to ensure that the feebleminded person had a suitable home and a means of support and would not break the law or become a public charge. In short, she had to show that sterilization following a period of "training" in the state institution could transform "defectives" into the deserving poor.

The Supreme Court's famous phrase "three generations of imbeciles are enough" captures eugenicists' antipathy toward allegedly feebleminded families, but in reality families played a significant role in the sterilization and supervision process. Of the first thousand patients sterilized at Faribault, more than half were released to members of their immediate family—parents, siblings, or spouses—and probably returned to their homes. Thomson's superiors at the Board of Control preferred at-home supervision, even though they assumed that most of the families were feebleminded, because releasing inmates was less expensive than institutionalization. In addition, state officials may have sympathized with respectable working-class parents who struggled to manage sexually delinquent "feebleminded" daughters but still wanted to care for them at home. Mildred Thomson, however, thought that family care was problematic. As the person responsible for the day-to-day supervision of feebleminded wards in the community, she worried that at-home care would be difficult to monitor and there would be a "higher percentage of failure in successful adaptation." Thomson favored sending sterilized individuals to a nonfamily destination, such as a Board of Control clubhouse or a state-approved boarding home. Nearly 40 percent of those sterilized during the program's first four years were released to a clubhouse or directly to the board.[26]

As we saw in chapter 2, the clubhouse program formally began in 1924, when the Women's Welfare League of Minneapolis joined forces with the Board of Control and turned one of its clubhouses for wage-earning women into a transitional residence for women "on parole" from Faribault. The Harmon Club was well established by the time the state's sterilization law went into effect, and the board naturally turned to the welfare league to help it supervise sterilized women in the community. By the summer of 1926, thirty-eight women had stayed at the Harmon Club. They toiled in laundries, restaurants, factories, and private homes, like other working-class girls, and spent evenings at the clubhouse doing housework and other domestic pursuits, such as sewing, lace making, and planning parties. "The girls are on the whole contented and happy with the pleasures which are possible for them," Thomson reported, and there was an economic benefit to the state. In twenty months, the women earned nearly $17,450, out of which they paid board, bought their own clothing and movie tickets, purchased presents for family and friends, and opened savings accounts. The state paid less than $2,400 toward the women's supervision, which was far less than the monthly per capita cost of $8,000 if they had remained institutionalized.[27]

Thomson recalled that the board's emphasis on community living in the early 1920s brought on "discussion of the need for sterilization." In 1926, the first year the sterilization law was in effect, the board announced a new regulation that all women had to undergo sterilization before parole to a clubhouse. Thomson wrote in her 1928 biennial report that sterilization made "possible many paroles which could not otherwise have been planned for" and announced two new clubhouses for feebleminded women. The Lynnhurst Club opened in St. Paul in July 1927 and the Duluth Club a year later. Unlike the Harmon Club, a partnership with the private Women's Welfare League, the Board of Control operated the Lynnhurst and Duluth Clubs on its own. Even so, it enlisted private charities and women's groups, such as the welfare league and the House of the Good Shepherd, to help with the supervision of feebleminded women. That these women's agencies did not run any equivalent residential facilities for men surely contributed to the sterilization program's emphasis on women.[28]

Thomson expended "great interest and much time" on the clubhouses and would remember them with fondness. A teacher and psychologist by training, she took pleasure in her professional relationships with Twin Cities social workers and in the personal ties that she developed with clubhouse residents. The clubhouses were not unlike social settlements and other social service agencies with a working-class female clientele, and they provided relatively privileged middle-class women like Thomson with meaningful work, a sense of community, and adventure. Thomson recalled the excitement of getting ready to launch the Lynnhurst Club: the pleasure of finding a large house in a good neighborhood, purchasing attractive furnishings, and inviting women's clubs, child welfare boards, social workers, and Faribault's superintendent to the open house. She spent many hours at clubhouse meals and parties, or "just sitting with the girls to get to know and understand them," and hosted parties for the women at her home. "When I got to know these girls and to see them in relation to the unhappy and sometimes tragic experiences of early life, I marveled at how well most of them adjusted rather than despaired at failures," she recalled.[29] As these examples illustrate, Thomson took a personal interest in her charges and reveled in the certainty that sterilization had provided these feebleminded women with the possibilities of a better life.

Thomson saw the clubhouses as a positive alternative to permanent institutionalization and viewed parole through the lens of social casework. She also fervently believed in eugenics, although how she viewed its practical application differed from Charles Dight, Minnesota's most vocal eugenics campaigner. Thomson assumed that the state needed to protect citizens from the procreation and antisocial acts of the feebleminded, but she also believed that it had an obligation to the feebleminded person, who "through no fault of her own" was unable to handle the complexities of life. The social worker, she wrote, should be a "sympathetic friend who is interested in the likes and dislikes, joys and sorrows" of her feebleminded clients and tries to ensure that their lives have some pleasure. "WE ARE PRIMARILY THE FRIENDS OF THE FEEBLE-MINDED," she declared in a memo to the county child welfare boards, "MADE SO BY LAW AND ALSO BY OUR NATURAL SYMPATHIES, I BELIEVE."[30]

The tensions between eugenics and child welfare shaped the sterilization program from the beginning. In the earliest reports on the parole program, the social work side triumphed. Thomson and the Women's Welfare League emphasized the similarities between feebleminded and "normal" working-class girls, as well as the need to help the former make personal and community adjustments. A visitor to the Harmon Club would be "quite unprepared" for what she would see, league secretary Elinor McIntosh explained. Instead of dim-witted idiots, there were ordinary girls engaged in ordinary activities, such as sewing, lace making, having a dancing lesson, and listening to the radio. The women's rooms were "models of neatness and orderliness," McIntosh boasted, "and all things considered there is very little friction." Harmon Club residents looked "like any group of normal girls in any boarding home," and their daily routine was the same as that at any working girls' residence. They were learning to adapt.[31]

Sterilized feebleminded women were also represented as normal in another way: their ultimate objective was marriage. Despite the legal prohibition on feebleminded and epileptic persons from marrying, the Board of Control had a policy of permitting and even encouraging women under guardianship to marry—if they were good housekeepers, had a fiancé who met the state's approval, and had been sterilized. Several Harmon Club residents got married, according to Women's Welfare League reports, and the club hosted a bridal shower and at least one wedding (when a resident chose to marry at the club, with her relatives in attendance). Of course, marriage meant something different for sterilized women than for those who could be mothers. The "normal" woman was supposed to stay at home with her children and depend on a breadwinning husband, whereas the sterilized wife was supposed to be self-supporting. Even so, the idea that a feebleminded woman would get married must have challenged the preconceptions of league donors, as Elinor McIntosh urged members to trust in the professionals' expertise. "No matter what our individual opinions may be on this subject," she said, "it is only fair to presume those who have specialized in this work with the feeble minded, know best."[32]

The clubhouses were the cornerstone of Minnesota's sterilization program in the 1920s, and these institutions shaped the profile of the sterilized population. When choosing which Faribault inmates to sterilize and parole, Thomson looked first for attractive, compliant women who were efficient workers, could get along with the other clubhouse residents, and would put the best face on the parole program. When the Lynnhurst Club opened in St. Paul, she asked Faribault superintendent Guy Hanna to refer women who were stable and adaptable and had IQs in the 60s. The girls should be "of the very best type in order that the Club House get a good name to start with," she wrote, even if they were not (yet) sterilized. Thomson's insistence on nice-looking, reliable women was a way to forestall community opposition. When the Duluth Club opened in a working-class residential neighborhood at a time when job opportunities were drying up and "neighbors were 'up in arms' at the intrusion," Thomson and Hanna's successor, J. M. Murdoch, tried to quell the discontent by ensuring that the first eight girls who arrived in April 1928 were "especially nice-looking and well-behaved."[33]

Physical attractiveness and tractability were beneficial, but the ability to do low-wage work without getting into trouble was far more important in deciding who should be sterilized and released. The search for satisfactory workers is a common theme in Thomson's correspondence with the Faribault superintendents. For example, a November 1927 list of girls "sterilized and available for parole" focused almost entirely on their capacity for work. The superintendent at the time, J. M. Murdoch, described two sisters in their midtwenties as similar in their "working ability." They were slow but cooperative, though the older one was more industrious and "particularly good at cleaning and assisting in housekeeping." Another woman was an experienced worker in the institution kitchen and had waited on tables. A fourth, a married mother of three whose husband had deserted her, was said to be a "fair worker" in the institution hospital. In order to be chosen for sterilization and release, it seems, a woman had to be considered a good worker.[34]

Not all women were so easily pigeonholed, however, and the many references to troublesome behavior illustrate the difficulties officials encountered when determining respectability outside the institution. Alma Dupont, for instance, was judged competent at a variety of jobs, including running the power machine in the tailor shop, but Murdoch worried about her behavior. Alma had been admitted to Faribault at the age of seventeen, possibly for sexual delinquencies, and then paroled to a Minneapolis welfare home. Before long, however, she was returned to Faribault for riding around with boys. Desperate to leave the institution, Alma assaulted the night watchman in an escape attempt. Nevertheless, Murdoch wanted to give her another chance (or to get rid of her). A week before her twenty-fourth birthday but five years after her initial admission, Alma was sterilized with her father's consent and paroled to the Lynnhurst Club. She was back at Faribault within the year. When the paper trail ends three years later, Alma was living outside the institution in a "suitable home."[35]

Thomson enjoyed working with Murdoch and felt that he shared her interest in a "total program" that linked the Faribault School with the wider community, but as we saw in chapter 2, she did not like his predecessor, Guy Hanna. He did not share the board's interest in parole and (in Thomson's view) cared mostly about cutting Faribault's budget. She could barely contain her fury when Hanna failed to inform her that several women released from the institution and paroled to a clubhouse had physical disabilities or were ill. Olive Mattison, she wrote, was a "sweet, docile little girl," but her dwarfism made it nearly impossible for her to get work, and Greta Acker, an incest survivor, kept losing weight. "It seems to me," she exploded to Hanna, "if the eating of a girl has had to be watched in order that she not become anemic, or she is particularly likely to suffer from constipation or has an unusual[ly] difficult time during her period of menstruation," her office ought to be notified so it could take special care.[36]

Thomson much preferred Murdoch's " 'team' approach," which she felt gave "zest to all planning." Murdoch took seriously residents' desire to leave the institution and worked closely with Thomson to find the "right" placement. In their seemingly endless ruminations about particular candidates for sterilization and parole, we can see a genuinely sympathetic if patronizing concern for the well-being of the women intermixed with disapproval of, frustration over, and even disgust with their behavior. For example, Murdoch agonized over whether Anna Coffey was physically ready for release. Two years after she was sterilized during a hernia operation, he told Thomson that Anna "has poor health, does very little work but gets along very well with others." She was too frail for an ordinary job, he conceded, but she might be able to manage "in a home where she would not be expected to do very much and if the family would take a sympathetic interest in her." Murdoch occasionally even recommended paroling women who were too weak for sterilization or who would be difficult to supervise but were "very anxious to get out." Thomson generally resisted releasing those cases. Although she got along well with Murdoch, she was responsible for supervising feebleminded people in the community and did not want to be liable for likely failures.[37] Ultimately, Thomson's correspondence with the Faribault superintendents shows that most sterilization decisions had little to do with abstract notions of hereditary feeblemindedness and were shaped instead by a mishmash of economic, administrative, and professional concerns.

Thomson initially assumed that sterilized women would be easier to supervise if they lived in a clubhouse instead of with their families, but she was wrong. Of the first thousand sterilizations, those discharged to a clubhouse were returned to the institution more than any other group. Clubhouse residents were younger and had higher IQs than the sterilized group as a whole, and they were more defiant. The large number of women who ran away from the clubhouses and had to return to Faribault indicates both the importance state officials attached to controlling women's behavior and their utter failure to exercise that control. Take Joyce, who was pretty and poised and started working as a prostitute at the age of twelve. Thomson did everything she could to dampen Joyce's rebellious spirit. Joyce had a brother and sister in the Red Wing and Sauk Centre correctional schools, but because she had an IQ of 72, she went to Faribault instead. Joyce was paroled to several different clubhouses and private homes, but she was unable to "adjust" and had to be readmitted to Faribault a number of times. Even after she had a baby and Thomson took the unusual step of letting her have contact with her child, Joyce again disappeared. The last Thomson heard of Joyce, she was courting two brothers who, unbeknownst to each other, were giving her money and expecting to get married. "Had Joyce been born into a respectable family—and had had perhaps a wee bit more intelligence—she would certainly have been the belle of the town," Thomson chuckled. "She had personality plus!"[38]

Joyce's winning ways may have made her defiance easier for Thomson to swallow, but most women's slip-ups were not as amusing. Clubhouse residents toiled long hours at low-paying jobs, if they were lucky enough to find employment, and many suffered from serious medical problems as well as psychological distress. The physical condition of the women was "nearly as poor as the mental," the welfare league observed in 1930; the residents struggled with "eye, tooth, foot, stomach trouble, nerves, operations in almost endless succession." The clubhouse was hardly the happy solution to the problem of the feebleminded that the Board of Control and Women's Welfare League had hoped it would be. In the first group of thirty-eight Harmon Club residents, three had tuberculosis and four returned to Faribault for nonmedical reasons: two stepped out with men when they were supposed to be at work, one engaged in "homosexual acts," and the fourth found life outside the institution so difficult that she begged to go back. This woman, named Mary, "wept because the matron had not told her where to find the darning cotton and, going out alone for a distance of only two or three blocks, she got lost." Thomson wrote in her memoirs, "I did not then realize that this dependence had been fostered at Faribault," but the policy of eugenic segregation required residents to be "kept childlike and satisfied with the simplicity of life in an institution," and Mary could not cope with the absence of a strict routine.[39]

Thomson boasted that Mary eventually returned to the community and made an excellent adjustment, but her history of institutionalization was not unusual. More than one hundred people—an astonishing 10 percent of those sterilized in the first ten years—bounced in and out of the state institutions. Eighty-three of the first thousand sterilization patients were returned after their initial discharge, and ten were readmitted twice. In addition, twenty-one women were transferred to other state institutions, such as the Cambridge Colony for Epileptics and the St. Peter State Hospital for the Insane.[40]

The behaviors and circumstances that led to long-term institutionalization were varied. Dorothy Williams, a twenty-five-year-old single woman released eight months after a sterilization operation, lasted less than a month before being readmitted because of her "inability to control her temper and cooperate with others." Dorothy was a conscientious seamstress in the Faribault School tailor shop, but as her mental state deteriorated, the staff felt they could not handle her outbursts, and she was transferred to the St. Peter Hospital for the Insane.[41] Amelia Prescott also suffered from spells, but she was stuck in the St. Peter State Hospital for a different reason: her family made no effort to secure her release. The Board of Control wanted to discharge Amelia after sterilization, and her parents initially agreed, but then they disappeared without leaving an address. The caseworker wrote scornfully that Amelia's parents did not seem to be of a "high order of intelligence and probably have about all they can do to look after themselves." Four months later, the board decided that nothing could be done to obtain Amelia's release. She was still in the institution when she died fifteen years later.[42]

These sad cases were the exception. The vast majority of sterilized Minnesotans returned to their communities and lived relatively ordinary lives. By removing their ability to have children, the state turned unfit feebleminded women into the respectable deserving poor, albeit at considerable emotional cost. Years later, Thomson admitted that the board's emphasis on making the clubhouse girls self-supporting, rather than facilitating their transition to community life, was a mistake. Nevertheless, she continued cheerfully, "hindsight is better than foresight," and in the context of the early 1920s, the clubhouse plan was "a great advance—a beginning of a gradual change in attitudes." Thomson evidently saw sterilization, which removed the possibility of pregnancy and thus increased the likelihood that a woman could be self-supporting, as part of that great advance.[43]

The Multiple Meanings of Consent

The final factor that the Board of Control had to consider when making a sterilization decision was the matter of consent. Under Minnesota's "voluntary" sterilization law, the operation could not be performed legally unless the spouse or nearest kin provided their written consent. If no relative could be found, the Board of Control or another duly appointed guardian could give consent. Historians have generally disparaged sterilization consent requirements, rightly noting that the legal loophole of "if no spouse or near relative can be found" made it easy to circumvent the consent requirement. Also, consent could be coerced. The statutory provisions for third-party consent for the feebleminded and even patient consent (for the insane) do not meet the standards of informed consent which emerged after the end of World War II. In Minnesota, the very idea of uncoerced consent is fallacious because the sterilization process began with *compulsory* court-ordered commitment and institutionalization.[44] Nevertheless, the existence of a statutory provision for consent was significant, and it requires us to rethink the one-dimensional view of sterilization as unilaterally imposed by the state on reluctant families. However flawed the consent requirement was, it gave families a critical if ambiguous part in the eugenic sterilization process. No doubt, some families consented to sterilization for their own ends: to control a difficult or misbehaving adolescent, to relieve the family of another mouth to feed, to hide the shame of sexual abuse or illegitimate pregnancy, or to free a loved one from the institution. Still, the very fact that their consent was required before the sterilization could proceed underlines both the limits of state power and the crucial role that families played, both in enforcing eugenics policies and in resisting them.

Minnesota officials took the consent requirement seriously, at least in the sterilization program's early years. Both the consent of kin, which was required by law, and the personal consent of the patient, which was legally unnecessary for the feebleminded, were listed in the Faribault register of sterilization cases. The board's efforts to secure personal consent, a meaningful but technically unnecessary act given that people under guardianship lacked the legal authority to consent to surgery, show officials' commitment to the law's "voluntary" aspects. Personal consent was recorded for 97 percent of the first thousand sterilizations.[45]

Relatives consented to sterilization in the vast majority of cases. As table 4.4 shows, the authorities recorded the written consent of a relative in 75 percent of the first thousand cases. One or both parents approved nearly half of the operations, while mothers on their own consented to almost one-quarter. Husbands

TABLE 4.4
Written consent to sterilization at Minnesota School for Feebleminded, 1916–1937

Consent given	Number	Percentage of total
Mother	233	23.37
Father	135	13.54
Husband	126	12.64
Parents (both)	119	11.94
Guardian	98	9.83
Sister	54	5.42
Brother	34	3.41
Other	30	3.01
Wife	23	2.31
Aunt	15	1.50
Board of Control	8	0.80
Uncle	7	0.70
Consent not recorded	149	15
Total number of patients[a]	997	100.00

Source: Record of Sterilization Cases, 1916–1937, Faribault State School and Hospital, Miscellaneous Medical Records, Minnesota Historical Society.

[a] Total number of "consent given" is greater than "total number of patients," as some patients had more than one relative give consent.

also figured prominently, even though most sterilization patients were probably unmarried. Thomson obtained consent from aunts, uncles, grandparents, numerous other relatives, and guardians. It is significant, however, that members of the immediate family—parents, spouse, or siblings—gave consent to 72 percent of the first thousand cases. Consent of kin was not recorded in 149 instances, or 15 percent of the sample, but this figure includes clerical errors and unnamed guardians and does not necessarily mean that no consent was given. Indeed, half of the patients sterilized without a relative's consent—77 people—were discharged to family members following the surgery. Clearly, families participated actively in the sterilization process even when they did not legally consent.[46]

Of course, the recording of consent does not necessarily mean that consent was freely given, or that it was given at all. Parents sometimes pressured a daughter who was sexually active or had a baby out of wedlock to consent to sterilization, and a husband could approve a sterilization operation for his wife, regardless of her own views. At least two young women who initially objected to sterilization apparently relented after pressure from their mothers. A mother of five institutionalized during a bitter dispute with her husband gave her personal consent to sterilization because she was afraid of losing child custody. Coercion also came from the state. Officials sometimes threatened to withhold institutional discharge or economic assistance, such as a mother's pension, until a sterilization consent form was signed. Thomson claimed that the state would never force citizens to violate their "religious and moral convictions" and consent to sterilization against their will, and she insisted that the state would never "make a bargain" and grant institutional release in exchange for sterilization. Yet she did not hesitate to inform families that release from the state institution would come "more easily and satisfactorily" after sterilization. Sterilization was not a condition of discharge, she said, but families should know that it was a valuable "aid to the reconstruction of their lives outside the institution."[47]

In a few cases that we know of, the official record of consent was false. A comparison of the Faribault sterilization register to other sources reveals some discrepancies, from either careless errors or a deliberate effort to mislead. To take but one example, the husband of twenty-eight-year-old Nathalie DeLong is listed in the register as consenting to her surgery, but we know from other sources that Nathalie spent most of her life—and became pregnant—at the Faribault School. Officials anxious to avoid a scandal had Nathalie transferred to the Rochester State Hospital to have her baby and may have invented a husband to sign the consent form. Perhaps they thought that such subterfuge was in Nathalie's interest. Superintendent Murdoch wanted to give her the opportunity to live outside the institution and discharged her to the Harmon Club six weeks after surgery.[48] What happened to Nathalie's baby is unknown.

Patients in state hospitals for the insane had to provide written consent to their own sterilization, and the evidence suggests that in the 1920s the Board of Control aggressively solicited patients' personal consent. During a visit to the Fergus Falls State Hospital in May 1929, for example, board member Blanche La Du interviewed seventeen patients, probably all women, to obtain their consent to surgery, reporting with satisfaction that only one person, a mother of six, said no. With a median age of thirty-one, the patients La Du interviewed at Fergus Falls were older than their soon-to-be-sterilized counterparts at Faribault. Fourteen were married, and only one did not already have a child. Several interviewees had large families. Seven patients had four children or more, and one, a thirty-nine-year-old divorcee, had nine. The next year, La Du interviewed fifteen more Fergus Falls patients. She admitted that "some of them changed their minds about wanting the operation," but she was confident that they would "change back as they had already signed their consent prior to the interview." Yet aside from La Du's visitation reports and a brief reference in the Fergus Falls State Hospital's 1930 biennial report to a surgeon who rendered "invaluable assistance by doing sterilization operations," I found no documentation of sterilizations performed at Fergus Falls. Whether the absence of an evidentiary record reflects sloppy record keeping, the deliberate disposal of evidence, or the intentional disregard of the statutory requirement that a "complete record" be kept of each case, the absence of a paper trail hints at the secrecy and stigma surrounding mental illness and the indignities many sterilization patients had to bear.[49]

Even though Minnesota's consent requirement was a sham in many ways, its significance should not be downplayed. Coercion was a central fact of life for poor women (and men), especially if they were labeled feebleminded, and involuntary sterilization must be seen in the context of the totality of their lives. Low-wage workers in laundries, factories, or private homes frequently faced employers who drove them too hard, stole their wages, or made sexual advances. Those who had physical or mental disabilities, or who had been committed to state guardianship as feebleminded, were exploited and marginalized, both in the state institutions that relied on their unpaid labor and in the private homes where they often worked. To be sure, motherhood or the dream of motherhood was fundamental to the identity of most working-class women. Having children was one of the most joyful and rewarding parts of their lives, and unwanted sterilization caused deep and lasting emotional as well as physical harm. Still, the infertility following surgical sterilization was only part of a larger set of injustices which included indefinite institutionalization, unremunerated labor, unnecessary medical treatments, lost custody of one's children, and sexual abuse.

As involuntary as Minnesota's "voluntary" sterilization law undeniably was, the statutory requirement of written consent to sterilization gave poor people some leverage in their dealings with state authorities. Thomson's correspondence makes clear that the job of tracking down families and "bring[ing] them to the point of consenting to the operation" was time-consuming and often unsuccessful. Relatives who refused to sign were often able to keep their loved ones from being sterilized. Faribault admissions records reveal several instances of patients who were admitted "for sterilization" but apparently never had the operation, either because doctors determined that surgery would be medically dangerous or because relatives refused their consent. The consent requirement was likely also a factor in the relatively small percentage of sterilizations performed on men and patients classed as insane. Catholics who had a moral objection to sterilization were often able to prevent their allegedly feebleminded relatives from undergoing the surgeon's knife. Catholic opposition to sterilization became more vigorous after the pope's condemnation of eugenics in 1930, and although some social workers said privately that Catholic opposition was overstated, more than a few Catholic welfare workers had "conflicting feelings" about the sterilization program, as did priests who regularly obstructed the board's plans. Statements such as "no action because of religion" were common in field reports of the 1930s and 1940s.[50]

Even when sterilizations occurred, the consent provision helped poor families in their negotiations with welfare officials. A Twin Cities social worker who considered sterilization a "questionable remedy" admitted that it "has worked out well in families where there were already enough children and the mother and father were convinced that there should not be any more."[51] The case of Sam and Lena B. provides a good illustration. The couple had two children when they were committed to state guardianship in 1934. Although the child welfare board wanted the pair sterilized immediately, relatives objected, and three years passed before the couple was taken to Faribault to have the operation. A daughter was born in the intervening period, and the couple's fourth child, a son, was born at the Faribault School. The family was reunited a few months after the parents were sterilized, and the social worker reported that they were happy: "Sam said he thought he had the right size family and was glad that they did not have any more children," she explained. The family resisted the state's sterilization plan when the couple had only two children, but they were content to stop at four.[52]

As Sam and Lena's story suggests, it can be difficult to untangle "eugenic" sterilization from the quest for birth control. Poor women did not all have the same interests and desires, and some actively sought sterilization as a form of birth control. As Johanna Schoen has observed, "Rather than being the victims of coercive eugenic programs, they used those policies and programs for their own ends." During the peak years of Minnesota's sterilization program, the distribution of birth control information and supplies was illegal, and although physicians in Minnesota could lawfully prescribe contraceptives in certain circumstances, many poor women were desperate for reproductive health care. During the Depression, in particular, institution records show a number of women who went to Faribault for sterilization and expected to return home as soon as they recovered from surgery. Annie Schroeder, a relief-dependent mother of ten children, Ida Nelson, who bore thirteen children in fifteen years of marriage, and thrice-married Violet Novak, who had three children and depended on public relief, were among them. In these cases, poor women's need for contraception converged with social workers' aim of providing humanitarian assistance and reducing relief costs and eugenicists' wish to reduce the birth rate of those they considered unfit.[53]

Yet women who consented to eugenic sterilization because they wanted contraceptive care were extremely vulnerable. They had to allow themselves to be declared a ward of the state, submit to a period of "training" in the state institutions, and, since feebleminded women were considered unfit mothers, risk losing their children. Some women had to spend more time at Faribault than expected when outbreaks of influenza or the measles caused surgical delays or when a family member would not sign the consent form. (A feebleminded ward of the state could not legally sign for herself.) In at least one case, the result was near disaster. Alice Clifford entered the School for the Feebleminded for sterilization in late 1932 but was stranded in the institution because a flu outbreak caused a temporary halt to all surgery. As her husband grew restless and the agencies caring for their children asked to be "relieved of their responsibility" so they could address other needs, the couple's friends worried that the delay was concealing the state's nefarious intentions. Six months passed before Mrs. Clifford finally had the operation and was able to return home.[54] These stories in different ways illustrate the difficult decisions that poor women seeking contraception faced: continue to risk their health in unwanted pregnancies and have children they could not afford, or forfeit their legal rights and submit to state guardianship as feebleminded and unfit.

Resistance

There is surprisingly little documentary evidence of opposition to Minnesota's sterilization program in the 1920s. In the correspondence of the Faribault School, I found only one letter protesting a planned sterilization. The writer was upset that the sister of a feebleminded woman had signed the sterilization consent form against the wishes of the girl's parents. Charlotte was "no more feeble mind then I or you," the woman asserted, and it was wrong "to ruin a girl like that because her sister —— wants to get a little smart."[55] This silence on sterilization contrasts with the many complaints on behalf of individuals who felt unjustly institutionalized and the numerous legal appeals for discharge from guardianship, the first step to getting out of the institution. The odds of a court challenge to guardianship succeeding were certainly greater than a challenge to sterilization, which was an administrative decision. Yet it is also possible that institutionalization—which, unlike sterilization, did not require the consent of kin—was the more urgent concern. Regardless of whether the "fix" was surgical or institutional, the feebleminded person's right to reproduce was denied.

Poor people rarely put their views about sterilization on paper, but they voted with their feet and got help from friends and family. Parents refused to return loved ones to Faribault after a vacation at home. Boyfriends helped women plan their escape and drove the getaway car. Sixteen escapes show up in the sterilization register, and the runaway problem was a major theme in Thomson's correspondence. She lamented the difficulty of getting women to stay at the Harmon Club and sulked when the brightest ones ran away. Making excuses for her disappointments, she blamed the women's disreputable families or the bad influence of the Minneapolis underworld. But she also tried to rationalize the women's actions. For example, she told Murdoch that Ellen Clancy, a prostitute "among the colored men of Minneapolis," had tried "to be satisfied and to make good" at the clubhouse, "but partial liberty without full liberty was too much for her." After a particularly devastating loss in April 1928, Thomson wrote despairingly that the "whole Club House idea is a failure, as three of our younger and best girls ran away without coming [home] from work yesterday."

She wondered if it was "all worth while." Ever resilient, Thomson purchased a car and thereafter spent many hours behind the wheel searching for those who had fled.[56]

The state's hold on feebleminded women was always shaky, but as we shall see in the next chapter, its control grew even more tenuous after the clubhouses closed during the 1930s. State appropriations for the parole program had always been meager, and the clubhouses depended on support from various constituencies: the Women's Welfare League and other private agencies, which provided housing and services in partnership with the state; the counties, which were legally obliged to support dependent residents; and the feebleminded women who paid room and board. The system worked reasonably well when work was plentiful, but it fell apart when farm prices plummeted. Just a few years after the Harmon Club opened, the building needed a new furnace and other repairs the welfare league claimed it could not afford. Then spiraling unemployment "played havoc" with clubhouse plans. League secretary Elinor McIntosh complained that the dramatic increase in joblessness made it "well-nigh impossible" for feebleminded women to be self-supporting. By 1931, only nine of the eighteen women living at Harmon Club had any work, and together they earned just $7,961, a paltry sum compared to their earnings in previous years. To make matters worse, many counties refused to subsidize feebleminded women at a clubhouse if space was available at Faribault. The counties' preference for institutionalization was "not wholly based on economic aspects," Thomson observed in her memoirs, but "placement in an institution was not only a solution, but a final one, unless self-support or family care was possible." Counties' insistence on institutionalization was rooted in the philosophy of the poorhouse and the punitive attitudes toward the undeserving poor.[57]

The women's resistance also contributed to the clubhouses' collapse. Thomson observed frostily that unemployed women "created conduct problems and formed habits that were not conducive to their later success." Residents' discontent had reverberated through the clubhouses from the beginning, but it worsened during the Depression. "It has been a sick, restless, runaway year," McIntosh despaired in 1930, and the clubhouse had its "poorest showing" since it opened. To make matters worse, she said the runaways were invariably the liveliest women with good jobs who could pay board, while those left behind were less capable mentally and therefore more likely to remain unemployed.[58]

The Harmon Club was stuck in a vicious circle. The Board of Control tried to fill the vacancies with women who had lower IQs, but these women had difficulty finding employment, and their joblessness aggravated the clubhouses' budgetary woes. Increasingly open opposition to sterilization added to the clubhouses' problems, for many women with the highest IQs would not "consent [to sterilization] readily, therefore are kept in the school and we must take the less intelligent." It was becoming more and more difficult for the Women's Welfare League to "relieve the School, fill our quota and help us pay our overhead." In December 1931, after three women ran away and a fourth took up with the ice deliveryman, the league concluded that the Harmon Club was a "rather useless piece of work—that time, energy and money could be more profitably spent on some constructive work." It turned the Harmon Club over to the Board of Control.[59]

Soon the whole clubhouse program collapsed. The Duluth Club closed in July 1931, and the Harmon Club shut down six months later. Although the Lynnhurst Club limped along until 1939, it functioned more as a temporary shelter and convalescent home than a residence for institutionalized women making the transition to community life. Reflecting on the clubhouses thirty years later, Thomson admitted that the Board of Control "failed to think clearly" about their function. State officials viewed the Harmon Club as a way to reduce costs and ease institutional overcrowding, but "should not its fundamental purpose have been helping girls to make a personal and community adjustment regardless of self-support? To a limited extent this was what it did. However, we hoped and spoke as though we expected the club to be self-supporting except for the cost of staff and supervision, and we found after a time this was not the case."[60] Writing in the early 1960s after she had retired, Thomson intended her remarks to contrast the enlightened attitudes of the postwar years with the archaic 1920s, but her recollections call attention to two central features of Minnesota's "eugenic" sterilization program: the primacy of the welfare objective and the iron grip of fiscal concerns.

As Thomson's remarks make clear, the everyday operation of Minnesota's sterilization program tells a different and more complicated story than the writings of eugenicists would suggest. In Minnesota, worries about bad heredity and preventing the birth of "socially inadequate offspring" were secondary to the more prosaic—and, sadly, more enduring—concerns about sex, illegitimacy, "bad" parenting, overcrowded public institutions, and the cost of relief. Thomson and other administrators were hardly all-powerful, and whether sterilization patients and their families resisted the operation or "consented" to it because they needed contraception, understood surgery to be the price of freedom, or literally had no other choice, they asserted their own needs and viewed sterilization in the context of the totality of their lives.

Thomson's own ideas about feeblemindedness changed distressingly little between the 1920s and the 1940s, but by the time the clubhouses closed the myth of the menace of the feebleminded had faded away. The poverty, dependency, and casual sexual styles that seemed to set young mentally deficient women apart from the mainstream in the 1910s and 1920s seemed almost normal by the 1930s, and the once-powerful rhetoric about the menace of the feebleminded was supplanted by intense political battles over communism, labor radicalism, and the New Deal. The women who lived in the clubhouses contributed to the shift in attitudes by showing that "mentally deficient" women were not so very different from other working-class women, and that discharging them from the institution would not endanger public safety. Yet despite the diminished fear of hereditary feeblemindedness, Minnesota's sterilization program peaked during the 1930s, and Thomson would look back on the era of the clubhouses as a lighthearted interlude when compared to the turmoil of later years. The next chapter explores the routinization of eugenic sterilization as a welfare policy during the 1930s, when the gap between eugenics discourse and welfare bureaucracy was especially marked.

STERILIZATION AND WELFARE IN DEPRESSION AND WAR

In May 1940, Mildred Thomson touted the social work benefits of sterilization in a paper she presented before the American Association on Mental Deficiency (AAMD). Drawing on Tena and Stewart as examples, she said that while the couple had "many good traits and were fond of their children," they could not handle the stress created by the Depression and unemployment. He drank, and she was "stepping out" as she had before her marriage, even though she was pregnant with her fourth child. Their children appeared neglected and abused. Although the couple had been committed to guardianship in 1934 after IQ tests found them to be feebleminded, three years later their behavior had not improved. The county welfare board decided to take action. With Thomson's help, it sent both parents to Faribault for sterilization and placed the four children (including the baby, who had been born in the institution) in boarding homes. Stewart returned home after two months, but Tena remained institutionalized for a total of eight months because, according to Thomson, her parents had "caused" her operation to be delayed. When she was finally sterilized and allowed to return home, a social worker got Stewart a Works Progress Administration (WPA) job so he could support his family, helped Tena develop her "latent sense of responsibility" as a mother, and reintroduced their children into the home.[1]

It is revealing that Thomson's paper made no reference to the eugenic rationale for sterilization, even though her audience was a professional association dominated by institution officials. Thomson's point was that the couple's economic circumstances and parenting skills could be improved with positive social work intervention and surgery. She treated sterilization as a routine welfare practice that, in the context of the Depression, made sure feebleminded parents did not have any more mouths to feed or rear children who got into trouble. Although she criticized the "over zealous" claim that sterilization was "wholly justified by the eugenic factors," Thomson never doubted the merits of Minnesota's program of "selective" sterilization when there was a "socioeconomic justification." When sterilization was based on individual casework, she believed, it had a rehabilitative function that could bring "tangible and immediate" benefits to both the sterilized individual and the state. Through sterilization, dependent and delinquent families could be made respectable and self-supporting.[2]

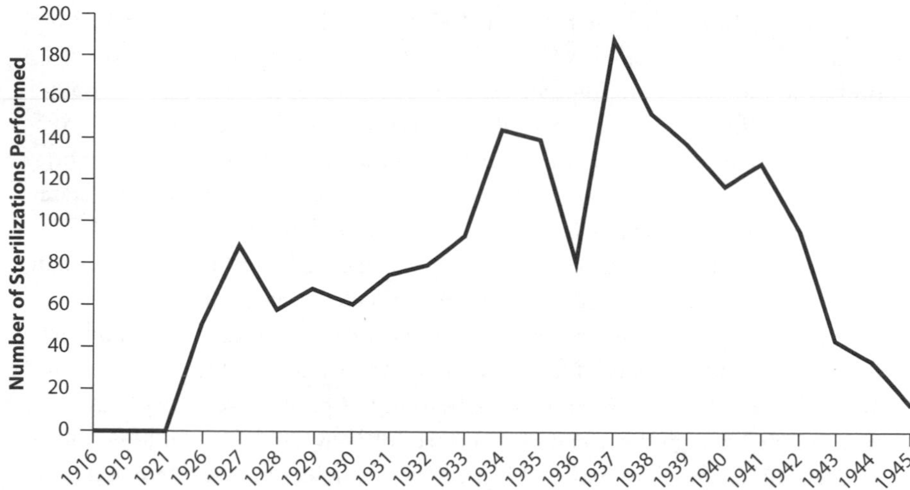

Figure 5.1. Sterilizations performed at the Minnesota School for the Feebleminded, 1916–1945. *Source:* E. J. Engberg to Carl Swanson, June 22, 1946, Faribault State School and Hospital, Superintendent Correspondence, Minnesota Historical Society.

Eugenic sterilization became a vital part of Minnesota's public welfare system during the Depression, and in the late 1930s the number of sterilizations reached an all-time high. As figure 5.1 shows, the Faribault sterilization program was active in the relatively prosperous 1920s, but the number of operations performed annually jumped after 1933. Significantly, the increase coincided not with the economic collapse, but with the influx of federal funding. More than one-third of Minnesota's 2,350 recorded sterilizations were performed between 1933 and 1938, the peak years of the New Deal. The largest numbers of operations occurred over a two-year period when Farmer–Labor governor Elmer Benson, an early critic of Nazism and strong proponent of social welfare entitlements, was in power. Although the number of recorded operations fell slightly when the Republicans regained control of the state house in 1939, Minnesota's policy of institutionalizing and sterilizing the so-called feebleminded remained an important part of public welfare practice until World War II, when surgical nurses were needed elsewhere.[3]

Why did sterilizations accelerate during the 1930s? Most historians attribute the increase—which occurred across the nation, not just in Minnesota—to the broad acceptance of eugenics beliefs and to budgetary pressures on the public purse; a few see a causal relationship between the expanding state and eugenics abuse. Yet the economic collapse had a paradoxical impact on policies and popular thinking about feeblemindedness and eugenics. On the one hand, the

Depression blurred the line between "feebleminded" and "normal" by making conditions once associated with feeblemindedness seem ordinary (pauperism, broken homes, and tramping, for example). On the other hand, the economic crisis intensified entrenched fears about social degeneration and decline. MES president Charles Dight was one of many who worried that unemployed workers' growing dependence on public welfare and charity put the United States on the verge of drowning in a "sea of mental and moral degeneracy." Still, Thomson recalled that "general interest in the mentally deficient was less than it had been for a time" and the Progressive Era belief that feebleminded women were inherently immoral receded. The gulf between eugenics rhetoric and sterilization routines widened during the 1930s. To explain the Depression-era increase in sterilizations, one must look beyond the public discourse of eugenics to examine how, amid the chaotic processes of New Deal state building, older ideas about local welfare responsibility and the undeserving poor were built into the structures of America's semiwelfare state.[4]

At first glance, it seems ironic that eugenic sterilization programs expanded as public acceptance of government's responsibility for social welfare was taking hold. In Minnesota, the new era began in 1930, when voters shook off sixty years of Republican rule and elected the charismatic Scandinavian American attorney Floyd Olson as their first Farmer–Labor governor. Both Olson and President Franklin Delano Roosevelt, who was elected in 1932 on a promise to rest his economic plan on the "forgotten man at the bottom of the economic pyramid," pledged to use the power of government to defend the interests of the common people. Once in office, Roosevelt moved quickly to alleviate hardship, and by 1934, 22 percent of the American population benefited from federal relief.[5]

The distribution of relief was a mammoth and messy undertaking shaped philosophically and administratively by a contradictory mixture of old and new. Historically, poor relief had been a local responsibility, but in the early 1930s county and state governments lacked the resources and administrative capacity to respond effectively to the ballooning crisis. When federal funds finally began to flow, the need to move quickly meant that national relief efforts relied on existing welfare agencies. This arrangement had many advantages, especially outside the South. It encouraged grassroots participation and, in the words of Minnesota historian Jerome Tweton, brought the cooperation of "small-town, rural America where people cherished the virtues of self-reliance and self-determination." At the same time, as many historians have pointed out, the New Deal's emphasis on cooperation with the states left local prejudices unchallenged and allowed racial discrimination to fester. In Minnesota, where the Board of Control and county child welfare boards were assigned the task of distributing emergency relief, the influx of federal funds greatly increased the power of local welfare boards, at least in the short term. Despite their new power, many welfare boards viewed economic hardship through an old lens. Even though nearly one in five Minnesotans received federal emergency relief, they continued to blame mental deficiency for joblessness, vagrancy, and welfare dependency. As Mildred Thomson stated simply, there was a "definite relationship between the persons receiving direct relief and work relief from the state and federal governments, and feeble-mindedness."[6]

New Deal welfare policies were also shaped by cultural ideas about what was fair. Historian Alice Kessler-Harris argues that an embedded belief system, or "gendered imagination," shaped the boundaries of what New Deal policy makers thought politically possible, desirable, and fair when the social welfare functions of the federal government were expanding. The primacy placed on gendered ideas about dependency and the right to work, based on the assumption that the "worker" was a (white) man with a dependent wife and children, led to the development of a two-track welfare state. Work-related entitlement programs, such as unemployment insurance and social security, generally excluded women and racialized men, while Aid to Dependent Children was means tested and structured to reinforce women's and children's dependency. At the time, this disparity was considered reasonable and just. Extending Kessler-Harris's argument to disability allows us to see how gendered and racialized ideas about work and dependency also framed discussions around policies for the so-called feebleminded, who were considered to be permanently unemployable and a drain on the public purse. New Deal policy makers, convinced that relief was (in Roosevelt's words) a "narcotic, a subtle destroyer of the human spirit" that could turn once-independent workers into paupers, designed federal relief programs to preserve the dignity of employable but temporarily jobless (white) male adults. But public assistance for "unemployables"—dependent children, single mothers, and people considered to have physical and mental disabilities—remained the responsibility of local authorities.[7]

The New Deal had an ambiguous effect on eugenics policies in Minnesota and across the nation. On the one hand, it federalized the child welfare programs established during the Progressive Era, replaced the poor-law tradition of local responsibility with a national commitment to social welfare, and used the power of the federal government to protect poor people from the worst effects of the economic collapse. On the other hand, New Deal policy makers won the support of racist southern Democrats by accepting legislation that excluded most African Americans from work-related entitlements and wrote gender, race, and sexual inequities into the structures of the US welfare state. As political scientist Ira Katznelson writes, the "ugly and lasting consequences of this Faustian bargain" shaped social policy for the rest of the twentieth century. In northern states, too, local prejudices influenced determinations of relief eligibility, and welfare boards used their increasing authority to try to "fix" the poor. Yet if the

Depression and New Deal strengthened the hand of the state's eugenics abusers, it also planted the seeds of resistance. The federal government functioned to some extent as a bulwark against local prejudice and discrimination, and New Dealers' emphasis on administrative "standards," along with the new vocabulary about economic rights and the forgotten man, gave ordinary people new tools for contesting eugenics and state programs for the feebleminded.[8] After the return to prosperity in World War II, Minnesota officials no longer viewed eugenic sterilization as a poverty policy. Instead, they launched a new era of reform.

"Lousy with Politics": The Economic Crisis and the Board of Control

When the stock market crashed in October 1929, few Minnesotans imagined that Wall Street's crisis would ravage the Upper Midwest. The region had been deeply affected by the drop in agricultural prices in the 1920s, but the impact of the Great Depression was far worse. The price of wheat fell to 36 cents per bushel in the early 1930s, down from $2.96 in 1920. Milk prices were also down, bringing just two cents a quart. An ecological disaster exacerbated the farm crisis, as dust storms, grasshoppers, and drought destroyed crops, starved cattle, and blackened the sky. Driving through the "droughty" counties of western Minnesota, journalist Meridel Le Sueur described once-independent farmers descending into the "abyss of pauperism." People were not supposed to starve in America, she wrote, but "the whole country cracks and rumbles and cries out in its terrible leanness, stripped with exploitation and terror."[9] The fear, resentment, and growing militancy of midwestern farmers and workers shook Minnesota politics to the core.

The economic crisis affected every part of the economy. City dwellers who had thrived in the 1920s found themselves jobless or underemployed a few years later. One-quarter of Minneapolis factories disappeared during the Depression's early years. During the worst of the crisis, about one-quarter of Minnesota men were unemployed. People who were still working, including state employees like Mildred Thomson, faced deep salary cuts. Prior to the Depression, most people on public assistance were deemed unemployable: children, single mothers, the aged and infirm, and the so-called defectives and inebriates disparaged as the undeserving poor. Now able-bodied men and their families also turned to charity and public relief. "The man is helpless now," Le Sueur wrote bleakly. "He cannot provide. If he propagates he cannot take care of his young." Pauperism, homelessness, and family disruption, once seen as signs of hereditary feeblemindedness, were commonplace.[10]

The Depression sucked up the budgets of local governments and private charities and put enormous pressure on state welfare institutions. "In a period of economic stress . . . it is always the weakest who are the first to fail in making the necessary adjustments and who become an increasing burden," Board of Control chair Blanche La Du told a meeting of social workers in 1932. The inmate population in prisons, mental hospitals, and the School for the Feebleminded soared as economic stress pushed individuals and families to the breaking point, and people could not be released on parole because they had so little chance of supporting themselves. La Du was particularly worried about the children. Citing the principle first articulated at the 1909 White House Conference on the Care of Dependent Children that "home life is the highest and finest product of civilization; . . . [and] except in unusual circumstances the home should not be broken up for reasons of poverty," she warned that the alarming jump in the number of dependent and neglected children sent to the state orphanage at Owatonna "reveals a deterioration in the social fabric that if continued will be a menace to society." The large number of children in state care should be "a matter of grave concern for us all."[11]

For families with a mental deficiency designation or disabled relative, the economic pressures were even worse. Many "feebleminded" women lost their jobs or faced wage cuts when factories and laundries closed or the families who employed them could no longer afford domestic help or extra farm hands. The combined impact of the closure of the Board of Control clubhouses and poor families' inability to care for dependent relatives at home increased the demand for institutional placements, even though institution budgets were cut back. As a result, many who would have been discharged in the 1920s were forced to remain in—or return to—the state institution. Referring to one such woman, Thomson reported glumly that even though Letta Gerber was sterilized and "as good as she can be," she could not earn enough to be self-supporting and her family could not care for her. Letta would have to return to Faribault. Still, Thomson declared hopefully, "I am sure that although she probably will weep for a while after being returned, she will soon be contented in the Institution."[12]

The budget collapse weakened the social welfare shift away from institutionalization and toward community placement, provoking an intense debate within professional circles. The issue crystallized at the 1934 meeting of the AAMD. On one side, Thomson recalled, several social workers argued that it was better to keep feebleminded patients institutionalized than to release them into slavery-like placements where they worked long hours for room and board, but no pay, doing farm labor or domestic chores for private families. On the other side, New York superintendent Charles Bernstein maintained that institutional discharge, even if it meant working as a domestic servant without any pay at all, was always preferable to institutionalization because it allowed feebleminded individuals to "live in the world as normal people do" and opened up much-needed space in the institution. Unlike Bernstein, Thomson was based in the community, and she stood firmly on the social work side. "I always feared that wards might be exploited and felt that the state must protect them," she wrote in her memoirs, noting proudly that she rebuffed a request from an elderly couple who felt they were entitled to a live-in housekeeper from Faribault because of the taxes they paid.[13]

Thomson's claim that the state had to "protect" the feebleminded was rooted in eugenics discourse, but her concern about exploited labor also reflected the mood in Minnesota, where workers were unionizing and even the governor protested the unequal distribution of wealth. Governor Floyd Olson, the son of poor Norwegian and Swedish immigrants, had earned a reputation for toughness when as Hennepin County Attorney he confronted the Ku Klux Klan in the 1920s, and as governor in the early 1930s he was a leading proponent of government action on poverty and unemployment. "The old pioneer idea of government as confined to police power has passed off the stage," Olson declared in 1932. "The present economic system has shown its inability to provide employment and even food or shelter for millions of Americans. Only government can cope with the situation." Olson moved quickly when federal relief funds became available and was a strong, though not uncritical, supporter of Franklin Roosevelt's New Deal. Before he died in office from cancer in 1936, Olson oversaw a major expansion of public relief, set up a system of old-age pensions, passed a moratorium on farm foreclosures, abolished labor injunctions, and established the state's first income tax.[14]

Olson's economic agenda faced both a hostile antitax legislature and intense pressure from the Left. Shortly after his inauguration in early 1931, unemployed workers marched on the state capital, and nearly ten thousand people joined a union-led rally for economic relief. Farmers pushed back against foreclosures, and the militant Farm Holiday Association went on strike, withholding produce from the market in the fall of 1932. Even Mildred Thomson was caught up in the spirit of the times. She wrote in her memoirs that a growing number of social workers began to "wonder whether a political system that permitted such a depression could be the right one." She went to several communist-led meetings of the unemployed. "At that time I was quite naive and did not realize who organized these meetings, although pictures of American communists were on the walls," she wrote coolly during the Cold War, but although she found the presentations "more vitriolic than reasonable," she could understand the desperation of people who lacked the means to care for their families. Yet while Thomson was pulled to the left, other social workers worried more about the pauperizing effects of public relief. Their opposition to federal "make-work" projects and demand for tax relief revealed the polarization of New Deal politics and entrenched disagreements over the government's welfare role.[15]

Federal and state politics were dramatic, but the cruel inadequacy of America's poor relief system was laid bare at the local level. In law, every legal resident of Minnesota was entitled to basic subsistence, but in reality, local jurisdictions with declining tax bases could not meet the need. In 1932, fifty-five Minnesota counties operated on the county system of poor relief, but thirty-two still operated on the archaic township system, which left each small town or village responsible for supporting its own poor. In Otter Tail County, for example, relief for a population of fifty thousand fell under the jurisdiction of sixty-two township boards, seventeen village councils, and a city council, each of which funded and distributed aid as it saw fit. The assistance given to poor families varied dramatically according to the wealth and size of the local community and the personal inclination of local officials. While some county commissioners considered the protection of public funds to be their chief duty, others used bonds, overdrafts, and private donations to distribute as much aid as they could. In the early years of the crisis, variation and uncertainty in relief distribution were the only things poor Minnesotans could count on.[16]

Relief measures were particularly complicated in northern counties with large Ojibwe populations, where racial tensions and disputes over jurisdiction shaped the distribution of aid. Indigenous communities had been deprived of their homelands and means of support since the nineteenth century, when wars, treaties, and legislation pushed them onto reservations, regulated their behavior, and marked them as dependent, delinquent, and undeserving. After the 1889 Nelson Act authorized the division of Ojibwe lands into individual "allotments," ostensibly to encourage assimilation and self-sufficiency, members of the White Earth Reservation lost more than 90 percent of their lands.[17] As a result of allotment, intermarriage, and economic hardship, many Ojibwe lost their status as tribal members and federal wards. In some cases, their children were placed under state guardianship through the probate courts, making the local (non-indigenous) government responsible for their economic support. Poverty and health conditions were so dire that the secretary of the interior commissioned a review of federal Indian policy, and in 1928 social worker Lewis Meriam issued a scathing 847-page report called *The Problem of Indian Administration*. "An overwhelming majority of the Indians are poor, even extremely poor," Meriam began, and they were stuck in a "vicious circle of poverty and maladjustment." Meriam admitted that allotment was a disaster, denounced the scandalous mistreatment of children in boarding schools, and lamented the federal government's policy of child removal and family breakup. Yet even though he blamed federal policy for making indigenous people dependent on federal support and holding them in a "condition of perpetual childhood," Meriam criticized what he called Indians' "pauper point of view." In reality, Ojibwe families survived through a creative combination of wage labor, traditional fishing and rice cultivation, public relief, and federal payments. But to white social workers and policy makers, "Indians" embodied the undeserving poor. "Social workers are accustomed to dealing with people who have been pauperized," one social worker observed, but "we are not often faced with an entire community . . . demanding relief as a right."[18]

The Depression brought new urgency to the problem of indigenous welfare, at least in the minds of Minnesota officials. For one thing, as Board of Control representative Blanche La Du explained in 1931, the trust fund established by the federal government from the sale of Ojibwe lands was diminishing. At the current rate of depletion, there would be no federal monies for Native American education, medical care, poor relief, and per capita payments by 1939, and it might be "necessary for the state to assume full responsibility for Indian welfare." To make matters worse, several Minnesota counties with the largest indigenous populations had discontinued their child welfare boards because, they maintained, they could not manage the additional tax burden of assisting the indigenous poor. While Minnesotans were sympathetic to the problems of the aged, the sick, and children, La Du explained, they resented able-bodied Indian adults, who they felt took the "lion's share of that which is provided for the needy." Outside of Minnesota, too, county officials objected that the "federal government is trying to unload a lot of Indians on us. Our white taxpayers can't and won't stand it. They are already taxed to death." The solution, social workers always believed, was individual casework, and in 1932 La Du helped arrange a federally funded pilot project that sent trained social workers to the Consolidated Chippewa and Red Lake Indian Agencies to teach homemaking skills, work with sex delinquents and unmarried mothers, and conduct home investigations to ensure that relief recipients were truly needy and deserving.[19]

Worry about pauperization also shaped the Board of Control's handling of federal aid. In 1932, when President Hoover made emergency loans available to the states, Olson asked the board to help him prepare applications for federal funds and administer the aid. After Roosevelt became president and passed the Federal Emergency Relief Act (FERA) in May 1933, the Board of Control became the State Emergency Relief Administration (SERA), the agency solely responsible for allocating FERA funds. Henceforth, the board was in charge of federal relief, on top of its responsibilities for child welfare, the so-called feebleminded, and the state institutions. It distributed food and surplus commodities to people in drought-scarred counties, operated transient camps for unattached migrant men, and worked with the county child welfare boards to select nonindigenous recruits for the Civilian Conservation Corps (CCC). (The federal Indian agencies helped with the CCC Indian Division and managed relief on the reservations.) Relations among the state, county, and federal governments would never be the same.[20]

Working at lightning speed to ease the humanitarian crisis, relief administrators naturally relied on local welfare boards and personnel. Each county was required to organize a County Emergency Relief Committee that included two members of the child welfare board. The field representatives of the state children's bureau, which was responsible for child welfare and feebleminded wards, acted as the liaison to St. Paul. The Board of Control had long been frustrated by what it considered the unprofessional practices of county poor commissioners and tried to use its new power to impose modern social work methods, such as home investigations and confidentiality, on skeptical local officials. Determined to make sure that recipients of federal relief were deserving of aid, the state board insisted that county welfare workers inspect applicants' homes, inquire into their economic resources, and interview their relatives, former employers, and friends. "To be a 'deserving case,'" a federal investigator remarked scornfully, "a family has got to measure up to the most rigid Nineteenth Century standards of cleanliness, physical and moral. As a result, a woman who isn't a good housekeeper is apt to have a pretty rough time of it. And heaven help the family in which there is any 'moral problem.'" She was talking about Maine, but her comments applied equally to Minnesota. Such intrusions were standard fare for single mothers and the so-called feebleminded, but they were a new experience for recently unemployed nonindigenous men and a "painful ordeal to many families, often serving the final stroke to loss of morale and self-respect."[21]

To be sure, the emphasis on undeservingness did not go unchallenged. In Minneapolis in particular, many social workers rejected home investigations as paternalistic, denounced the delays in processing applications, and decried the inadequate amount of aid. Those who joined the radical "rank and file" social work movement insisted that their clients' problems were not psychological but economic. Their clients were already oversupervised, they maintained; poor people needed economic assistance—they did not need to be fixed. On the other side, more conservative social workers worried that mass relief "fostered greed, a grab-for-myself 'gimme' attitude." The "truly forgotten man," quipped a Ramsey county welfare official, "is he who struggled along on an income less than our inadequate relief budgets without a word of protest."[22]

The Board of Control was committed to both modern social work methods and the principle of local responsibility, and it gave local units considerable freedom to apply—or not apply—for federal funds. The result was tremendous inconsistency in access to federal relief funds. Lorena Hickok, a former *Minneapolis Tribune* reporter who traveled around the country as an investigator for FERA chief Harry Hopkins, had a "pretty poor impression of the relief show in Minnesota." Six months after FERA went into effect, most Minnesota counties had "no relief set-up," and less than one-half had received federal aid. She blamed foot-dragging at the county level and the state board's inefficiencies for delaying the start of work-relief projects in the northern part of the state.[23]

In Hickok's view, Minnesota's relief problems were political. "The whole set-up in this state was—pardon the vulgarity—lousy with politics," she told

Hopkins. Olson, a Farmer–Laborite, and La Du, a Republican, were "at loggerheads and always had been." The Democrats were weak, "most of the money and the press are Republican and hostile," and Governor Olson—despite being a "remarkable man" and "about the smartest 'Red' in this country"—had his "finger too much in the pie." La Du's supporters, mostly Republicans, alleged that the governor wanted to staff the relief agencies with patronage jobs, yet Hickok told Hopkins that the state welfare agency was also to blame. The Board of Control was "an institutional organization, not a relief organization," she explained; it was created to run prisons and mental hospitals, and it functioned "rather badly" as the state relief agency. When a frustrated Olson stripped the board of its responsibilities and made himself the state relief administrator in December 1933, Hickok was sympathetic. "There will be politics in it," she conceded, "but, gosh, there was plenty of that in Mrs. La Du's set-up, apparently. And very little efficiency."[24] As the Depression destabilized the localism and deserving/undeserving distinction that shaped traditional relief practices, new welfare policies gave rise to a new kind of administrative state. It was the beginning of the end of the Board of Control.

The Most Feebleminded-Conscious State: Dependency and Delinquency in the New Welfare Era

In the early years of the Depression most county child welfare boards tried to carry on as they had in the past. At first they attempted to assist "deserving" families by using existing programs such as mothers' pensions, where administrative procedures and funding mechanisms were well established. Yet county mothers' aid was at best a partial solution to the relief crisis. The size of the allowance depended on the county's revenue (the state made no financial contribution), and recipients had to be the children of "proper" mothers. Grant levels varied according to the local judge's "attitude toward relief in general, whether it be liberal or conservative," and his views of proper (and improper) mothering. There was also strong disagreement about aid to mothers with low IQs. In rural counties, maternal unfitness—often associated with mental deficiency—accounted for 15 percent of ineligibility rulings, compared to only 3 percent in the urban counties. Yet although psychologist Frederick Kuhlmann was adamant that allowances should never be granted to women who were "definitely mentally defective," two-thirds of probate judges in one survey said they would not disqualify a mother on the grounds of low intelligence alone.[25]

The preoccupation with mental deficiency is a common theme in the minutes of the county child welfare boards. For example, during the first years of the Depression, the child welfare board in Chisago County spent much of its time trying to stop fathers from drinking away their wages and girls from staying out late with men. Board members investigated recipients of mothers' pensions, filed paternity claims, arranged placements for the children of unmarried mothers, and sent feebleminded wards to Faribault. Yet by late 1933, the county poor fund was more than $11,000 overdrawn, and fiscal considerations increasingly impinged on the board's moral assessments and welfare plans. Board members urged several unmarried mothers to put up their babies for adoption so that the county would not have to pay child support, and they advised a young woman not to file paternity charges against her baby's father because he was married and they feared that his entire family would wind up on relief. Increasingly, they ordered mental tests for unwed mothers and for parents who depended on relief or had been accused of child neglect, knowing that committing county residents to the Owatonna orphanage or Faribault School lowered the cost of supporting them.[26]

As in the 1920s, the child welfare board spent months trying to fix a few hard-to-manage families. The stories of Helen and Eva Lidstrom, two "feebleminded" sisters who had babies out of wedlock, are illustrative. Board members placed their babies in boarding homes, pressed the putative fathers to pay child support, and made arrangements to have the women committed to state guardianship and sterilized. Sterilization plans proceeded smoothly for thirty-four-year-old Helen, who had an IQ of 47, but the board had more difficulty sterilizing her sister. For reasons that are unclear, the probate judge delayed Eva's commitment hearing for more than a month, and then her mother's refusal to consent to sterilization delayed the process further. Mrs. Lidstrom only relented when her daughter became ill. Eva was taken to Faribault in the summer of 1937, purportedly "for her own protection," and a tubectomy was probably performed eleven months later.[27]

This welfare board's priorities and aggravations were nothing out of the ordinary, at least in Minnesota. Thomson believed that Minnesota social workers were more aware of the "relationship of low mentality to social problems" than their counterparts in other states. If so, the reason was largely structural. In rural counties especially, the same child welfare board members who watched over unwed mothers and the so-called feebleminded also helped families with mothers' allowances, old-age assistance, and work-relief jobs. In Thomson's view, the mixed caseload was advantageous. In fact, it reinforced the notion that poor people who seemed less than respectable were feebleminded and that surgery was the only fix.[28]

A similar attitude affected Minnesota's indigenous communities. Although the Indian Reorganization Act of 1934 had reversed the policy of allotment, federal subsidies for state-run medical, education, and welfare programs serving Native Americans kept indigenous families under scrutiny and monitored their adjustment to white Christian norms. At least nine indigenous women were among the first thousand sterilization patients at Faribault. Like their nonindigenous counterparts, these women tended to be unmarried mothers (that is, they had children outside of legal Christian marriage) or women with large families who allegedly drank and neglected their children, prompting a probate judge to commit them to state guardianship.[29]

Jurisdictional questions about federal, state, and county responsibility complicated the sterilization approval process. While the Consolidated Chippewa Indian Agency sent several feebleminded women to Faribault for sterilization, authorities believed that Minnesota's sterilization law did not apply to members of the Red Lake Band. (The Red Lake Band had resisted nineteenth-century allotment policy and thus retained sovereignty, along with the federal government, over tribal members—the state had no jurisdiction.) The Red Lake Indian Agency sent some "promiscuous" feebleminded girls to Faribault and paid their school fees of $25 per month, but since Minnesota's sterilization law only applied to persons under state guardianship, the Red Lake girls had to remain in the institution indefinitely, which was "very unsatisfactory to them, and their parents, as well as being very expensive for the Indian Agency." After twenty-four-year-old Annie Austin ran away from Faribault for the third time in three years, social worker Mary Kirkland reported that her office faced "much opposition" from parents whose daughters remained at Faribault for a long period and could not understand "what the difference between the status of Red Lake Indians and Consolidated Chippewa Indians is in the matter of sterilization." While federal jurisdiction "protected" some Ojibwe women from unwanted sterilization, it did not protect others. For indigenous and white families alike, the state's handling of feebleminded individuals was confusing and unpredictable.[30]

Throughout Minnesota, the Depression and the New Deal brought fiscal and administrative pressures that intensified social workers' concerns about clients they considered feebleminded. In the Twin Cities, where the child welfare board distributed relief and caseloads reached as high as five hundred families per worker, many social workers complained that too much time, effort, and money were expended on families where feeblemindedness, not unemployment, was the main problem. In 1934, the Ramsey County Child Welfare Board organized a committee of experts to develop a coordinated strategy. The overcrowding at Faribault had created a "more and more serious problem" on the front lines, a St. Paul social worker explained. The institution could only accommodate a fraction of the feebleminded, but since feebleminded guardianship was lifelong, the case could never be closed. "The number of children, their doings, the whole thing piles up so terribly that one cannot face it," another social worker despaired. "We don't know what the answer is. I think now it is not so much a matter . . . of getting the feebleminded committed, but of what to do with them after they are committed, or catching the feebleminded girls and boys before they can marry and establish homes."[31]

Questions of money and jurisdiction were always central to decisions about commitment and sterilization. Feebleminded commitment cemented the state's power over hard-to-manage families, institutionalization had the potential to close the file on a difficult case, and sterilization reduced the chances of yet another child on the dole. For that reason, county welfare boards often ordered IQ tests for parents and children living in "deplorable conditions . . . and in many instances whole families were then committed to guardianship as feebleminded." Thomson thought that placing entire families under guardianship made harried judges and welfare workers feel "satisfied that they had taken some kind of action," even though they still had to help find child care and work relief. However, she observed with characteristic understatement, "some of these families were difficult to work with; not all those tested and committed to guardianship under the circumstances proved to be really feebleminded and their frustrating experiences made them resentful. Tests and decisions had been made too hurriedly."[32]

Eugenics propagandists continued to talk about curbing reproduction among the unfit, but for Thomson and many other social workers, the drive to sterilize was largely bureaucratic. In her professional correspondence and written reports, Thomson rarely mentioned eugenics, *Buck v. Bell*, other states' sterilization programs, or even the world beyond her department. Thomson wrote numerous histories of Minnesota's program for the feebleminded, but they almost always began with the treatment of the feebleminded in pioneer days and traced the state's broadening enlightenment. Even when she attended national meetings, she usually returned home secure in her conviction that Minnesota's community-focused program for the feebleminded was better than the institution-based programs of other states. She proudly called Minnesota the most "feebleminded conscious" US state.[33]

Thomson's narrow focus belied the fact that ideas about mental deficiency were changing. Although most Minnesota welfare officials still believed that feeblemindedness was a permanent impairment and was usually inherited, they were also aware that societal definitions were shifting. In the Progressive Era, the fast pace of urban-industrial life and new diagnostic tools such as the IQ test had raised the bar for mental normality, leading to a feebleminded diagnosis for many individuals who would have been considered normal in the past. During the Depression, the bar was raised yet again. In the new low-employment economy, experts believed, feebleminded people who had been self-supporting a decade earlier were rendered permanently unemployable, not because their disability got worse, but because high unemployment brought more competition. Thomson and her colleagues were convinced that the feebleminded unemployed would never again be self-supporting. They assumed that mechanization, automation, and employers' rising insistence on efficiency would limit feebleminded workers to low-paid farm labor and domestic service, where the number of jobs was declining. The resulting poverty and idleness would lead to serious behavior problems and heighten the menace of the feebleminded. The large numbers of seemingly sexually dangerous men on the road and in Depression-era transient camps only reinforced their fears.[34]

In Minnesota, the most forceful Depression-era challenge to the eugenicist idea of a feebleminded menace came not from Catholics teaching about intrinsic human worth, but from secular critics of exploited labor and concentrated wealth. John Rockwell, who was Thomson's classmate at Stanford and became Minnesota's education commissioner in 1934, scoffed at psychologist Frederick Kuhlmann's insistence that everyone with an IQ below 75 should be committed to state guardianship. Rockwell pointed out that many people with low test scores were socially well-adjusted. If they were more prone to delinquency and dependency than other people, it was because feebleminded children were given a poor education and then made to compete in a glutted labor market. Feebleminded people were capable of being good employees, Rockwell insisted, but they either could not get jobs or were paid such "exceedingly low wages" that they dragged down the salaries of everyone else. The problem, in his view, was that government had no control over private industry and therefore could not prevent such exploitation. Unlike Thomson, who saw the feebleminded person's inclination to delinquency as a basic instinct to be controlled, Rockwell moved toward a social interpretation: delinquency was an understandable attempt to satisfy basic human needs for food, clothing, and entertainment in an intensely competitive capitalist world. "Society has never undertaken to give the lower social economic groups any degree of economic security," he declared, and until it did so, a relationship between defectiveness, delinquency, and dependency could not be assumed.[35]

Rockwell was making a relatively modest social critique, but his was the minority view. More common were the beliefs of a social worker with the St. Paul Community Chest, who objected to what she saw as the troubling trend toward treating the feebleminded as an "'exploitable' group." In the new welfare order, she warned, "literally thousands" of poor mothers would have to be permanently subsidized, resulting in "nothing short of developing a program to preserve the unfit." For many social workers, the New Deal expansion of relief heightened the urgency of identifying individuals and families who were habitually dependent and delinquent—the undeserving poor.[36]

Despite their different views on the source of the feeblemindedness problem, social workers generally agreed on the utility of counting and classifying clients and supported Kuhlmann's long-standing goal of a statewide census of the feebleminded. Enacted in April 1935, the census law required doctors, nurses, hospitals, school authorities, and child welfare boards to report the names, addresses, and personal information of anyone believed to be feebleminded and directed the state to file petitions for commitment whenever advisable. This sweeping law exemplified new state mechanisms of observation, normalizing judgments, examination, and control, but ironically, it also revealed the political weakness of eugenics hard-liners in 1935. The Board of Control apparently struck a panel to administer the law but made no effort to get an appropriation. Thomson flat out rejected Kuhlmann's plan to have census administrators (psychologists) decide the disposition of cases based on their IQ scores. To "persons actually working with individuals," she wrote, it was obvious that making a determination on paper and placing a name on a census roll would accomplish nothing. The census law was out of step with the board's social casework orientation, and Thomson considered it irrelevant.[37]

Kuhlmann did everything he could to put the law into effect. He secured WPA funding to create a card database of the twenty thousand persons his office had tested over the years, but the funding ended before they reached the end of the alphabet. He did manage to take a census of the feebleminded in southwestern Redwood County, where an enthusiastic county attorney obtained FERA funds to test all the county's schoolchildren. Yet although the results confirmed eugenicists' assumptions—families with a feebleminded child were two and a half times more likely than those with normal children to be dependent on relief—nothing was ever done with the study.[38]

If the census law was a symbolic but ultimately shallow victory for eugenics, two other less noticed developments were far more significant in extending the state's power over the bodies of those deemed unfit. First, a major revision of the probate code in 1935 tightened the state's grip over those considered feebleminded and extended compulsory commitment to people with epilepsy for the first time. The new law eliminated the residency requirement for filing a commitment petition (permitting welfare boards or police officers in the Twin Cities to file a petition against a legal resident of another county) and made discharge from guardianship more difficult. Worse, because experts could not agree on a definition or classification method, the statute did not define a "feebleminded person." This made the adjudication of feeblemindedness even more arbitrary and subjective than it had been before.[39]

Second, a sweeping opinion issued in late 1936 by Attorney General William S. Ervin drastically loosened the Board of Control's relatively restrained sterilization practices. Ervin determined that a feebleminded ward did not have to be institutionalized prior to sterilization and that the surgery did not have to be performed at a hospital under the board's jurisdiction. The patient's institutional residence did not matter as long as he or she was lawfully committed to state guardianship and other procedural requirements were followed. The upshot was that eugenic sterilization operations could now be performed at any hospital, and the state could transfer feebleminded wards from one institution to another for sterilization (usually Sauk Centre to Faribault) and then send them back to finish their sentences. The attorney general's opinion also strengthened the previously unofficial link between sterilization and parole by clarifying the board's authority to make sterilization a condition of parole. In a separate opinion issued four months later, the attorney general said that Faribault's superintendent did not need to conduct a personal examination of patients being considered for sterilization, but could base his recommendation on written reports. The last seven sterilizations in the Faribault casebook were recorded nine days later. With no further documentation extant, the full consequences of the attorney general's decisions are unknown. It seems clear, however, that these largely bureaucratic legal opinions had farther-reaching consequences for the bodies of the feebleminded than many more public eugenics victories.[40]

Party Politics and Sterilization Routines

By the late 1930s, Minnesota's sterilization program was propelled largely by bureaucratic momentum and party politics. In the first half of the decade, Thomson's bureaucratic disposition, and the fact that because her department "had no money grants, it was somewhat remote from political theories about relief and the rights of the individual," kept the program for the feebleminded out of the political fray. By 1936, Thomson was president of the Twin Cities chapter of the American Association of Social Workers. She spent the rest of the decade consumed by political intrigue, professional rivalries, and patronage battles.[41]

In her memoirs, Thomson recalled the years from 1936 to 1939 as a time of "change and also of considerable stress." Her morale was affected by dramatic changes to state government and the Board of Control. First, Carl Swendsen, a Board of Control member since 1911, died in late 1933, and Olson decided not to reappoint Blanche La Du, the board's chair and a Republican, when her term ended in 1936. Then Governor Olson died suddenly in August 1936, and Elmer Benson, a leader of the Farmer–Labor Party's left wing, became governor five months later. Benson was associated with the Popular Front, the Communist Party strategy of forming alliances with noncommunist organizations (such as the Farmer–Labor Party) to fight against fascism, and his political opponents relentlessly attacked him. They accused him of corruption, of being a closet communist, and of packing the growing state bureaucracy with patronage appointments. Some of his opponents waged a nasty anti-Semitic whispering campaign, alleging that Benson's wife was Jewish and that Jewish communist advisors influenced his decisions. Benson's Farmer–Labor Party was defeated in the 1938 election, and Harold Stassen, a thirty-one-year-old moderate Republican, replaced him. The impact on Thomson was palpable.[42]

The intense partisanship created mayhem in the state bureaucracy. Thomson recalled "an atmosphere of intrigue" and "sense of uneasiness" in the state agencies; "there was a feeling that anyone might lose his job at any time and that 'spies' for the governor or those around him, would report words or actions out of line with the policy of the administration." Thus, when Faribault superintendent J. M. Murdoch resigned suddenly in May 1937, Thomson assumed that a former friend, the left-leaning Laura Halse, was involved. In the 1920s, Thomson regarded Halse as a vivacious and "very bright—indeed, brilliant—person with a real interest in the underdog in general and the feebleminded in particular," but by the late 1930s Thomson's views had changed. She became convinced that Halse was fostering employee dissatisfaction with working conditions at the Lynnhurst Club (where the clubhouse staff demanded an eight-hour day), and the two women disagreed over whether the clubhouse, which was beset by economic problems and residents' unrest, should be closed. When in 1937 St. Paul psychiatrist Edward J. Engberg replaced Murdoch as superintendent of the Faribault School and Halse went on the payroll, Thomson assumed that her ex-friend was plotting to take over her job. Those were "trying days," she recalled, not only because of the economic situation but also because she had to worry about being "double-crossed." Yet it was Halse, not Thomson, whose employment was terminated when Stassen became governor.[43]

Thomson was adept at navigating the changes in the state bureaucracy, but her program did not entirely escape the anticommunist smear and anti-Semitic insinuations that clouded state politics in the 1930s. For example, a highly partisan complaint lodged against the matron of the Lynnhurst Club accused her of letting her husband and son stay at the clubhouse and eat for free on the taxpayer's dime. The complainant alleged that the clubhouse matron refused to let the residents buy new clothes at Christmastime, instead forcing them to buy stolen dresses from a "Jewish woman," and that her son was a sex maniac to boot. As the menacing image of the female feebleminded sex delinquent lost its power, political scare tactics focused increasingly on male sex offenders, communists, and Jews. Now a left-leaning clubhouse matron was denounced as "not fit" to care for the "unfortunate" feebleminded girls.[44]

Thomson's program was also affected by the "drastic administrative changes" that accompanied two major reorganizations of state agencies in 1937 and 1939. The first reorganization was necessary to comply with the 1935 Social Security Act, which required states to meet certain administrative standards before they could receive federal grants. The county child welfare boards, which were optional and staffed mostly by volunteers, fell far short of national standards. To comply with federal guidelines, an otherwise deadlocked legislature agreed in 1937 to abolish the child welfare boards and create new mandatory "county welfare boards" with salaried executives. The welfare boards retained their responsibilities for dependent and illegitimate children and feebleminded wards but were also in charge of "all forms of public assistance and public welfare, both of children and adults."[45]

In 1939, Governor Stassen abolished the State Board of Control in a sweeping reorganization of state agencies. The board was replaced by a three-member Social Security Board composed of the directors of three newly created departments: the Division of Public Institutions, the Division of Social Welfare, and the Division of Employment and Security. The Division of Public Institutions took over managerial responsibility for the state's eighteen public institutions, including the School for the Feebleminded, while the Division of Social Welfare took over the other duties once held by the Board of Control, including child welfare, guardianship of the feebleminded, the licensing of maternity hospitals and child-caring agencies, services for people with physical disabilities, recruitment for CCC and WPA projects, surplus commodity distribution, and the administration of old-age assistance. Thomson's bureau (now called the Section for the Feeble-minded and Epileptic) initially followed the state children's bureau into the Division of Social Welfare, but in 1941 her office was moved to a new Mental Health Unit within the Division of Public Institutions, making her community-oriented program subordinate to the state institution.[46]

Stassen was elected on a promise to restore honesty and efficiency to state government, which Governor Benson's opponents claimed had become corrupt when the Farmer–Laborite was in power. A reorganization of state government was certainly necessary in the wake of the hurried, and often haphazard, expansion of the state bureaucracy during the New Deal, and a civil service system for government employment was long overdue. Patronage had a long history in Minnesota, but the practice of rewarding party loyalists with government jobs was particularly contentious in the 1930s because of the rapid increase in government jobs at a time of high unemployment. From Thomson's perspective, however, the Republican regime was not very different from the one it replaced. More than two thousand Farmer–Labor appointees were purged in the six months between Stassen's inauguration and the day the civil service bill went into effect, and one thousand new employees were hired to replace those who were let go. The " 'purge' of farmer–labor carryovers" hit the social welfare sector particularly hard, for Farmer–Labor appointees had been in charge of relief distribution and were chiefly responsible for building the New Deal welfare state.[47]

Tired and depressed that so many colleagues had been fired, Thomson turned to the site of her greatest comfort: the rules. In memo after memo, she recounted the history of Minnesota's program for the feebleminded, described sterilization as a step to community placement, and advised county welfare boards on commitment procedures and sterilization routines, which had changed appallingly little over the years. She repeated the old saws that feebleminded commitment was not a punishment (despite the fact that the police usually escorted the person to the institution) and that no one was pressured to consent to sterilization (although patients were often kept in the institution until after the operation). To be sure, there were a few procedural changes. Faribault medical staff now discussed patients being considered for sterilization at their regular case conferences. In addition, Thomson interviewed those recommended for sterilization, and a Faribault School social worker made sure that the consent form was signed in the presence of two witnesses.[48] But for the hundreds of Faribault patients who understood sterilization to be their ticket to freedom, the new procedures were superficial at best.

The Eugenics Program under Attack

The impassive prose in Thomson's official memos and reports masked an uncomfortable truth: by the late 1930s, Minnesota's program for the feebleminded was under assault. Across the country, experts questioned the basic premise behind eugenic surgery. Lawyer Jacob Landman, in an important 1932 critique, and psychiatrist Abraham Myerson, in an influential 1936 study for the American Neurological Association's Committee for the Investigation of Sterilization, averred that scientists did not know enough about the transmission of mental deficiency to support a policy of compulsory eugenic sterilization. The Myerson report was so persuasive on this point that even the snobbish *New York Times* penned an editorial "against sterilization" in 1936. "The hereditary effect in feeble-mindedness cannot be denied," the *Times* declared, "but to argue, as the eugenists do, that we are likely to be swamped by the untypical Nams, Kallikaks and Jukes, is to substitute fear and emotion for science and reason." The Myerson report was sharply critical of Minnesota's supposedly voluntary sterilization law, which made surgery the "price of freedom" from the state institution, but ironically its chief recommendation—that sterilization should be voluntary and each case should be judged on its individual merits—reflected the policy that Minnesota already had, at least on paper.[49]

Sterilization also faced growing opposition from the Left. Journalist Meridel Le Sueur, whose stepfather represented a few families challenging feebleminded commitment in court, described Minnesota's sterilization program, like police harassment and social work intrusions, as punishment for young working-class women who acted on their sexual desires. "The police are pretty hard on a lone girl," Le Sueur wrote in a 1934 article; "When the police see you wandering they always think you are bad if you are a girl." Le Sueur told the story of Mabel, a pretty farm girl who had a baby out of wedlock. Mabel was given an IQ test after her baby was born, and "of course, she failed pretty thoroughly." In a trenchant critique of IQ testing, Le Sueur wrote, "She was scared stiff anyway, and it was about forests and she has never seen more than one tree at a time in her life, just growing between the sidewalk and the curb. . . . If they had asked her how a wolf gets by in a city, where to get the best hand-outs, how to catch a guy that will take you to a show maybe, and a feed after, and how to get away without giving him anything, she would have passed one hundred percent. They asked her about the wrong kind of jungle."[50]

Le Sueur fleshed out her critique in *The Girl*, a novel written mostly in the 1930s but not published until 1978. *The Girl* tells the story of an unnamed country girl who was driven off her family's farm by poverty and her father's brutality and found work at a speakeasy in St. Paul. Her lover beat her, but he also awakened her sexually and got her pregnant. After the boyfriend dies following a bungled bank robbery, the rest of the story centers on the community of supposedly disreputable working-class women—a prostitute, a communist, and an unwed mother—who sustained one another in their struggle with the capitalist state.

The first reference to sterilization comes on the first page. Clara, the prostitute, tells the narrator how to avoid getting picked up by the police who "give you tests and sterilize you or send you to the woman's prison." Le Sueur portrays sterilization as the embodied violence of capitalism, male supremacy, and a child welfare system that purported to protect poor women and children but actually degraded them by taking away their fertility, a principal source of pleasure and power. A social worker who pretended to be the girl's friend betrays her confidence. Summarizing the girl's case in the callous language of psychology, the social worker wrote, "*The girl is maladjusted, emotionally unstable, and a difficult problem to approach. . . . She should be tested for sterilization after her baby is born. In our opinion sterilization would be advisable.*" Although the social worker described signing the sterilization consent form as "just a little routine matter," the girl knew otherwise. "They don't need any more children from workers," the communist organizer Amelia told her; "They don't need us to reproduce our kind." Amelia helped save the girl from sterilization, but they could not save Clara, who died from the electric shock treatments forced upon her. Still, the novel ends with the girl giving birth to a daughter, proving that women acting together could defy the heartless bureaucrats, stop the state from institutionalizing and sterilizing sexually active girls, and preserve the power of working-class motherhood.[51]

Poor women and men resisted eugenic sterilization in real life too. In the first years of the sterilization program, Thomson expended considerable energy on convincing the relatives of purportedly feebleminded women to consent to sterilization and searching for those who escaped. Ten years later, the bureaucracy was more commanding and the system of surveillance more adept, but social workers had to contend with a much more vocal community of critics and an increasingly skeptical public. Although federal relief programs initially increased the problematic power of the county child welfare boards, the political trends of the 1930s mostly went the other way. President Roosevelt defended the common man against the established interests, left-wing social workers criticized welfare department paternalism, and political adversaries of the governing party leveled charges of mismanagement and corruption in the state institutions. In the process, they created a space for more open rebellion against eugenics policies. Thomson's correspondence from the late 1930s and 1940s is packed with references to local resistance, less-than-cooperative county welfare workers, and courtroom disasters. In one county, welfare board members refused to commit an allegedly feebleminded woman they thought should be institutionalized because they feared that their homes might be set afire! Kuhlmann complained bitterly that social workers who attributed the delinquency and dependency of people with low IQs to their environments, not heredity, repeatedly asked him to reexamine borderline cases. "There are 'I. Q. shoppers' who take their cases from clinic to clinic hoping to get the report they want, and often succeeding," he lamented.[52] Still, most Depression-era challenges to Minnesota's eugenics program focused on saving particular individuals from the state's grasp. Except for Le Sueur and a handful of radicals, midcentury critics of eugenic sterilization rarely expressed concern for poor people's personal freedoms or reproductive rights.

The loudest protests were motivated by partisan resentment. Minnesota's most vulnerable citizens became a political football in the battle over Farmer–Labor patronage and expenditures at the Faribault School. A month after Stassen's inauguration, the state legislature allocated the substantial sum of $50,000 to a joint committee charged with investigating corruption in the Farmer–Labor government. The Benson administration was accused of handpicking government workers, wasting thousands of dollars in state funds, and forcing employees on the state payroll to contribute a percentage of their salaries to the party. The investigation focused in part on the Faribault School. State senator and committee chair A. O. Sletvold alleged that the school spent thousands of dollars on renovations of the superintendent's residence but had no money to repair the antiquated plumbing. He accused Superintendent Engberg of using public funds to pay for two private servants, entertain guests at his home, and have a chauffeured car drive his son to and from school. Sletvold also maintained that there had been a "spirit of unrest" at the institution and that employees were threatened with reprisal if they did not contribute a portion of their salaries to the Farmer–Labor Party.[53]

The committee also criticized the mistreatment of patients. While Engberg lived in luxury, the committee contended, inmates did not have enough milk or butter, and their medical needs were not met. It cited the appalling treatment of Blanche Harkner, who broke both legs and injured her spine in a fall but had to wait several days before being transferred to a Minneapolis hospital, as an "outstanding example" of medical neglect. In fact, Faribault's internal reports show that what happened to the twenty-one-year-old patient was much worse than the Sletvold committee said. Shortly before midnight on February 2, 1939, at the institution hospital where sterilizations were performed, Mrs. Harkner and a companion tied some sheets to a bathtub, unscrewed a locked window, and climbed out. Her companion managed to get away, but Blanche fell two and a half stories to the ground, shattering both feet and injuring her spine. Her injuries were serious, and she was sedated and (after a delay of several days) placed in traction. Even so, Faribault medical staff did not ask surgeon George Eitel to make a special trip from Minneapolis. When Eitel finally examined the young woman during his regularly scheduled visit, he recommended immediate transfer to a hospital in Minneapolis. The Board of Control then consulted a different physician, who claimed that the treatment Mrs. Harkner was receiving at Faribault was satisfactory and advised delaying the transfer to give her more time to get over the shock. When the transfer was finally approved, a blizzard caused a delay of two more days. It was not until February 11, eight days after the original injury, that Blanche Harkner was taken by ambulance to Minneapolis. She returned to Faribault a month later in a full body cast, which was removed in June. The Faribault medical staff expected Mrs. Harkner's mobility disability to be permanent but saw no reason to criticize her medical care. They did, however, recommend bars on hospital windows to deter further escape attempts.[54]

Significantly, the Sletvold committee did not criticize the sterilization program at Faribault, even though a planned sterilization operation likely prompted Harkner's attempted escape. Superintendent Engberg reported 250 sterilizations performed at the Faribault School during Harold Stassen's first two years as governor, despite the committee's assurances that the "evils" wrought by the Farmer–Laborites were being remedied by the new Republican administration. In the end, the Sletvold committee found no conclusive evidence of wrongdoing at the institution, and Engberg stayed on as superintendent. The main impact of the investigation was the purge of Farmer–Labor personnel. Ironically, some of the discharged employees got revenge by testifying against the institution in a later scandal. Treating institutionalized persons as a political football was a bipartisan game.[55]

Thomson was not directly affected by the Sletvold investigation (her office was in the Division of Social Welfare at the time), but she was at the center of the allegations of incompetence and mismanagement leveled by two external studies of Minnesota's mental health programs. A 1939 US Public Health Service survey of mental hospitals by Grover Kempf and Samuel Hamilton condemned the poor condition of Faribault's facilities and the "very striking deficit" in the community program Thomson ran. Two dormitories for defective delinquent adults were like prisons, Kempf and Hamilton reported, and the "sterilization of defectives is a vigorously advocated procedure." Although some Minnesota officials still clung to the "crudely unscientific notion that by this means inferior hereditary strains can be terminated," the more common argument was economic: "sterilization for even one feeble-minded person may save the community the cost of supporting another one . . . [and] supervision is much cheaper if the morals of the person supervised are not a matter of concern." The investigators expressed particular concern that patients living in the community were not supervised by professionals trained to work with the mentally retarded, but by county welfare boards "utterly inadequate" to the task. "Standards change," they wrote sternly, "and what was excellent in the past may need extension or improvement today."[56]

A 1941 report by the American Public Welfare Association was even more critical. Author Milton Kirkpatrick, a psychiatrist affiliated with the National Committee for Mental Hygiene, concluded that the entire premise of the Minnesota program was flawed. "Feeblemindedness in itself implies no physical danger to the community," he wrote, challenging the basic premise of Thomson's program, and he argued that higher-grade defectives should be self-supporting. Kirkpatrick was especially critical of the Faribault School's admissions and discharge procedures, which were "entirely at the discretion" of the supervisor for the feebleminded (Thomson) and based largely on local welfare needs. Moreover, he said, since institutional discharge depended on the willingness of the county of residence to support the feebleminded ward but counties paid only $40 per year for institutional care, there was "little likelihood that they will stir themselves very violently" to help feebleminded wards return to their community, where the cost of supervision was much greater.[57]

Kirkpatrick said nothing about sterilization, but he sharply criticized Minnesota's policy of lifelong guardianship for failing to provide "any advantage to the individual which would not otherwise be available." About five hundred new commitments were made each year, and by 1940 the state had more than 7,300 feebleminded wards. Guardianship was "more theoretical than practical," however, since the state did not have the resources to supervise so many people. Kirkpatrick concluded that there was "little justification for the state assuming 'en masse' responsibility for so many people . . . when it has so little to offer." His recommendations basically involved removing Thomson from control. He proposed discharging from guardianship every feebleminded person who had lived satisfactorily outside the institution for one or two years, giving the Faribault School's medical director the authority to admit or discharge patients, and turning Thomson's department into a powerless "liaison agent" between the institution and the counties.[58]

Thomson was stunned. She later wrote that the release of the Kirkpatrick report in January 1941 "gave me a shock! It was more than critical—it was devastating—in its estimate of the program for the mentally deficient and epileptic." But she dismissed the criticism as a professional disagreement between psychiatrists who wanted to "re-create the feebleminded in the image of the mentally ill" and those like her who were more realistic. Kirkpatrick did not understand the extent and permanence of the feebleminded problem, Thomson complained; "he was assuming that if you refused to recognize a problem, it did not exist." Her own views had hardly changed since the 1920s. As late as 1942, she still described the feebleminded as a financial and emotional burden and insisted that "low mentality and delinquencies are bound together." Referring to the long waiting list for institutional placement and the difficulty in finding suitable boarding homes, she wrote that her office spent a "great deal of time at the expense of the taxpayers, trying to make plans that at best are very unsatisfactory! Nothing constructive can be done for a large part of this group." Reflecting on Kirkpatrick's criticisms twenty years later, Thomson concluded that the state's emphasis on "economy in spite of need" was at fault. Since the death of A. C. Rogers in 1917, she explained in her memoirs, the priority of the Board of Control had been keeping costs low. The Depression heightened the need to economize, but the state's tightfistedness continued even after the economy improved. Taxpayer stinginess shaped the treatment of Minnesota's most vulnerable citizens before, during, and after the heyday of eugenics.[59]

Thomson devoted four pages of her memoirs to the critical national reports but said nothing about an even greater blow: the Minnesota Supreme Court's stinging repudiation of feebleminded commitment and compulsory institutionalization. *In re Masters* (1944) centered on Rose Masters, the wife of a poor tenant farmer and mother of ten. The Masters family, although not prosperous, had a good reputation in their community until the mid-1930s, when they applied for county poor relief. Beginning in 1937, the family received regular visits from agents of the Martin County Welfare Board, who felt that the Catholic couple had more children than they could properly support and would benefit from sterilization. They committed both parents to guardianship, but as usual only Mrs. Masters was sent to Faribault in May 1942, seven months after the birth of her tenth child. Three months later, her neighbors petitioned for her release. The district court rejected their appeal, but the Minnesota Supreme Court reversed the lower court's decision.[60]

The *Masters* case, like so many others, centered on child welfare, dependency on relief, and bad mothering. The county welfare board was convinced that Mrs. Masters was a moron. Although the cause and first appearance of her "abnormal behavior" were unknown, the symptoms were clear: poor housekeeping and child neglect. Mrs. Masters was physically lazy and "apparently indifferent to the needs of cleanliness in her home," the board secretary stated flatly. "It may be the result of repeated child-birth which has exhausted her. . . . She should not have any more children from her health standpoint." The specific list of Mrs. Masters's supposed deficiencies was long. The family rarely attended church. Ten people squeezed into a run-down five-room house. There were never any proper meals; the only food on the table was bread and syrup, and the bread was never sliced, just torn off in the middle. The children looked dirty and tired. Their hair was long, their clothes were tattered, and their school attendance was poor. The beds were not clean. Rumpled garments were piled in the corners. Chickens roamed through the house. The welfare board had tried to fix the problem by placing a housekeeper in the Masters home, but when Mrs. Masters became pregnant with her tenth child, social workers resolved to break up the family. They sent five of the children to an orphanage and placed the youngest three in boarding homes. (The two oldest sons were in the army.)[61]

The *Masters* case revolved around that enduring question: who was feebleminded, and who got to decide? The parties agreed on the facts of the case, so the only question was whether the evidence proved, or failed to prove, that Mrs. Masters was a moron—and whose assessment of her mental abilities was most valid. Her neighbors and friends testified that Mrs. Masters was "perfectly capable," and her children were "just as normal as anyone's children." One neighbor observed that "she wasn't probably as good a housekeeper as some people, but she was a very good mother." Most of the neighbors viewed Mrs. Masters's removal to the state institution as "punishment for having ten children," Justice Thomas O. Streissguth wrote, and their reaction was understandable. Families used to "point with pardonable pride" to having lots of children, but "even in this modern age of birth control and social welfare agencies, the circumstance of being the mother of an unusually large family, as measured by present standards, should not label a woman as a moron." Still, he maintained, it was not the fact of her having so many children but her failure to properly care for them that led the welfare board to break up the family. The question of child neglect was separate from their mother's mentality. Even if Mrs. Masters were restored to capacity, her children would remain wards of the state. "Their welfare, and not their mother's, is supreme in determining who shall have their custody."[62]

While the neighbors and social workers clashed over Mrs. Masters's parenting skills, the lawyers on each side concentrated on asserting—or damaging—the credibility of the experts who evaluated her intelligence. A state psychologist testified that Mrs. Masters's IQ of 64 proved that she was a moron, and that her law-abidingness, good morals, and "creditable" court performance were thus irrelevant. A physician testifying on behalf of Mrs. Masters took a very different stance. He testified that Mrs. Masters did not have the large tongue, protruding lip, thickened skin, and excessive sexual impulse of a moron. "She may be a little sub-standard," he explained, "but there are a lot of people sub-standard." During cross-examination, the state poked holes in the doctor's outdated assumptions about the physical appearance and sex perversions of the feebleminded and exposed his ignorance on the subject of intelligence testing.[63]

In the end, the critical factor in deciding Mrs. Masters's fate was not the assessments of the experts, but her demeanor in district court. A photograph in the state archives shows that Mrs. Masters was an attractive blond woman, and in court she maintained her composure under pressure, demonstrated good knowledge of her multiplication tables, and even engaged "in occasional repartee with counsel." A letter that Mrs. Masters wrote while at Faribault and was introduced into evidence revealed that her spelling and penmanship were good, and she had a fair vocabulary. Both sides agreed that she was a model inmate at Faribault. She used a power sewing machine to make nightgowns and wrote letters for inmates who were unable to write for themselves. The state's lawyer tried to prove that Mrs. Masters was feebleminded by showing that she was happy and well treated in the institution. Unlike a factory operative, she was not forced to stand at her work. Nor did her chores extend to cleaning the toilet. "You like your work at the tailor shop," the lawyer asked, "and you have nice, congenial women to work with?" "Yes," she said. Her attorney, on redirect, then asked, "Would you rather be at home than where you are?" "Yes," she answered again, "I most certainly would."[64]

The court's unanimous 1944 decision was an unequivocal repudiation of the broad eugenicist understanding of mental deficiency which had led to large numbers of compulsory commitments. There were some procedural irregularities —for example, Mrs. Masters had no formal notice of the original hearing in probate court—but the decision focused primarily on the lower court's inflexible conception of feeblemindedness and errors regarding the burden of proof. The district court had treated feeblemindedness as a permanent, inherited birth defect that could be measured and diagnosed with certainty from the results of an IQ test alone. However, as Justice Streissguth pointed out, there was no statutory definition of feeblemindedness and no "hard and fast" test for determining its existence. The experts were not in agreement. IQ alone was insufficient evidence of mental deficiency for the purpose of commitment. "The statement frequently made that all persons with I.Q.'s below 70 are feeble-minded is not justified," he declared. "Intelligence is made up of too many factors to permit of such a dogmatic statement."[65]

The court further rejected the eugenicist claim that mental defectives needed perpetual care. "Feeble-mindedness, viewed from a sociolegal rather than a purely medical standpoint, is not necessarily a 'permanent' and 'incurable' condition, as stated by the trial court in its memorandum," and Mrs. Masters's "intelligent responses" on the stand constituted "persuasive proof . . . that, having been given the chance of complete physical and emotional convalescence at the state institution for more than a year, her condition has definitely improved." Finally, Justice Streissguth ruled that the lower court erred by making the burden of proof for petitioners too severe. A perfectly respectable woman should not be required to provide "clear and satisfactory" proof that she was normal. "Human liberty is too precious, the family home too fundamental, and mother love too sacred" to require that a mother seeking to "return to her home, her children, her neighborhood, and everything that is dear to her" should have to provide more than a fair preponderance of evidence to prove her mental competence.[66] With this ruling, the court narrowed the legal category of a feebleminded person, established that a mother who had a large family and was dependent on relief could be mentally normal, and ordered a new trial. Feeblemindedness, the court seemed to saying, was not a question of poverty and dependency, and the state needed a better set of rules to guide judges in deciding whether or not a person was feebleminded and ought to be deprived of rights, liberty, and the family home. Just how many poor mothers shared Mrs. Masters's fate is unknown. But the records of the state welfare department suggest that her situation was not unique.

War and Welfare: Rethinking Sterilization

Even before the *Masters* decision was handed down in March 1944, wartime exigencies and mounting criticisms had provoked significant changes to the state program for the feebleminded. Thomson now told county welfare boards not to press for commitment or institutionalization if the supposedly feebleminded person was not a "social problem" or if there would be opposition from family and friends. As a result, the number of commitments (and sterilizations) slowed. Thomson reported 696 new commitments in her 1944 biennial report, a drop of 40 percent from four years earlier. A staffing shortage led to a fall in the number of sterilizations as well. Faribault reported 155 women and 63 men sterilized during the 1941–1942 biennial period, but only 25 women and 10 men in 1945–1946. Female sterilizations dropped off faster than vasectomies because they required more nursing care. Although 70 percent of sterilizations were performed on women in 1941–1942, women accounted for just 55 percent of sterilizations in 1944.[67]

Thomson attributed the wartime drop in commitments to "better economic conditions and improved case work in the counties." But loosening attitudes toward premarital sexuality and birth control, as well as more effective treatment for venereal disease, also played a role. By 1936, when the United States Supreme Court overturned the federal ban on physician-prescribed contraceptives, many doctors already provided contraceptive advice to married women, and the Minnesota Birth Control League operated seven birth control clinics across the state. Access to contraception or abortion was far from universal, however, and as late as 1945, a few women still sought sterilization for contraceptive purposes at the Faribault School Hospital. For example, a mother of six, whose "sex delinquencies" and IQ of 74 got her committed in 1936, asked to be sterilized in 1945. But she was considered too bright and her children too well adjusted, and her operation was not approved.[68]

Wartime dislocation also brought new attitudes toward teen girls' heterosexual expression. Unwed motherhood was no longer seen as a sign of mental deficiency, at least if the unmarried mother was white; instead, single pregnancy was considered the unhappy result of emotional immaturity, which could be treated and even cured if the young mother was permanently separated from the child. As more and more "illegitimate" babies were put up for adoption, unmarried motherhood no longer signaled a permanent condition; most unwed mothers could "move on." Now girls' illicit sexuality, even if it resulted in pregnancy or venereal disease (now treated with sulfa drugs or antibiotics), seemed to have no permanent ill effects. The Progressive Era strategies of eugenic segregation and sterilization appeared on increasingly shaky ground.[69]

The booming war economy also brought about new thinking about mental retardation. Men and women who had been disparaged as permanently unemployable defectives during the Depression were now recognized as perfectly capable of supporting themselves and their families in war industries and military service. Even Mildred Thomson had to admit that "many of our wards were more competent that we had thought them to be." After 1944, male veterans who had been considered feebleminded during the Depression were able to use the entitlements of the GI Bill to further their education, buy a home, and enter the middle class.[70] For the "high-grade" feebleminded, the war brought significant new opportunities and respect.

The war also had consequences for those who remained in the institution. Many state employees, including sixteen Faribault staff members, Thomson's assistant, and Governor Stassen, joined the military. This aggravated the problem of understaffing just as skyrocketing prices, a scarcity of supplies, and the fact that many institutionalized persons lacked ration cards made it difficult to maintain the institution's already low medical and dietary standards. The war thus worsened the isolation and dismal conditions of supposedly lower-grade individuals who remained in the institution, even as most mentally deficient Minnesotans were better off.[71] In this way, the war redrew the boundaries between the "good" feebleminded persons who deserved a chance at a normal life and the "bad" ones who had to remain institutionalized.

The creation in 1945 of two new residential facilities reinforced the divergent tracks separating the "good" and the "bad." The State Public School at Owatonna, no longer needed as an orphanage because the New Deal created a social safety net and welfare officials were less inclined to break up poor families, became a residential school for mildly retarded children who could eventually return to the community and be self-supporting. The Annex for Defective Delinquents at the St. Cloud Reformatory was established for men and boys who had serious behavior problems and, officials believed, ought to be institutionalized for life. As these two very different groups of "physically well" patients were transferred out of Faribault, they were replaced by children and adults who had severe disabilities and required more care. Although economic prosperity and new welfare entitlements had softened popular attitudes toward the "mentally retarded," making it possible for many to live in the community, officials never stopped believing that some defective, dependent, and delinquent individuals should be institutionalized for life.[72]

In 1946, yet another election-year scandal about conditions at Faribault showed just how much—and how little—attitudes and institutional conditions had changed. This time it was former Farmer–Labor governor Hjalmar Petersen, now running for governor in the Republican primary, who condemned the "long and savory record of brutality, mass sterilization and mismanagement" of the politicians in power. Under the Republican administrations of Stassen and Edward Thye, the Petersen campaign alleged, Faribault patients were beaten, tied to toilets for twenty-four hours at a time, served food unfit for human consumption, and forcibly sterilized as their "price of freedom" from the institution.[73]

For the first time, sterilization was deemed sufficiently troubling to earn a place in political discourse. Newspapers printed allegations of mass sterilization and other abuses. One report featured a doctor who claimed that 240 sterilizations had been performed *each year* between 1939 and 1941, many more than had been performed under the Farmer–Labor administration (and nearly twice as many as Engberg reported privately). Other ex-employees testified to other abuses: patients working fourteen-hour days at unpaid institution work, women getting pregnant in the institution, and brutal beatings with broom handles and wooden coat hangers. At least one "child" (an elderly woman) died from her wounds. A grand jury was ordered and Thomson was called to testify, but no charges were laid. Sterilizations were certainly performed at Faribault, the grand jury concluded, but they were done in compliance with the law. The local newspaper, noticing that allegations of mistreatment at Faribault usually only came up in election years, condemned the cynical use of the state institution for the feebleminded as a political football.[74]

As the 1946 scandal suggests, fifteen years of depression and war had had a paradoxical impact on Minnesota's program for the feebleminded. Although the economic crisis and subsequent influx of federal funds created the conditions for a more aggressive sterilization program by strengthening the power of state and county welfare authorities, the combined effects of the program's overreach, new federal welfare measures, and New Deal administrative standards opened the door for more successful resistance and reform. The Minnesota Supreme Court did not overturn the eugenic commitment law in *Masters*, but it did hold that having a large family and being dependent on relief did not make a woman a moron, and World War II further widened the boundary of who was considered deserving of government aid. The mounting criticisms of Minnesota's program for the feebleminded reflected new ideas about poverty and welfare as much as the disapproval of eugenics.

Thomson testified at the grand jury, but her attention was elsewhere. After the war, she devoted her considerable energy to supporting the middle-class parents of "retarded" children. As we shall see in the next chapter, Thomson played such an important role in the formation of the Minnesota Association for Retarded Children that its president praised her "enlightened concern for the retarded that was far ahead of her time."[75] Her retirement in 1959 opened the door for even farther-reaching reforms. The next chapter explores the interwoven histories of eugenics and welfare in the postwar era of reform.

CHAPTER SIX

FROM FIXING THE POOR TO FIXING THE SYSTEM?

Hjalmar Petersen's election-year allegations of mass sterilizations at Faribault signaled the end of an era in Minnesota. In less than six months, the trial of doctors at Nuremberg began, and eugenics would be forever associated with Nazi war crimes. As New Deal–era social programs and unionization reduced extreme poverty and a booming economy made it possible for "mentally deficient" Minnesotans to be self-supporting, institutionalization was increasingly limited to those believed to require confinement for life: the severely disabled and the thoroughly depraved. As we have seen, sterilizations also decreased. State officials reported only two sterilizations in 1946 and just five sterilization operations over the next two years. Although surgeries increased in the early 1950s, Minnesota never again treated sterilization as a solution to the problems of the poor. At the same time, the bitter political struggles of the 1920s and 1930s gave way to the liberal centrism of the postwar years. In the 1950s, Minnesota leaders no longer found political advantage in partisan battles over patronage, public welfare spending, and corruption in the state institutions. Instead, both parties found common cause in their support for New Deal welfare entitlements, mental health reform, and civil rights.[1]

This chapter explores the changes and continuities in Minnesota's program for the "mentally deficient" after 1945, when the idea of protecting society from the feebleminded menace gave way to helping the innocent mentally retarded child. It explores how the growing acceptability of New Deal entitlements, the new prominence of medical genetics, and middle-class parents' activism on behalf of "retarded children" weakened the purported connection between poverty, race, and low intelligence. The mental health reforms of the early postwar years and the federal government's "wars" on mental retardation and poverty in the 1960s lay the foundation for disability activism and the reproductive rights movement of the 1970s. Yet, despite growing demands to fix the system, the basic framework of US welfare policy, with its emphasis on local responsibility and protecting taxpayers from the undeserving, remained in place.

Historians have engaged in a vigorous debate about World War II's impact on eugenics. Until recently, most assumed that eugenics declined in response to the Holocaust. Although eugenics had already been weakened by Catholic opposition, new research on genetics, and the passing of leaders such as Charles

Davenport, these historians argue that Nazi horrors "brought a recoil in America against race doctrines and naturally placed the eugenics movement under suspicion." In the postwar years, most Americans dismissed eugenics as a Nazi pseudoscience, and even eugenicists denounced the Germans' "Perversions of Eugenics," but recent developments, such as new reproductive technologies and the decoding of the human genome, threaten a return of eugenics, and the "specter of better breeding is thrust upon us once again."[2]

Since the 1990s, a new generation of scholars has emphasized the durability of eugenics ideas and institutions in the postwar years. Eugenicists remained committed to their cause, these historians argue, although they often promoted it under a different name. International family planning organizations, the development of human genetics as a scientific field, and even the pronatalist culture of the baby boom are seen as evidence of the eugenics movement's success. State sterilization laws remained on the books. Most states saw a modest increase in surgical sterilizations after the war, as the medical facilities in public institutions returned to normal. In several southern states, surgeries increased dramatically in the postwar years. Nationwide, at least 18,551 eugenic sterilizations—nearly 30 percent—were recorded in the years after 1945.[3]

Yet despite the obvious continuities, the 1940s were a watershed in the history of eugenic sterilization, not only in Minnesota but across the nation. For one thing, the United States Supreme Court decision *Skinner v. Oklahoma* (1942) ruled that the compulsory sterilization of criminals was unconstitutional. The decision did not overturn eugenic sterilization, but it recognized procreation as "one of the basic rights of man" and held the application of state sterilization laws to a stringent standard of strict scrutiny. Equally important, the 1940s accelerated broad intellectual, economic, and political shifts that redrew the line between "good" and "bad" people with mental disabilities and made sterilization on eugenic grounds seem anachronistic, at least in Minnesota. White unmarried mothers were much less likely to be labeled feebleminded than they had been in the past; in the postwar years, teen pregnancies were blamed on psychological neurosis or a bad environment. At the same time, male sex offenders who were considered defective or degenerate and thus incapable of rehabilitation were confined to the prison-like Annex for Defective Delinquents or—if their IQs were in the normal range—committed as psychopathic personalities to the St. Peter State Hospital Ward for the Dangerously Insane. While defective delinquent men remained institutionalized because they were thought to pose a danger to the innocent child, "mentally retarded" white women who got pregnant out of wedlock were portrayed as innocent children themselves.[4]

On an intellectual plane, two interrelated developments helped sever the tight conceptual link many eugenicists drew between race, class, and low intelligence: social scientists' repudiation of biological racism and the development of medical genetics. Both of these intellectual challenges to scientific racism had been building for years. Columbia University anthropologist Franz Boas laid out his relativistic understanding of culture and critique of Anglo-Saxon superiority in his 1911 opus *The Mind of Primitive Man.* While never disputing the significance of individual heredity, Boas rejected the notion of inherent racial characteristics, including differences in intelligence, and showed that the differences between "primitive" and "civilized" humans were cultural. Boas and his students dismissed eugenics as "Nordic nonsense" and questioned the validity of IQ testing. By the interwar years, the majority of American social scientists strongly rejected eugenicists' racial typology. Instead, they sought cultural and environmental explanations for academic failure, low socioeconomic status, and the supposedly weak family structure of African Americans and other groups. In 1944, Gunnar Myrdal's influential *An American Dilemma: The Negro Problem and American Democracy* demolished the purportedly scientific claim that African Americans, as a group, were genetically inferior. Myrdal described the weaknesses he saw in African American culture—unstable families, poor education, high crime rate, and so on—as a "distorted development, or a pathological condition" of the wider American culture. Myrdal, who was a leading advocate of eugenic sterilization for people with intellectual disabilities in his native Sweden, was clear: America's "race problem" was caused by white prejudice and discrimination, not black biology.[5]

Geneticists also repudiated simplistic ideas about race, while retaining a commitment to eugenics. In 1935, the socialist eugenicist Hermann Muller (winner of the Nobel Prize in 1946 for his work on radiation-induced genetic mutations) complained that eugenics had become "hopelessly perverted" by class and race prejudices. Four years later, twenty-three scientists signed his Geneticists' Manifesto, an unequivocal refutation of Nazi scientific racism. Although most geneticists remained agnostic on the question of whether there were any inherited mental differences among races, many readily endorsed the 1951 UNESCO Statement on Race, saying that there was no firm scientific evidence for racial differences in intelligence. Outside the political arena, medical geneticists emphasized the dangers of atomic mutation, not just heredity, and worked for the amelioration of individual suffering as well as population-level genetic improvement. Like social workers' emphasis on individual casework, their orientation toward the individual patient softened the hard edge of eugenics discourse while retaining its basic assumptions about intelligence and normality.[6]

By the 1940s, even some prominent eugenicists denounced scientific racism and coercive governmental programs designed to weed out the so-called unfit. With the deaths of Harry Laughlin, Charles Davenport, and Charles Dight between 1937 and 1944, eugenics organizations were increasingly represented by "reform eugenicists" who tried to distance themselves from their predecessors' openly racist ideas. Frederick Osborn, who became president of the American Eugenics Society in 1946, set out the "new" eugenics doctrine in his 1940 book *Preface to Eugenics*. Osborn argued that innate intelligence was not a racial characteristic and that variations in heredity were much greater within groups than between them. Still, he remained convinced that genetics played a significant role in mental deficiency and advocated a three-pronged eugenics program: compulsory sterilization for the feebleminded, "voluntary" sterilization and birth control for individuals of below-average intelligence, and an expanded welfare state, including family allowances, to ensure "freedom of parenthood" for the most intelligent.[7]

The intellectual currents leading away from eugenic sterilization as a poverty policy were also bolstered by national economic and political developments: an expanding economy, urban growth, massive federal investment in biomedicine and social welfare, the political realignments of the Cold War, and demands for civil rights. Although mental institutions fell on hard times during the war, in 1946 the National Mental Health Act and Hill–Burton Hospital Survey and Construction Act brought massive federal funding and oversight to biomedical research and hospital construction, raising expectations that mental illness and even mental retardation could be treated and eventually cured. In Minnesota, feebleminded commitments dropped significantly, and individuals who remained under guardianship were no longer viewed only as a "potential menace or financial burden from whom the community must be protected, as was true in the past."[8] Even Mildred Thomson turned her attention away from the so-called defective, dependent, and delinquent classes, the traditional focus of Minnesota's eugenics program, and concentrated instead on helping respectable parents who had a mentally retarded child. Her retirement in 1959 opened the door for further reforms, and in the 1960s federal initiatives such as the President's Panel on Mental Retardation and the War on Poverty took a step toward fixing the system that bound eugenic sterilization to public welfare. Yet the persisting tradition of local welfare responsibility and the political difficulties of assisting the "undeserving" poor ensured that eugenic-style efforts to "fix" the poor would continue.

The Politics of Liberalism and Mental Health Reform

The dramatic political realignments that shook Minnesota in the 1940s also had consequences for state eugenics programs. The 1944 merger of the Democratic and Farmer–Labor Parties (known as the DFL) and subsequent defeat of DFL communists in 1947–1948 brought Farmer–Labor radicalism and the open class conflict of the 1930s to an end. Now the leaders of both political parties were liberals who combined an unyielding anticommunism with support for New

Deal social programs and civil rights. They agreed that government should provide for its weakest citizens, but they rejected the Farmer–Laborites' critique of concentrated wealth. More and more, Minnesota's business and political leaders focused their attention on issues that seemed to be above politics: good government, mental health reform, and civil rights. All three Republicans who served as governor from 1939 to 1951 supported basic civil rights initiatives, as did juvenile court judge Edward F. Waite and social worker Catheryne Cooke Gilman, who had served together on the 1917 Child Welfare Commission that recommended the eugenic commitment law. Likewise, Hubert Humphrey, America's future vice president who was then Minneapolis mayor, appointed a Council on Human Relations to combat racial discrimination and anti-Semitism and enact a fair employment practices ordinance.[9]

In the late 1940s, two Minnesota politicians won national attention for their outspokenness on human rights. At the 1948 Democratic National Convention, Humphrey gave his famous civil rights address urging his fellow Democrats to "get out of the shadow of states' rights and to walk forthrightly into the bright sunshine of human rights." Although Senator Strom Thurmond's southern Dixiecrats walked out of the convention in protest, Humphrey's star, along with northerners' attention to civil rights, was on the rise. Meanwhile, Minnesota's Republican governor Luther Youngdahl launched his own rights campaign on behalf of the "forgotten souls" in the state's mental institutions. He later made national headlines by setting fire to a huge pile of straitjackets and manacles at the Anoka State Hospital. Given the political animosities of a decade earlier, it is remarkable that the 1948 DFL convention endorsed the Republican governor's platform on the grounds that mental health reform was "non-political and non-partisan." (Echoing the state's eugenicist past, the DFL also warned that handicapped persons could become "an even greater problem" if they were not rehabilitated.)[10]

If civil rights and human rights were controversial nationally, in Minnesota they were not. The state's black population was small, especially outside the Twin Cities, and the somewhat abstract idea of improving race relations brought Minnesota's political leaders together across political and ideological lines. (In this regard, their relative inattention to Minnesota's much larger indigenous population is striking.) "Although ultimately shallow," writes historian Jennifer Delton, "attention to 'the Negro' formed an oasis of cooperation between once quarrelling groups of Minnesotans, bringing together Catholics and Lutherans, Jews and Christians, Yankees and eastern Europeans, and labor and management." Delton's analysis of civil rights holds equally true of mental health reform. The crusade to improve conditions in the state's mental institutions did a lot of "ideological work. It created a sense of unity. It provided a new sense of political morality after issues of economic justice were unable to." These politicians were "acting out of principle," she observes, "but their actions fulfilled a political need."[11]

Ironically, dismantling Minnesota's eugenics program and extending citizenship rights to people with intellectual disabilities was abetted by the World War II–era crisis in the state institutions. Despite the general prosperity of the war years, World War II was the nadir for state institutions. Administrators struggling to cope with escalating costs, high staff turnover, and a scarcity of supplies postponed critical building repairs and relied on patients' unpaid labor. After the war, a varied group of mental health reformers, including psychiatrists, journalists, parent activists, and conscientious objectors who had worked in the institutions as an alternative to military service, publicized the shameful conditions. Many drew an analogy with Nazi Germany. Albert Maisel's shocking photo-essay "Bedlam 1946" for *Life* magazine described mental hospitals as a shameful "man-made hell" and showed patients naked, locked in restraints, kept on a starvation diet, and toiling at unpaid labor for years on end. "Through public neglect and legislative penny-pinching," Maisel wrote, psychiatric hospitals have degenerated into "little more than concentration camps on the Belsen pattern." Similarly, in *The Shame of the States*, journalist Albert Deutsch challenged Americans repulsed by the Nazis' "mercy-killing" of people with physical and mental disabilities to question their own policy of "euthanasia by neglect."[12]

The gruesome conditions at Faribault were well known, as a result of the politically motivated scandals discussed in the previous chapter, but in the late 1940s a series of damning reports on the state's mental hospitals presented such conditions as a nonpartisan humanitarian crisis for the first time. In 1948, the Minnesota Unitarian Conference published an influential report stressing the chasm between modern psychiatric knowledge and the archaic treatment of the state's mental patients. Not one Minnesota hospital met the minimum standards of the American Psychiatric Association, the report lamented. Food and clothing were grossly inadequate, patients had no toothbrushes or soap with which to clean themselves, and restraints such as mitts, ankle cuffs, straitjackets, and (in one hospital) chains substituted for treatment. More than half of the patients in one hospital ward were completely idle. Investigators saw "unkempt patients vegetating" and people treated worse than the livestock on the institutions' grounds. Like Progressive Era eugenicists, but with a different purpose, reformers used visual images that dehumanized the "insane" and "defective" to goad the public into action.[13]

Also like the Progressive Era, but in contrast to the 1930s, postwar reformers blamed public ignorance—not the party in power—for the appalling institutional conditions. "Science has made progress," the Unitarian conference reported, but the public still treated the mental patient as a "criminal or a brute."

Governor Youngdahl, calling for a "new attitude" and the removal of words like *crazy* and *lunatic* from popular parlance and the statute books, declared that "these unfortunate people are human beings; they have souls," and urged all Minnesotans to recognize that they too were "at least partially responsible for allowing these conditions to exist." In Youngdahl's view, the "core of the problem [was a] lack of understanding on the part of the public. We need publicity to give people the facts."[14]

Journalists took up Youngdahl's challenge. In 1948, reporter Geri Hoffner and photographer Arthur Hager published "Minnesota Bedlam," a ten-part series documenting the horrific conditions in the state's mental hospitals, which described mental patients as being "crowded like animals" into overfull institutions and showed that the "tragic results of three-fourths of a century of penny-pinching and public indifference" were grievously clear. Hoffner also wrote a scathing critique of the Sauk Centre Home School for Girls, where administrators imposed such a "regimented, disciplined, hard-working life" on wayward girls that they effectively reproduced the policies of a bygone era. The girls were not allowed to wear makeup, their letters were censored, and they were forced to do backbreaking work like waxing the floors. Those caught breaking the rules or trying to escape were locked in their rooms and put on a diet of bread and water. Hoffner reported that 90 percent of the inmates were committed for sex offenses, such as prostitution or incest ("each one more damning to the girl's parents than to the girl herself"), but Sauk Centre had no social worker or psychiatrist on staff. She was told that the most troubled inmates (and those most likely to run away) were "feebleminded" girls with IQs in the low 70s. Although they were too high-functioning for the permanent segregation of Faribault, the superintendent explained, these girls "just do not have enough to battle the world." A decade earlier, these young women would have been sterilized. They were not sterilized in 1948, but they were still not considered fit to be mothers. Those who were pregnant were forced to put their babies up for adoption.[15]

This negative publicity and the governor's frank admission of the need for improvement empowered a growing number of Minnesotans to complain about conditions in the Faribault School. Most of the complainants protested unexpected monetary charges or the difficulty of getting a discharge from guardianship or the state institution. A few objected to plans for sterilization. In 1948, for example, Bridget O'Grady complained about the "awful mess" in the state institutions. She had been confined at Faribault for three years and seven months and was sterilized against her will. Although Bridget was released after the operation, she was "maimed for life because she is unable to bear children." She asked, "How can anyone say I am feebleminded? There is nothing wrong with my mind."[16]

As in the past, the most poignant letters focused not on sterilization, but on the injustice of being institutionalized indefinitely for a minor sexual offense.

The letters also reveal family members' deep anger and frustration at officials' callous response. One woman wept that her daughter, who once had a steady job, was kept a prisoner at Faribault for almost two years and denied the opportunity to earn a living simply because she was the innocent victim of an immoral man. A Catholic family objected that their daughter was kept in the institution only because her religion meant that she could not be sterilized, and pleaded for her release. Others complained that they were not allowed to visit family members. A woman who thought that her daughter had been sentenced to six months "for discipline" objected that the girl was still at Faribault two years later. Despite weekly trips to the institution, her mother was never allowed to see the superintendent. It was an "awful thing" to force a girl to do unpaid work in the Faribault School's tailor shop for eight hours a day, the mother complained, "for just a little mistake she made in picking up some wrong company."[17]

Being confined in an institution was bad enough, but many families were sickened to learn of the forced labor and physical abuse their relatives endured. This was especially true when loved ones suffered violent attacks from attendants or fellow inmates. The Nelson family complained to the governor that their twenty-one-year-old daughter had not been outdoors in seven months. Her legs and feet were so swollen she could barely walk. The school was "not handling her right," they cried; it was not fair to lock her up for the rest of her life for something she did not do. Their daughter had been normal before she went to Faribault, but she was likely to "go febal mined—just watching the others in there." The siblings of a young woman with epilepsy and tuberculosis were also frantic with worry. Astrid Helsin had been transferred to Faribault from the Cambridge Colony for Epileptics without her family's knowledge or consent. She was forced to sleep in a locked room with a slop jar, but with no bell or light to call for help, and she had to listen to other patients crying and singing all night long. After Astrid's epileptic spells recurred because she was exhausted and scared, her family begged the state to move her to a tuberculosis sanatorium. An official noted coolly that the Helsin family might have some cause for concern, but they seemed "somewhat querulous in their manner."[18]

If midlevel officials were dismissive, Governor Youngdahl was not: he made mental health reform his "No. 1 objective" for 1949. The son of Swedish immigrants and a devout Lutheran, Youngdahl traced his interest in mental health to his days as a municipal court judge, when he had to sentence alcoholics and petty criminals to jail or the workhouse, even if they had an intellectual disability or were mentally ill. But he also saw mental health reform as part of the Cold War struggle for human rights. Americans did not agree with the "totalitarian" view that people unable to serve the state should be discarded, Youngdahl proclaimed; "The human being is an individual whose values cannot be measured adequately in terms of materialism, usefulness to the state, physical fitness or mental capacity." His landmark mental health reform bill, passed in 1949, promised "dignity and hope" to mental patients and a "radical change" (and an increasingly medical orientation) in state policy. The new law doubled the state's mental health budget, providing for twelve hundred new employees and increasing per-patient expenditures. The legislation also required staff to put "modern methods" of psychiatry and medicine into practice and serve the same meals to patients and employees alike.[19]

When the *Minneapolis Morning Tribune* reporters reprised their tour of state institutions in 1950, they found that the new monies were making a difference. The state was halfway to its goal of providing treatment for every patient, Hoffner reported, and patients who were considered incurable were no longer left naked and chained in the back wards. Faulty plumbing fixtures, dilapidated fire escapes, and leaky roofs had been fixed. Minnesota became the first state to require that patients and institution staff be given the same diet. In 1948, the reporters had "struggled to get down" a supper of sauerkraut, boiled potatoes, and watery stew. Two years later, patients dined on roast beef and peas, and the tin cups of 1948 had been replaced with utensils and colorful plastic dishes. Still, as the title of their article suggested, "Much Remains to Be Done."[20]

Although journalists were enthusiastic, Mildred Thomson found the new regime stressful. She resented the press coverage of mental hospitals as snake pits and grumbled that Governor Youngdahl gave "free rein" to militants who demanded "immediate and drastic action." Indeed, her 1963 memoir seethes with anger at the state's first commissioner of mental health, Ralph Rossen. Although Rossen would be remembered as a visionary who rejected the "mass care" of the past and brought a new philosophy of individual treatment to Minnesota state institutions, Thomson complained that he undermined established procedures regarding Faribault's waiting list and was dismissive of her concerns. The idea that "a mere social worker, should question his decision was preposterous!"[21]

Thomson eventually resolved her difficulties with Rossen, but their disagreements reveal deeply ingrained differences of gender, generation, and professional orientation. When Thomson began working for the state of Minnesota in 1924, the department for the feebleminded was part of the children's bureau of the State Board of Control, and her all-female staff worked with the county child welfare boards to support and supervise unmarried mothers and feebleminded wards. Thomson's outlook was shaped largely by the children's bureau's social work perspective. Twenty-five years later, Thomson worked at the same job, but now her program was just a small section of a large bureaucracy at the Division of Public Institutions. She still took pride in her close working relationship with the county welfare boards, but the (male) psychiatrists and administrators who were now her superiors viewed her community welfare approach as unscientific and out of date.

The mounting criticisms of Thomson's program added to her defensiveness. Her uneasiness was clear when in 1950 Governor Youngdahl, having been asked about his position on sterilization, passed the question on to Rossen, who in turn asked Thomson to draft a response. Unable to tell whether the governor was for or against the policy, she covered all the bases. In her first draft, Thomson presented the policy within a eugenics framework. Although administrators had no plans for "wholesale sterilization and release to the community," she said, sterilization allowed some mentally deficient persons to live outside the institution and was "from a genetic standpoint, advisable, and from a social standpoint of advantage not only to the community, but to the individual in that it gives the protection needed." In a subsequent draft, she stressed the social work argument. Although the "question of heredity" might be a factor in some instances, she admitted, this was not true in all cases, and the "inadequacy of the person to exercise the responsibilities of a parent" was also a basis for sterilization. She also stressed the professionalism of the program's administrators: sterilizations were authorized by the director of public institutions, with the assistance of a team of specialists; they were performed by a "surgeon of standing"; and social work supervision continued after the patient left the institution. She concluded by nervously reiterating her hope that the governor "really does believe in the law that we have in Minnesota and in the way in which it is administered."[22]

As Thomson's painstaking justifications suggest, by 1950 attitudes toward eugenic sterilization were in flux. Several bills to repeal the sterilization law were proposed, and although they never made it to the floor of the state legislature, the drop in surgeries which began during the war continued into the postwar years. Faribault's biennial report for the period ending July 1948 listed no female sterilizations and only four vasectomies. Four years later, the number of operations had increased—to twenty-three and two, respectively—but "large numbers of wards were never again even considered for sterilization." In her memoirs, Thomson attributed the decline to a shift in attitudes that had begun during the war: "The success of wards in industry during the war had helped to bring about the change, perhaps somewhat unconsciously. If they were able to show greater ability and better judgment than we had expected, perhaps we need not be so concerned about the possibility of their having offspring. Moreover, some of the knowledge of human genetics gained during these later years had ended the idea that mental deficiency was inherited as an entity. Thus sterilization could be considered on a more selective basis."[23]

Thomson even began to rethink her own deeply held assumptions about the inability of the feebleminded to be good workers and parents. In the late 1940s, she and her assistant Phyllis Mickelson reviewed the case files of more than five thousand persons who were under guardianship, with the result that many were discharged. Mickelson also published a pioneering study entitled "The

Feebleminded Parent" (1947), which examined ninety families to determine the impact of mental status on successful or unsuccessful parenthood. Mickelson divided parental care into three somewhat arbitrary categories. Satisfactory care meant that the children were fed and clothed and attended school; questionable care was inconsistent, but not so bad as to require the intervention of child protection authorities; and unsatisfactory care was so bad that the child should be removed from the home. She found that 42 percent of the feebleminded parents provided satisfactory care, while only 26 percent provided care that was so unsatisfactory as to justify neglect proceedings. Mickelson's study signaled a major attitudinal change: mental ability was not the sole determiner of adequacy of care. Sterilization might have helped these families by reducing the number of pregnancies, she observed, but the family income, the mother's mental health and relationship to her husband, and the number of pregnancies and children in the home were also important. With counseling and social services, many feebleminded women could be satisfactory parents. Mickelson's paper signaled the beginning of a major change.[24]

Few welfare officials shared Mickelson's optimistic view of the feebleminded parent, but by the early 1950s most of them considered the state's aggressive eugenic sterilization program a relic of the past. The director of a St. Paul foundation, ignoring the broad bipartisan support that the sterilization program had once enjoyed, wrote in 1952 about "our then, so-called voluntary sterilization policy," by which social workers committed women with low IQs to state guardianship "whenever possible" and refused to release them if their families objected to the surgery. IQ test results had been the "sole criteria" for determining the disposition of poor youngsters, he complained, and guardianship was used as a way to "shift care costs from local tax budgets to the State." He continued, "Now, of course, sterilization seems to have passed completely from the program of our State hospitals, due no doubt to pressures from religious groups," and professional social workers no longer viewed mental deficiency commitment as a step toward sterilization.[25] In postwar Minnesota, plentiful jobs and an expanding social safety net meant that eugenic sterilization was no longer deemed necessary or viable as a welfare strategy.

Good Families, Bad Genes: Sheldon Reed, Parent Associations, and the "Retarded" Child

While institutional reform dominated the headlines, two behind-the-scenes developments reinforced the new thinking about mental retardation: the formation in 1946 of the Minneapolis Association of Parents and Friends of the Mentally Retarded, and the appointment of Harvard geneticist Sheldon Reed as the director of the University of Minnesota's Dight Institute for Human Genetics in 1947.

The Minnesota Association for Retarded Children (MARC), a statewide parents' group formed with Thomson's support, emerged in the postwar years as a significant force for reform. MARC members, most of whom had children with intellectual disabilities, worked to reduce the stigma of mental retardation by redefining individuals with intellectual disabilities as innocent children; they also lobbied for special education and community-based services so that mildly retarded children could live at home. Thomson helped them navigate the welfare system. Reed provided them with scientific legitimacy and a conceptual framework, medical genetics, which explained how respectable middle-class families could have retarded children. Working with Thomson, Reed, and reform-minded politicians, MARC made middle-class families key clients of the welfare state and laid the foundation for the disability rights movement of the 1970s. Yet the image of the innocent middle-class retarded child they created did little to dislodge negative stereotypes of those with severe disabilities or "bad" retardates who were undeserving and poor.[26]

At first glance, it may seem surprising that Thomson, the longtime administrator of Minnesota's eugenic commitment and sterilization program, and Reed, the Dight Institute's director, contributed so much to the parent reform movement. In fact, as we have seen, Thomson had always taken pride in being a "friend" of the mentally retarded and their families. By the late 1940s, moreover, she was hurt and alienated by the increasing medical orientation of the state's mental health bureaucracy, the lack of attention given to mental retardation in comparison to mental illness, and the fact that the negative publicity and criticisms of the state's mental health program invariably seemed to strengthen the power of male medical professionals, especially psychiatrists, over the mostly female social workers who were blamed for past abuses and the system's current problems. In contrast, parent activists, many of them women, seemed appreciative of Thomson's community–social work perspective. They shared her frustration with doctors' arrogance and with the belittlement of mental retardation as an important policy concern. They were grateful that Thomson encouraged parents to start their own organization and helped arrange the first meeting of the National Association of Parents and Friends of the Mentally Retarded (later the National Association for Retarded Children) in Minneapolis in 1950.[27]

Reed's insistence that "good" parents could have "bad" genes also facilitated the growth of parent associations by reducing the shame of mental retardation. Reed, who served as director of the Dight Institute from 1947 until his retirement in 1978, was a pioneer in the new field of genetic counseling, a term he invented to distinguish his medically oriented counseling from a coercive eugenics program, and his compassionate message about "bad" genes found a welcome audience with middle-class parent groups. Before Reed came to Minnesota, Mildred Thomson later recalled, the state's medical and welfare establishment did not question the assumption that "mentally deficient parents produced mentally deficient children." Reed's insistence that mental deficiency was not inherited as an entity and "anyone may have a retarded child" gave parents "new understanding and hope." As Reed explained in his first report as Dight Institute director, "Mendel's laws of heredity . . . have no respect for the social or economic status of the family concerned." Inherited disabilities could strike people of any background.[28]

Reed's medical therapeutic approach to eugenics resonated with middle-class parent groups. The Dight Institute had been established in 1941 with a bequest from MES president Charles Dight and a mandate to promote eugenics through instruction, research, and a consultation service for individuals with specific genetic concerns. In contrast to the institute's first director, Clarence Oliver, who favored pressuring people with undesirable traits to stop reproducing, Reed prided himself on providing genetic information in a manner that was "compassionate, clear, relaxed, and without a sales pitch" so that families could make their own reproductive decisions. In his view, couples who knew their genetic histories could decide for themselves whether to avoid pregnancy or—more commonly—take the risk of having more children, knowing that the chance of disability was small. In an article in *Eugenics Quarterly* Reed admitted that nondirective counseling could lead to the births of more disabled children, but he thought that couples "who are sufficiently concerned to come for counseling have commendable concepts of their obligations as parents and these laudable characteristics should be transmitted to the next generation."[29]

A complex figure, Reed was both postwar Minnesota's most prominent eugenicist and an outspoken liberal on civil rights. He was a member of the American Eugenics Society and the pro-sterilization Human Betterment Association of America, but he consistently rejected the most extreme class and race manifestations of eugenics. Reed routinely used his status as Dight Institute director to denounce the "pernicious perversion of Darwin's ideas . . . by the Nazi criminals." He hailed *Brown v. Board of Education*, the United States Supreme Court case that overturned racial segregation in schools, and was an early advocate of transracial adoption (he believed that mixed-race children were the best genetic risk). "The hereditary racial differences are, like beauty, only skin deep," he proclaimed; "All men are brothers under the skin!"[30] At the same time, Reed used familiar eugenics arguments in support of sterilization. He described Minnesota's voluntary sterilization law as a humane measure that allowed mentally deficient individuals to leave an institution where they were "deprived of all freedom" and reside in the community without being "encumbered with children." The "population 'explosion' and the automation 'explosion' " made the need for eugenics greater than ever, he wrote in 1965. Since it was unrealistic to expect the "more intelligent" people to have more children, it was "imperative" for the "less intelligent" to have fewer.[31]

The hard edge of Reed's eugenics outlook was most visible in his writings about those he considered less than deserving—the poor and the disabled. He drew a sharp distinction between the middle-class family with genetic defects which sought his advice and the "common garden-variety of moron family" which was unlikely to seek help. His class-based eugenics approach is evident in *Mental Retardation: A Family Study* (1965), a seven-hundred-page follow-up study to the eugenics family study that A. C. Rogers initiated and ERO field-workers Saidee Devitt and Marie Curial conducted in the 1910s. Sheldon's wife and coauthor Elizabeth Reed, who was also a geneticist, tracked the descendants of 289 of the original patients and eventually gathered information on more than eighty thousand people. They concluded, unsurprisingly, that the greatest predisposing factor for mental retardation was a mentally retarded relative, regardless of whether the disability was primarily genetic or environmental in origin. To the Reeds, the solution was clear. "When voluntary sterilization becomes a part of the culture of the United States," they declared, "we should expect a decrease of about 50 per cent per generation in the number of retarded persons."[32]

Even within the middle-class family, Reed privileged the normal at the expense of the defective. A large portion of the Dight Institute's work in the 1940s and 1950s involved evaluating newborns for adoption placement, and despite Reed's liberal views on race and women's rights, he did not hesitate to recommend removing babies from unmarried mothers or advising white families not to adopt infants of African American ancestry when he thought their skin tone would be too dark. Nor did he question the then-common view that a child with severe disabilities should be institutionalized. A "drooling idiot" could be an embarrassment to siblings, Reed explained harshly, and "an invitation to improper sexual exploitation by ill-mannered neighbors." Such a child would be better off in an institution. Not unlike Faribault superintendent A. C. Rogers around 1900, Reed felt that lifelong custodial care was beneficial because "the child will find himself among his equals and he will be able to compete with them, whereas in the home community he will always be either overprotected or cruelly rejected from social contacts." Middle-class families who put up illegitimate infants for adoption and institutionalized their mentally disabled children could feel they were acting selflessly. The mentally retarded child would be with her "own kind," and normal children could have a normal family life.[33]

Many parent activists shared Reed's views, including the distinction he drew between respectable parents who had a retarded child and the "common garden-variety of moron family." In the early 1950s, the "innocent" retarded child of respectable parents replaced the "common garden-variety of moron family" in the public discourse on mental retardation. When Nobel Prize–winning author Pearl Buck disclosed the long-kept secret that she had a mentally retarded daughter who lived in an institution and TV star Dale Evans went public with the short life of her severely disabled daughter, they gave new visibility to an issue many families had once kept secret and began the process of extricating intellectual disability from delinquency and dependency. In 1962, Eunice Kennedy Shriver, the president's sister, put to rest the simplistic association between mental retardation and bad heredity by writing about their institutionalized sister in the *Saturday Evening Post.* "Like diabetes, deafness, polio, or any other misfortune, mental retardation can happen in any family," Shriver explained. "It has happened in the families of the poor and the rich, of governors, senators, Nobel prize winners, doctors, lawyers, writers, men of genius, presidents of corporations—the President of the United States." With increasing public awareness and investment in research and education, "the years of indifference and neglect are drawing to a close." The families of retarded children now had hope.[34]

It is no accident that this hope developed after the New Deal, when social welfare entitlements were well established and expectations for government support were rising. Across the United States, parent volunteers raised funds for medical research and operated community programs for individuals with disabilities. But they also emphasized their own families' entitlement to services, challenging both the stigma of intellectual disability and the shame of dependency on government programs. MARC (specifically the Minneapolis chapter) established the nation's first Boy Scout troop for boys with mental retardation and one of the first day care programs for children with severe disabilities. It operated a summer camp, held weekly dances and recreational programs, and worked closely with staff from the county welfare boards and state institutions.[35] Like the clubhouses for feebleminded women funded and operated by Women's Welfare League volunteers in the 1920s, MARC's social service activities illustrate the private–public partnership that has long characterized the US welfare system and succeeded in large measure because they claimed to help children. Unlike the welfare league, however, MARC members were also making claims on the state for middle-class families.

Sociologist Allison C. Carey has demonstrated that parent activists created both a "need-based narrative depicting their offspring as 'eternal children' and a human-rights narrative stressing the obligation of the state to provide for its members, regardless of their abilities." Yet the economic argument was always front and center. Parent activist John L. Holahan made this clear in a 1952 speech, which contrasted Depression-era parents, who were pressured to institutionalize children with intellectual disabilities because the money spent in caring for them was "literally bread taken from the mouth of some normal member of the family," with the prosperous families of the postwar years. These families could carry the extra cost of a retarded child, Holahan acknowledged, but it was not fair to expect them to shoulder the whole burden. The parents of retarded children were responsible citizens. They were intelligent, paid taxes, fought in wars, and contributed to society, he explained; they needed to know that their children were safe in school or day care so they could continue to make a contribution to society. Furthermore, he warned, echoing the arguments of an earlier era, denying services to the families of the retarded could be costly. The stress of caring for a disabled family member without any help could turn the mother into a "household drudge" and lead to antisocial traits among the normal children; welfare records were filled with such families. "We don't want the mentally retarded set up in style, at great expenses to the taxpayers," he maintained. "Nor, do we want them ignored, left to their own devices, withdrawn from the social scene." Parents of retarded children only wanted that to which they were entitled.[36]

Parent groups ultimately had an ambiguous impact on mental retardation policy. As historian Katherine Castles has observed, their efforts to prove that they were "nice, average Americans" helped disentangle intellectual disability from the stigma of hereditary taint, racial inferiority, and lower class status. Yet it may have perpetuated another type of class and racial divide. As disability rights activists would later point out, parents' interests and priorities were not necessarily the same as those of their children, and their powerful lobby sometimes obscured the wishes and even negated the rights of adults with developmental disabilities. Moreover, by presuming to speak for all retarded children, middle-class activists inadvertently heightened the invisibility of those whose families were not white, educated, or middle class. Many educated parent activists drew a line between their own respectability and the undeserving feebleminded of old. Rejecting the idea of hereditary feeblemindedness and searching for a cure, they defined intellectual disability as a medical problem, rather than a matter of social welfare or human rights.[37]

Yet their impact on attitudes toward and policies on intellectual disability was significant. By the mid-1950s, Minnesota welfare officials seldom referred to mentally deficient paupers or criminals; instead, they presented themselves as helping the innocent middle-class child. This shift is evident in a 1954 booklet, *You Are Not Alone*, written by Phyllis Mickelson. Prior to the war, Thomson sent regular communications to probate judges and county welfare boards, but not to parents, who were generally presumed to be feebleminded themselves. *You Are Not Alone* was her agency's first direct communication to parents, and MARC's influence was clear. The pamphlet's chief message was that "mental deficiency can—and does—happen to anyone," regardless of race, education, or income. "Perhaps you thought—mistakenly—that it was due entirely to heredity or to 'bad blood' in the family," the pamphlet explained, but in fact, there were many causes of mental retardation. At a time when most Minnesotans associated the county welfare boards with poor relief or eugenic institutionalization, *You Are Not Alone* made a point of telling parents they had a legal right to welfare services and that many "equally capable" parents were using these services too. The social worker did not have a ready-made agenda, but was simply there to help with individual planning.[38]

The new emphasis on middle-class families required a certain amount of deception, since Minnesota's program for the mentally deficient had been designed for the poor. Nearly forty years after the Child Welfare Commission asserted the state's need for legal control over a "serious public menace," state policy toward those considered mentally deficient still rested on the principle of court-ordered guardianship—that is, the legal removal of the child from its parents' custody. Guardianship was encouraged when people with retardation were living at home (a holdover of the eugenics assumption that their families were also unfit), but it was a legal requirement for placement in a state institution. A 1956 pamphlet called *Looking Ahead* described guardianship as a way for the state to "protect your child in any way necessary," even after the parents were gone. Guardianship did not mean giving up parental rights or responsibilities (except in cases of child neglect), *Looking Ahead* explained; it simply allowed the state to exercise parental authority and assure "lifetime service" to the child. "He is Still YOUR Child."[39]

In law, those comforting words were patently untrue: the Minnesota Supreme Court had ruled in *In re Wretlind* (1948) that the very act of signing a petition to place a child under guardianship made a parent the legal adversary of her child. The case revolved around Bernetta Wretlind, an "illegitimate" child committed to guardianship and sent to Faribault in December 1943 at the age of twelve. Bernetta's mother, like many other women in similar circumstances, soon changed her mind about her daughter's institutionalization. When Bernetta was released for a two-week visit home in the summer of 1945, her mother petitioned for her daughter's release. Her petition was denied on the grounds that the girl was still feebleminded, so the family made its challenge on procedural grounds. They alleged that the original commitment was invalid because there had been no notice of a hearing. (A hearing had been held and attended by Bernetta, her mother, stepfather, and the county attorney, but the petitioners claimed that their presence at the hearing did not constitute a waiver of Bernetta's constitutional right to notice.) In an important decision with complex implications, the court ruled that Bernetta's mother became her daughter's legal adversary when she signed the original commitment petition, but the lower court's failure to appoint a guardian ad litem to protect the minor child's interests in court invalidated the proceedings. Since a guardian ad litem had not been appointed, the guardianship was void.[40]

To Thomson, the *Wretlind* decision showed that the court did not understand the purpose of guardianship. Without mentioning the case by name, she wrote in her memoirs that it involved a "truly neglected, illegitimate child—a girl—who needed protection." After Bernetta was released from guardianship, she became pregnant out of wedlock and was placed under guardianship again. According to Thomson, this proved the court's failure to see that guardianship was "basically protective." By ruling that the child was entitled to a guardian ad litem, the court forced commitment proceedings to become more formal and thus "more difficult for the families." Many parents hesitated to commit a child to state guardianship, knowing that the law, when "interpreted literally," gave them no control over the planning for their children. Thomson never wavered in her belief that state guardianship was essentially benign. She understood the benefits of guardianship and institutionalization, even if parents and the courts did not.[41]

Thomson's continuing faith in the benefits of institutionalization is astonishing, given how awful the state institutions continued to be. Conditions at Faribault were so bad that it lost its status as an accredited hospital in 1958. MARC, confessing its own "negligence for not spotlighting these inadequacies sooner," made adequate staffing of the state institutions for the mentally retarded its "number one objective" for 1959, declaring that "humane considerations must take precedence over the book-keeping approach."[42] Change proceeded rapidly in the next few years, as reformers, employees, and volunteers at the state and—for the first time—federal level attempted to fix a broken mental health system. By the mid-1960s, President Kennedy's mental retardation legislation and President Johnson's War on Poverty toppled long-standing eugenics-based assumptions about sex, race, and the undeserving poor. By the end of the decade, a new generation of activists challenged state sterilization practices and, ultimately, the institution itself.

State Officials Rethink Sterilization and Mental Retardation

The 1960s brought major changes to attitudes and policies affecting poverty and mental retardation, at both the state and federal levels. Mildred Thomson retired in September 1959 after thirty-five years as supervisor of the Section for Mentally Deficient and Epileptic, and the next year, David J. Vail, a Harvard-trained psychiatrist and advocate of mental patients' rights, became director of medical services at the Minnesota Department of Public Welfare. Vail soon launched a full-scale attack on "dehumanizing practices" in Minnesota's mental institutions. Until his untimely death in 1971 at the age of forty-five, Vail worked to wrest administrative control from the old-time medical superintendents, break down the rigid separation between institution and society, and undo the cruel traditions of what sociologist Erving Goffman called the "total institution." Within months of his appointment, Vail demanded that every Minnesota superintendent embrace the goal of accreditation and the concept of an Open Hospital, which had unlocked doors and a therapeutic, rather than custodial, environment. Criticizing hospital practices that benefited staff but not the residents, Vail proposed to end degrading procedures, such as having the police transport patients to the institution and forcing patients to do unpaid work in superintendents' homes, minimize the use of seclusion and restraints, and respect patients' human rights.[43]

Thomson's retirement in September 1959 also brought change to the Section for the Mentally Deficient and Epileptic. Within a few months, Thomson's successor (and former assistant) Frances Coakley upended her predecessor's work. Coakley was president-elect of the AAMD, and she soon announced that the Section for the Mentally Deficient and Epileptic "accepted the new concepts of mental retardation." In the past, she explained, experts mistakenly believed that intelligence was fixed, that heredity was the main cause of mental retardation, and that mentally retarded people were a burden on their families and communities. However, new scientific research showed the complexities of mental retardation and raised the prospects for successful treatment. Even the AAMD defined mental retardation as a "term descriptive of the current status of the individual with respect to intellectual functioning and adaptive behavior" and recognized that a person's mental status could change.[44] The intellectual premise of Minnesota's eugenics program—that mental deficiency was permanent, inherited, burdensome, and menacing—had collapsed.

Vail and Coakley also took up the issue of eugenic sterilization. Although sterilization no longer attracted much attention from politicians or the press, operations had continued in small numbers throughout the 1950s. A Faribault psychologist told historian Philip Reilly that he had evaluated forty-six women and eight men between 1955 and 1960, and most of them were sterilized. As in the past, the majority of operations were performed on high-functioning women about to leave the institution, and officials frequently withheld release from the institution until a sterilization consent form was signed. Reilly reported that a few non-institutionalized women with illegitimate children were also sterilized, and table 6.1 suggests that a few patients in other institutions were sterilized as well.[45]

Vail raised the issue of sterilization at an open-ended meeting of institution officials in November 1960. With uncharacteristic diplomacy, he began by asking longtime Faribault superintendent Edward J. Engberg to describe the state's past and present sterilization practices. Engberg's answer shows how little the sterilization program had changed since the 1920s. Sterilizations, Engberg explained, were authorized after "very careful" study on three types of mentally retarded persons: (1) a man or woman likely to have retarded children owing to "hereditary factors," (2) a woman unable to provide "adequate care" for her children, and (3) a man who could not support his family because he was "inept

TABLE 6.1
Sterilizations officially reported in Minnesota, 1946–1970

	Feebleminded[a]		Insane[b]		Total		
Year	Female	Male	Female	Male	Female	Male	Annual total
1946	1	0	1	0	2	0	2
1947	0	0	1	0	1	0	1
1948	0	4	0	0	0	4	4
1949	3	3	1	1	4	4	8
1950	11	1	0	0	11	1	12
1951	13	0	2	0	15	0	15
1952	10	2	4	0	14	2	16
1953	11	2	0	0	11	2	13
1954	6	1	3	0	9	1	10
1955	5	1	2	1	7	2	9
1956	17	1	0	0	17	2[c]	19
1957	8	0	2	1	10	2[c]	12
1958	7	1	0	0	7	1	8
1959	5	0	1	0	6	0	6
1960–1961	6	0	4	0	10	0	10
1962	1	0	0	0	1	0	1
1963	0	0	0	0	0	0	0
1964	—	—	—	—	—	—	0
1965	—	—	—	—	—	—	0
1966	—	—	—	—	—	—	0
1967	—	—	—	—	—	—	0
1968	—	—	—	—	—	—	0
1969	—	—	—	—	—	—	1
1970	—	—	—	—	—	—	0
Total	104	16	21	3	125	21	147

Sources: Data for 1946–1963 are from "Sterilizations officially reported . . . 1946–1963," Association for Voluntary Sterilization Records, Social Welfare History Archives, University of Minnesota Libraries. Data for 1964–1970 are from Tricia Farris, "Sterilization: Use, Misuse, and Abuse" (St. Paul: State of Minnesota House Research Department, May 1974), Minnesota Historical Society; NB: no information on gender.

[a] "Mentally deficient" after 1951.

[b] "Mentally ill" after 1951.

[c] One male sterilization listed as "other" in 1956 and 1957.

at properly carrying out his role as a father and husband." Decisions about sterilization were always made in the context of institutional release, but Engberg insisted that "no pressure" was ever used to force relatives to consent. He added that patients who were not released after being sterilized often got upset or ran away.[46]

Most of those in attendance offered a cautious endorsement of a program they seem to have truly believed was voluntary and based on the patient's individual needs. Arnold Madow, the Faribault psychologist who assessed patients for sterilization, emphasized that eugenics was just one of several considerations and that he made a "careful evaluation and cautious determination in every case." Ralph Rosenberger of the Annex for Defective Delinquents remarked that sterilization was once common at his institution but was now quite unusual. He added, however, that he still thought the policy useful in cases where the stress of family responsibilities could lead a male defective into delinquency. Coakley expressed the strongest anti-sterilization view. Citing the influential 1958 study *Mental Subnormality*, by Richard Masland, Seymour Sarason, and Thomas Gladwin, she explained that intelligence was shaped by a range of "social, cultural, and psychological" (as opposed to strictly hereditary) factors and stressed the need to "avoid conclusions which are based on past practices." In her view, the sterilization program failed to differentiate between eugenics objectives and the "social management of irresponsible persons." In the past, she said, state welfare policies discriminated against people with developmental disabilities, but in 1960 public education and economic aid to the poor were more universally available, making eugenic sterilization unnecessary. The availability of social services, in other words, rendered sterilization anachronistic.[47]

Vail chose his words carefully, saying there was "no easy solution" to the sterilization question. Some institutions performed no sterilizations at all, while others required women to undergo sterilization before they could be released. He believed that tying sterilization to institutional release was "too arbitrary" and left too little allowance for individual consideration. There were, after all, significant fluctuations in mental functioning, and it was not always possible to predict whether a person with retardation would be a poor parent. Equally important, he added, sterilization went "against the human order" and should be used "with great caution," for, like lobotomy, it "removes something from the human body on a permanent basis. This is to be avoided if possible." In 1961, Vail ordered a halt to eugenic sterilizations in Minnesota public institutions.[48]

Similar discussions occurred nationally. While old-timers continued to defend sterilization as a "protection, not a penalty" and insist that mental defectives felt relief and even satisfaction knowing they would not be burdened with children, a new generation of psychiatrists, lawyers, social scientists, and social workers presented a very different picture. In 1962, the *Eugenics Quarterly* published a stunning challenge to the long-standing assumption that people did not mind being sterilized. Anthropologist Robert Edgerton and Georges Sabagh, a sociologist, conducted forty interviews with high-functioning, mostly white people sterilized and discharged from California's Pacific State Hospital between 1949 and 1958. More than two-thirds of the ex-patients disapproved of the operation and only one-fifth clearly approved. Young married women were the most likely to be unhappy and unmarried men the most likely to be content. Edgerton and Sabagh hypothesized that ex-patients were unhappy with the surgery because it kept them from "assuming the normal roles of motherhood or fatherhood" and "passing as normal." All the interviewees had suffered degrading experiences in the institution where they were sterilized and may have associated sterilization with that "punishment and humiliation." Infertility was an ever-present "symbol of incompetence" and a "permanent mark of the mortification that the patient had to endure." They quoted a thirty-year-old woman, who conveyed her feelings of incompetence and hurt: "Gee, I sure would like to have a baby. . . . They never told me that they were going to do that surgery to me. They said they were going to remove my appendix and then they did that other. They should have explained to me. . . . After they did that surgery to me, I cried. . . . I still don't know why they did that surgery to me. The sterilization wasn't for punishment, was it? Was it because there was something wrong with my mind?"[49] Edgerton and Sabagh conducted their fieldwork at the height of the baby boom, when the expectation that most women would be mothers was particularly intense, but their remarkable interviews represent one of the few times before the 1970s that "experts" asked sterilized individuals what they thought. That their findings were published in *Eugenics Quarterly* is a measure of the changing outlook.

The Federal Government Wages War on Mental Retardation and Poverty

Reform-minded administrators and parents got an additional boost in 1960: the election of President John F. Kennedy gave them a champion in the federal government. The Kennedy family's involvement with mental retardation was personal and long-standing: the president's sister Rosemary, who was considered mildly retarded, had to be permanently institutionalized after a botched lobotomy. But Kennedy's "war" on mental retardation was also politically advantageous. Just as Republican governor Luther Youngdahl and his political opponents found bipartisan mental health reform to be politically beneficial in the 1940s, Kennedy and his critics found much to gain from a dramatic expansion of social services that, for the most part, defined individuals with mental retardation as child-like dependents needing protection. Congress passed Kennedy's mental retardation bill, while civil rights legislation stalled. Unlike equality for southern African Americans, Kennedy's plan to "help" the mentally retarded was seen as humanitarian and nonpolitical. Few votes were at stake, and legislators found agreement easy.[50]

In reality, the new policy was highly political, for it greatly expanded the role of the federal government in an arena previously left to the states. The President's Panel on Mental Retardation, created in 1961, also reflected reformers' enduring faith in science and professional expertise. Most of the panel's twenty-seven members were doctors, educators, and natural or social scientists. Only NARC's Elizabeth Boggs represented parent groups (and she had a PhD in chemistry). There was not one civil rights leader, despite mounting concern about the number of African Americans erroneously labeled mentally retarded. The president's sister, Eunice Kennedy Shriver, although officially a consultant, was de facto chair. As in the past, the experts disagreed sharply over the nature of mental retardation and even who "the retarded" were. While some panelists understood intellectual disability to be a biomedical or neurological condition affecting people from every social and economic background, others maintained that people with retardation came primarily from disadvantaged backgrounds. They stressed the role of "adverse social, economic, and cultural factors" in causing mental retardation and the urgency of addressing social problems such as malnutrition, inadequate prenatal care, and cultural deprivation.[51]

The panel's report, *A Proposed Program for National Action to Combat Mental Retardation* (1962), tried to strike a balance between conflicting attitudes and ideas. At times it described mental retardation negatively, as a costly problem that caused "untold human anguish," but it also stressed the dignity and humanity of each person. It portrayed the disabilities arising from cultural deprivation as "a source of accumulating 'social dynamite' in our large cities," while also emphasizing the potential of individuals with mental retardation and their entitlement to "full human and legal rights." The panel stressed the need to prevent mental retardation, but in contrast to eugenics-inspired efforts to combat the menace of feeblemindedness by sterilizing the unfit, the President's Panel called for a sweeping welfare system that improved basic services for all people and instituted specific programs for people with retardation. These included maternal and infant health care and preschool education, to address the problem of cultural deprivation, and a system of comprehensive, community-centered services, to provide a "continuum of care" for people with special needs—education, day care, recreational programs, vocational opportunities, and so on—with the goal of encouraging the development of their "maximum capacity" and providing accommodations in cases in which disabilities could not be overcome.[52]

In October 1963, Kennedy signed two bills that made intellectual disability a federal concern for the first time. Both bills passed by a wide margin. The Maternal and Child Health and Mental Retardation Amendment to the Social Security Act provided grants to the states for prenatal and infant care to prevent intellectual disability and improved services for people with intellectual disabilities. The Mental Retardation Facilities and Community Mental Health Centers Construction Act provided federal funding for special education teacher training, university-based research centers, and clinical facilities. Minnesota was the first state to submit a plan to the US surgeon general and received $3.8 million in grants.[53]

The President's Panel also called for "a new legal, as well as social, concept of the retarded, including protection for their civil rights." It emphasized the urgency of moving beyond the traditional view that mental retardation was static and incurable, while also acknowledging the difficulty of writing a more complex understanding of mental retardation into law. As the Task Force on Law wrote in a separate report, the social effects of disability were unpredictable, but the law dealt in absolutes: an individual was competent or incompetent, innocent or guilty, a ward of the state or legally free. The Task Force sharply criticized the courts' overreliance on IQ scores and the use of "social incompetency as the single criterion of mental retardation." It recommended instead the dual criteria of "subaverage general intellectual functioning" and "impairment in adaptive behavior." At the same time, the Task Force also called for a broad expansion in social welfare entitlements, such as Social Security and public education. "The richer these general services, and the more easily available they are," it observed, "the less the need for special services for the retarded." While eugenics-era welfare policies simply tried to limit the number of births in "multi-problem" families with a history of mental illness, mental retardation, alcoholism, and so on, the Task Force emphasized the aggregation of disabilities. Since "each additional misfortune exacerbates the effect of the previous one, and each additional misfortune helps pave the way for the next," it said, the successful treatment of any one problem would make "the burden of mental retardation . . . easier to bear."[54]

At the same time, the Task Force backed away from a defense of marital and reproductive rights. It stated that marriage should not be "categorically denied to all retarded persons" and that mentally retarded wards should be permitted to marry with the court's consent. Its stand on sterilization was equally limited. More than half of US states then had compulsory sterilization laws, and the task force admitted that there were "serious questions about the validity of the scientific assumptions on which these laws were based and the way in which it is decided who should be sterilized"—in practice, the superintendent had "great discretion." But its conclusion was timid: sterilization decisions should not be based on scientific misjudgments or "inadequate opportunity for administrative and judicial review."[55]

Political scientist Julius Paul, reflecting in 1965 on the panel's tepid critique, speculated that the issue of sterilization was a "bit too hot," and the panel did not want to jeopardize its larger disability rights agenda on a policy that at the time affected relatively few. The Task Force was considerably less equivocal on guardianship, and on this issue it asserted the legal rights of people with intellectual disabilities in the strongest of terms: "It is a basic democratic principle that no diminution of human rights and human dignity can be countenanced by the law for any person—let alone any class of persons—except for good reason, following due process, and then to the minimum degree necessary and for the shortest period possible." The President's Panel made a point of distinguishing guardianship over property and guardianship over a person and recommended both limited personal guardianship and the possibility of institutionalization without the requirement of guardianship. Curiously, it also praised Minnesota's "unique guardianship program" as a model that "might well be studied by other states."[56]

The federal panel's positive view of Minnesota's program likely reflected the influence of NARC representative Elizabeth Boggs and the bond forged over many years between parent activists and social workers from Minnesota. Many reformers outside Minnesota viewed the state's guardianship program as "outstanding and unique" because it did not require institutionalization. Although legal guardianship was vested with the commissioner of public welfare (who succeeded the Board of Control), day-to-day duties were carried out by county social workers. To supporters, this distinctive and long-standing arrangement allowed the commissioner, the public institutions, and the county welfare departments to form an "unbroken triangle" that gave "effective service" to wards. Indeed, as late as 1966, Minnesota was the only state to provide "active guardianship" and counseling outside the institutions. For this reason, Boggs praised Minnesota's guardianship program as a "remarkably vigorous institution that has brought peace of mind to many parents and helped to maintain as many socially inadequate retarded persons outside public institutions as in them." It was not the law but the "*service of guardianship*" that was important, Boggs explained; successful guardianship depended on the hard work of "qualified and conscientious people" who cared about the retarded. She might have added that guardianship worked best when the parents were well educated and middle class, and when families and social workers saw eye to eye.[57]

Legal guardianship, and indeed intellectual disability policy more generally, did not work as smoothly when the client was poor. Even as middle-class parent activists demanded and achieved special education and program entitlements for retarded children, eugenics-inflected ideas about race, class, and low intelligence gained new life in the burgeoning social science literature on poverty and cultural deprivation. Anthropologist Oscar Lewis initially developed his theory of the "culture of poverty" in a series of ethnographic studies about Mexicans and Puerto Ricans, but he depicted poverty culture as a near-universal "way of life handed on generation to generation along family lines" which transcended regional and even national boundaries. Lewis was a liberal who supported an expansive welfare system, but his description of persistent poverty as a cultural phenomenon reinforced the common belief that something other than lack of money was wrong with the (undeserving) poor. Predictably, many of the traits Lewis identified with the culture of poverty—present-time orientation, lack of impulse control, dependency, weak ego structure, and sexual confusion—bore a depressing similarity to the supposed characteristics of feeblemindedness which Minnesota officials disseminated decades earlier. As a federal poverty researcher explained in 1963, some children "seemed destined to poverty almost from birth—by their color or by the economic status or occupation of their parents." Regardless of whether social scientists viewed persistent poverty as culturally determined or genetic, its markers were deeply gendered and embedded in long-standing antipathy toward the "defective, dependent, and delinquent" classes. By the 1960s, however, the emblem of degeneracy had mostly shifted away from poor rural whites like the Jukes. Instead, the focus was on urban black welfare recipients, who were purportedly trapped in a "tangle of pathology" involving dependency, illegitimacy, criminality, and the failure of youth.[58]

Lewis's theory of a culture of poverty was closely linked to the concept of cultural deprivation, which figured prominently in the report of the President's Panel on Mental Retardation. Deprivation theory held that children who grew up in poverty often suffered from poor health, malnutrition, and inadequate intellectual stimulation (e.g., poor parenting), which could have a devastating effect on a child's IQ and lead to learning difficulties or mental retardation. The concept of "familial mental retardation" applied to individuals who, like the "high-grade" feebleminded of the eugenics era, shared an intellectual handicap with other family members but had no identifiable organic disorder. Like the earlier theory of hereditary feeblemindedness, cultural deprivation drew on and reinforced negative stereotypes about the poor. Yet the shift from biology to culture was not inconsequential. Whereas mental deficiency was considered permanent and incurable, the damaging effects of deprivation and the culture of poverty could presumably be undone. Some postwar social scientists maintained that intelligence was manipulable and argued that compensatory programs like Head Start, which provided low-income preschoolers with early childhood education and nutrition, could raise student IQs. Despite the real success of a number of antipoverty programs, however, the failure to address the structural and systemic causes of welfare dependency left the notion of an undeserving poor intact.[59]

Historian Mical Raz observes that liberal reformers piggybacked on public support for programs that helped (white) "mentally retarded" children in order to win approval for federally funded services that benefited poor black youngsters who would otherwise be dismissed as the undeserving poor. The unfortunate result, however, was not a more generous system of social services and entitlements, but the overdiagnosis of racialized children as mentally retarded. In the postwar years, as in the Progressive Era, popular thinking about child welfare and mental ability ran along two tracks: intellectual disability was a medical problem for the innocent middle class and a problem of lower-class pathology.[60]

Fixing the Institution: A Major Minnesota Problem

While policymakers and politicians focused on preventing retardation by combating poverty and expanding health, education, and welfare services in the community, mental health reformers and administrators set their sights on fixing the institution. In 1961, soon after his appointment as director of medical services in the Department of Public Welfare, David Vail distributed Erving Goffman's book *Asylums* to institution staff and urged them to examine the ways they personally had participated in the erosion of patient dignity for bureaucratic convenience—for example, through regimented scheduling, institutional clothing, and toilets without doors. Writing in the 1960s, Vail did not imagine an end to the need for institutions. But his attack on dehumanizing practices was pathbreaking. He condemned the practice of treating mental patients as subhuman or animal, reminding staff that when they treated patients in dehumanizing ways, they also dehumanized themselves.[61]

Years later, psychologist Wolf Wolfensberger, whose theory of normalization transformed disability policy in the 1970s, credited Vail's book *Dehumanization and the Institutional Career* (1966) with helping him see the humanity and growth potential of people with intellectual disabilities. In the mid-1960s, however, Vail's "rehumanization" crusade was an uphill battle. Conditions at Faribault and other state institutions were dire. Although the expansion of community services had enabled many who would have been institutionalized in the past to live their entire lives in the community, this had led to significant underfunding and a shift in the institutionalized population: the majority of residents were now people with severe disabilities and complex medical needs. In the early 1960s, public institutions for the mentally retarded were desperately understaffed and overcrowded. Since most federal funding went to new programs and construction, the state was left responsible for Faribault's upkeep. Many legislators saw Faribault and other institutions—crammed with apparently hopeless defectives without any future—as a drain on the state budget. Parent activists, reform-minded administrators like Vail, and even the governor turned to the press to raise awareness of the humanitarian crisis and try to convince the legislature to increase funding.[62]

In 1965, *Minneapolis Tribune* reporter Sam Newlund published yet another exposé of the scandalous conditions at Faribault. He described patients with severe disabilities who were heavily drugged and lived "like animals" in the school's Dakota Building, where "human beings exist in shadows." Newlund challenged any lingering assumptions about hereditary feeblemindedness by opening his story with Tom, the twenty-three-year-old son of a Minneapolis research chemist who had two other "normal" children and was an active member of MARC. Tom had lived at Faribault since he was seven years old. Once strong, well coordinated, and a "very pretty child," he had become "homely and ugly" after years in the institution. He lost muscle control, toilet-training abilities, and his feelings of human warmth. Ironically, Newlund reported, a booming economy and the liberal social programs of the Great Society had left institutions in even worse shape than before. Because people with moderate disabilities could live at home and attendants could get better-paying jobs, Minnesota's public institutions had become the preserve of persons with severe disabilities and workers who had few other options. The state could no longer rely on patients' unpaid labor, and Faribault was terribly understaffed. One evening, Newlund wrote, a night-duty aide was left alone with 163 male patients. Newlund interviewed overworked staff members and portrayed them sympathetically, but the other human beings at Faribault—the patients—remained voiceless and in the shadows.[63]

Newlund's article prompted a flood of letters to the editor and calls for legislative change. Vail wrote, disingenuously, that the article appeared without "the connivance or the foreknowledge" of the Department of Public Welfare, which had to "scrupulously avoid actions which could be construed as bringing pressure to bear on the legislature." Many of the letters were written by parents of children with disabilities. Most were sympathetic. A few, however, reacted with disgust. A Minneapolis woman wrote that better staffing would make little difference to severely disabled patients. "The worst ones, who are merely breathing vegetables, should be gently put to sleep forever," she said. Another reader agreed: Faribault inmates resembled humans only in their superficial "physical characteristics," and families would be better off without the "misfortune of such a sub-being born to them." In *Dehumanization and the Institutional Career*, Vail referred to these letters as examples of the "*man as other* mode of dehumanization." Perhaps, he suggested, "we" (so-called normal people) were responding to the physicality of disability. The involuntary movements and bodily manifestations of difference contributed to a "perception of the unfortunate as *other than human*. . . . How else could we explain the ways in which the mentally disordered have been dealt with?"[64]

Dehumanizing practices at Faribault also affected institutionalized persons who did not have any physical disabilities or stigmata. In 1969, the depressing inarticulateness of even the highest-functioning residents at a total institution captured the imagination of Jean Brust, a Minneapolis socialist who wrote a sympathetic MA thesis on moderately retarded adult women at Faribault. When Brust did her field research, the school was an institution in transition, and the thirty-six women she interviewed were heading toward release. Within six months, all but three had left.[65]

Brust's interviewees lived the consequences of Minnesota eugenics. On average, each woman had lived more than twenty-two years at Faribault. Two-thirds had been committed after the age of fourteen, and their alleged deficiencies were inseparable from either their sexual adventurousness or their abusive families. Peony, for example, had been at Faribault since 1936 and had never been punished or tried to run away. The residents agreed that it was "all her mother's fault. Her mother didn't want her out." Garnet, a "pretty girl, thin, blond, looking and acting younger than her 24 years," was the rebel of the group. She had spent five years at Faribault in the mid-1950s, was discharged to her parents, and then was reinstitutionalized as a teenager when her "heterosexual activity broke the mores of her southern Minnesota hometown." While Brust was doing her field research, Garnet got in trouble: she was seen kissing her steady boyfriend and punished severely. (Patients were allowed to go for walks with their boyfriends twice a week, but hand-holding and kissing were strictly prohibited.) Forbidden to go to social functions for two weeks, Garnet hopped on her bicycle and tried to run away with her boyfriend. After being caught, she was banished to a lesser dormitory where she had to care for bedridden women with severe disabilities. When she returned to her regular cottage two weeks later, Garnet was thin and contrite. But she "inspired little sympathy" from the other residents, and her boyfriend was seeing someone else.[66]

Brust was appalled by the women's passivity and willingness to follow arbitrary rules. She observed no real cliques or friendship dyads and little casual socializing. One evening, when no aide was on duty, several women waited two hours for permission to smoke. Brust concluded that the women were devoid of their own culture apart from the institution rules. She argued that their social failures and repeated rejections, and the resulting low self-esteem, were to blame. "The women in this study have been defined as less-than-human, or lesser humans, by society at large," she concluded. "That they react somewhat like docile children should not be surprising."[67] The discipline and daily humiliations of institution life rendered them permanent children and, as Vail would say, added to the dehumanizing effect.

Vail died in 1971 before the deinstitutionalization movement took hold, but he and Gerald Walsh, MARC's executive director, were important figures in the international reform network that developed the theory of normalization, the idea that people with intellectual disabilities should be able to experience living conditions and routines as close as possible to the norms of mainstream society. Indeed, Sweden's Bengt Nirje first articulated the principle of normalization after a tour of the Faribault School. In the 1960s, Vail and his fellow reformers assumed that the institutions could be humanized, but within a decade many had concluded that dehumanizing practices could not be dislodged from the institutional structure. As Walsh observed soberly in the mid-1960s, even when administrators and superintendents wanted to provide humane, innovative, and individualized care, they were often prevented from doing so because of the dual "lacks of citizen interest and finances from tax funds." As in the past, people classed as dependent and defective were considered undeserving of public aid.[68]

Sterilization and Welfare in the Community

Vail suggested that dehumanizing mental institutions could be usefully compared to the other "singular nest of dehumanization," the welfare office. Community welfare work was much like institution-based psychiatry, he said. It was complicated by "public scorn for the poor, public distrust of the bureaucrats responsible for the work, niggardly budgets aimed at bare survival, and nasty local politics. The result is an impossible quagmire in which rules and regulations run wild; paperwork is burdensome to all concerned—truly unbelievable in its complexity; and deliberate efforts are constantly being made, through the pressure of public suspicion, to keep financial grants to a bare minimum." The very purpose of welfare, it seemed, was to force poor people to live at a "subhuman level." Writing at the height of the War on Poverty, Vail was angry: "A 'war' which is fought in little skirmishes by means of 'projects' scattered around the country is not the answer. The entire welfare system should be 'spaded up from the roots.' "[69]

While Vail waged war against dehumanizing practices in welfare offices and institutions, legal reformers took aim at the bedrock of Minnesota eugenics: the state's much-praised program of state guardianship for people with intellectual disabilities. In 1965, University of Minnesota law professor Robert J. Levy published a withering critique of the state's guardianship program and particularly the gap between the law on the books and the law in action. Levy began by saluting the lofty ideals of the President's Panel on Mental Retardation and the "great strides" in mental retardation research, treatment, and education. He acknowledged the useful protective function of guardianship when relatives were absent or abusive. At the same time, Levy declared, it was not enough to rely on the good intentions of state officials. Coercive legal authority should be kept at a minimum, and human rights should be preserved.[70]

Levy focused on three troubling aspects of Minnesota's guardianship program: the state's virtually unlimited guardianship power, social workers' reliance on outdated ideas about mental retardation, and ungenerous fiscal arrangements. First, Levy observed that despite lip service to individual planning and civil rights, the commissioner of public welfare who acted as public guardian had nearly absolute authority over his mentally retarded wards. Most Minnesotans were unaware of the full extent of the state's power, but the only judicial oversight was the initial hearing in probate court. Yet hearings were rushed and unrecorded, and there was no post-commitment review of any kind. In one fifty-five-minute session in a Hennepin County court, Levy personally observed thirteen persons committed to state guardianship for the rest of their lives. Since probate courts did not have court reporters, the hearings were not recorded. Even the commissioner was not free to restore the individual's civil rights.[71]

Equally disturbing, Levy found that commitments were often based on outdated views of mental retardation. Probate judges relied almost entirely on the assessments of county caseworkers, many of whom still believed the old dictum that mental deficiency was permanent, incurable, and accurately measured by an IQ test. On paper, Mildred Thomson's retirement had brought a major change to Minnesota's mental retardation program and a rejection of routine commitment in favor of open access to community services. In practice, many county welfare workers followed the policies Thomson wrote in the 1920s. Even after the President's Panel called for voluntary institutionalization without the requirement of legal guardianship, many counties still treated the parents of children with intellectual disabilities as if they were also feebleminded, and the DPW (Department of Public Welfare) Manual described voluntary institutionalization as an "injustice" to wards.[72]

Inexcusably, the two main grounds for a mental deficiency commitment—sexual delinquency and economic dependency—had not changed since the 1920s. Although the terminology was different (the word *moron* was no longer used), county welfare departments still treated sexual activity outside marriage—including rape—as a reason for guardianship, and commitments of unmarried mothers were common. Frequently, Levy reported, commitment was a step toward sterilization. If an unsterilized ward got married or became pregnant, the local welfare department might try to arrange emergency placement in an institution to pressure the family to consent to sterilization. In 1960 a woman in her twenties asked if she "had to have" the operation and was told that although "no one would insist" on it, release from the institution would take "longer" if she did not.[73]

One of the most egregious documented examples of abuse in the postwar years involved a Mexican American teenager, who was already under state guardianship as a neglected child when she became pregnant at the age of seventeen. The girl wanted to marry her boyfriend, a nineteen-year-old African American, and he was willing to take responsibility for the child. The caseworker tried to prevent the marriage on the grounds that the girl was underage. When that failed, she started proceedings to commit the teen to state guardianship as mentally deficient and epileptic. (Her IQ scores revealed her to be "dull-normal," and she had had one "epileptic" seizure, which was controlled with medication.) The social worker planned to put the child up for adoption "if and when found suitable."[74]

The teen mother's experience bore a depressing similarity to that of the protagonist in Meridel Le Sueur's Depression-era story "Sequel to Love." She spent three weeks in a locked room at a county hospital before being transferred to Faribault. Her baby was born in March 1960, and the county immediately moved to terminate parental rights. The difference from the 1930s was the response of state officials. The commissioner of public welfare (presumably Coakley acting on his behalf) filed a petition to restore the young woman to capacity and also opposed the termination of her parental rights. But the doctors at Faribault held on to their outdated eugenicist views. They claimed that the girl would pose a "serious problem" in the community (alleging that she was immature and lived in a poor environment) and insisted that she stay in the institution for a "period of training." In the end, the young woman was confined at Faribault for sixteen months before she was released from mental deficiency guardianship and allowed to marry her fiancé.[75]

As this pregnant teenager's horrific experience shows, the constitutional right to liberty and due process carried little meaning for pregnant women who were considered potentially unfit mothers. In fact, Levy declared, official state policy was irrelevant. As long as counties were responsible for welfare costs, "local government parsimony and legislative myopia" encouraged the establishment of guardianship. Counties bore the entire cost of casework services and foster care, which could total $1,800 annually, but when county residents were committed to a state institution, the county's economic responsibility for a "retarded" person dropped to as little as $120. Moreover, since placement on an institution's waiting list was based on the date of guardianship, county workers had a strong economic incentive to proceed with commitment. "Because the counties have tried to save money by maximizing institutional care of the retarded," Levy explained, "poverty has often been the effective reason for the establishment of guardianship." Welfare departments "have misused the guardianship program; many probate judges have completely abdicated their judicial responsibilities." Moreover, he continued, counties often manipulated the guardianship program to control people who were not disabled but simply had "problems."[76]

By the late 1960s, the chorus of opposition to local welfare officials who abused their authority was growing louder. There was also increasing public support for reproductive rights. The approval of the birth control pill in 1960, the family planning services provided through the Office of Economic Opportunity beginning in 1965, and two landmark Supreme Court decisions—*Griswold v. Connecticut* (1965), which upheld a married couple's right to contraceptive use, and *Loving v. Virginia* (1967), which overturned Virginia's eugenics-era antimiscegenation law—dramatically altered the context for sterilization practices and debates. By the end of the decade, the American Bar Foundation reported, only a handful of states averaged more than fifteen eugenic sterilizations per year. In Minnesota, writes historian Philip Reilly, the opposition to sterilization was so strong that in 1969 Faribault officials were unable to convince a judge to authorize the sterilization of a "mildly retarded" woman who had lost custody of her five illegitimate children after "repeated episodes of child abuse." The examining psychiatrist apparently agreed on the "social desirability" of her having no more children but objected to "infringing upon her civil rights through an intervening surgical procedure." He advised birth control pills instead.[77]

Reilly called the period from 1945 to 1970 the "quiet years" in sterilization's history. Public discussion of the issue was infrequent (and dominated by critics of eugenics), even though most states' sterilization programs continued to operate. In a few states, most notably North Carolina, the number of sterilizations actually increased after 1945. As has been mentioned, the targeted population shifted too: eugenic sterilization statutes were now deployed primarily against poor black women, who were labeled mentally retarded because they were unmarried mothers and depended on welfare. In an effort to widen the policy's reach beyond individuals with a mental deficiency designation, ten states drafted (but did not pass) new legislation that criminalized illegitimacy among welfare recipients. Had the laws passed, dependent mothers of two or more illegitimate children would have been potentially subjected to a fine, prison term, the termination of their parental rights, and possibly sterilization. In the most notorious case, the Mississippi legislature approved a 1964 bill that made having a second or subsequent illegitimate child a felony, punishable by three to five years in prison, but allowed those convicted under the law to opt for sterilization "in lieu of imprisonment." Public reaction exploded. The bill was widely condemned by civil rights groups, religious leaders, and mainstream news outlets, such as *Newsweek*, and the sterilization provision was withdrawn. Even the pro-eugenics Association for Voluntary Sterilization called the bill shocking. The Student Nonviolent Coordinating Committee circulated a compelling pamphlet, "Genocide in Mississippi," that underscored the bill's racist aspects. Civil rights leader Fannie Lou Hamer became one of the first women to speak publicly about her own experience of involuntary sterilization. Hamer contended that 60 percent of the women who passed through the hospital in her small Mississippi town had been surgically sterilized. The operation was so common that it was known as a "Mississippi appendectomy," a term that both called attention to the routine nature of sterilization abuse and located it in the segregated South, ignoring the long history of similar "appendectomies" elsewhere in the country.[78]

The proposed Mississippi law exemplified the "return of punitive sterilization proposals." As the pioneering critic of compulsory sterilization Julius Paul observed wryly in 1968, the steep decline in "eugenic" sterilizations had been accompanied by a rise in "voluntary" sterilizations performed on poor women by private physicians, and by a series of "noneugenic" sterilization statutes that tried to ward off rising welfare costs by targeting single mothers on Aid to Families with Dependent Children. Most of these states already had eugenic sterilization laws, and the new proposals were legally unconnected to eugenics. Still, Paul observed perceptively, "Efforts at punishing 'immorality,' 'grossly sexually delinquent behavior' and just plain illegitimacy are much akin to the efforts at the end of the last century and beginning of this century to sterilize criminals, sexual perverts, and other variously defined 'socially degenerate' persons." Although eugenicists had framed their arguments in terms of biological inheritance, and proponents of sterilization in the 1960s talked about morality and money—"the promiscuous poor will procreate us into oblivion"—both eras relied on "a notion of 'fitness' as a precondition for the right to procreate." The economic, racial, and sexual implications of eugenics-era sterilization were little changed, Paul observed; "History apparently *does* repeat itself in selective ways."[79]

At first glance, routine sterilization abuse in southern states and the punitive sterilization proposals of the late 1960s appear to be solid evidence of the eugenics movement's success. Eugenics-era superintendents like Engberg remained in power, and, as several historians suggest, new federally funded programs—specifically, family planning services and the War on Poverty—gave eugenics-minded physicians and welfare workers new tools to inflict mass coercive sterilization. A closer examination of state-level policies and welfare practices, however, tells a more complicated story. Liberal reformers and welfare officials were never as powerful as is often assumed. In the 1960s, as in the past, their ambitions were hampered by America's decentralized welfare authority, the constant struggle over government spending, partisan politics, and the perception of many Americans that the chronically poor and disabled were a drain on the public purse and undeserving of aid. Although reformers succeeded, to some extent, in enlarging the category considered deserving of aid, localism and taxpayer stinginess remained common themes.

Despite pockets of abuse, compulsory eugenic sterilization had few defenders by the late 1960s. As the country grew more and more divided over the Vietnam War, the War on Poverty, Black Power, and women's rights, Americans who agreed on little else found common ground in a deep revulsion over compulsory sterilization and "eugenics"—which they increasingly associated with southern racism and Nazi crimes. Even eugenics organizations expressed their opposition to "compulsory" measures (one even renaming itself the Association for Voluntary Sterilization), and sterilization administrators sought some form of patient consent. Yet the rhetorical repudiation of a seemingly faraway eugenics masked the durability of the social prejudices and economic pressures that drove American sterilization routines, and it deflected attention away from the fundamental issue of economic justice. The gap between eugenics discourse and welfare politics endured.

CONCLUSION

In 1973, a $1,000,000 lawsuit prompted by the sterilization of two young black girls at a federally funded family planning clinic in Alabama blasted the issue of forced sterilization into headlines across the nation. Readers of the *Minneapolis Tribune* learned that fourteen-year-old Minnie Lee Relf and her twelve-year-old sister, Mary Alice, were sterilized because social workers worried that "boys were hanging around the girls" and saw sterilization as the "most convenient" way to ensure they would not get pregnant. The girls' mother, who was illiterate, put her X on the consent form, thinking she was consenting to birth control shots.[1]

The Relf sterilizations exploded into the nation's consciousness after nearly a decade of struggle over civil rights, birth control, and the War on Poverty. The Relfs launched their lawsuit less than six months after the United States Supreme Court's landmark abortion decision, *Roe v. Wade*, and in the midst of congressional hearings on medical experimentation and the forty-year Tuskegee Syphilis Study, a US Public Health Service investigation into the effects of untreated syphilis on black men, which failed to offer the study participants penicillin long after it was found to be an effective treatment for the disease. Both the *Relf* case and the Tuskegee revelations raised troubling questions about official assumptions concerning the sexual behavior of poor Alabama blacks, exposed the tragic effects of medical indifference to informed consent, and evoked comparisons to Nazi Germany. *Relf* presented an opportunity for civil rights and welfare rights activists to bring the personal stories of sterilization survivors to public attention for the first time and exposed a nationwide "epidemic" of sterilization abuse. For many liberals, the realization that the United States had a eugenics-like program of "sterilizing the poor" despite a nine-year War on Poverty was gut-wrenching. As one *New York Times* reporter asked rhetorically, "How did it all happen?"[2]

Relf v. Weinberger is well known to scholars of reproductive rights, but until recently it has received surprisingly little attention from historians of eugenics. This may be because the Relf sisters were sterilized not under Alabama's eugenics statute, but under the auspices of a family planning clinic funded by the Office of Economic Opportunity as part of the War on Poverty. Still, the eugenic connotations of the Relf sterilizations are stunning. Many black activists saw their case as unquestionable proof of the "low esteem in which Black life is held and the genocidal nature of programs supposedly designed to help Blacks." They noted that at least eighty minors had been sterilized at federally funded clinics in the fifteen months before the story broke, and, like ten of the eleven minors sterilized at the Montgomery clinic, most of them were black. Most commentators agree that the Relf sisters' "race and poverty" made them candidates for birth control injections, but that racism was the "true motive" behind their sterilization. As Angela Davis observed in 1981, the "casual sterilization of two Black girls" was a "horrifyingly simple" tale of deception and abuse.[3]

The Relf family tragedy was not merely an expression of the racist or neoeugenic intentions of federal policy makers. Their story also reflected the deep-seated antipathies toward those once known as the defective, dependent, and delinquent classes. The press described Lonnie and Minnie Relf as illiterate black farmhands who had migrated to the city, where they lived in public housing with their six children, and had often been dependent on food stamps and public aid. Mr. Relf was unable to work because of a back injury resulting from a car accident. Both girls, like many children of uneducated southern blacks, were regarded as mentally retarded, a designation the family lawyers accepted for twelve-year-old Mary Alice, who also had a speech impediment and no right hand. As the Southern Poverty Law Center (SPLC) pointed out, "Mental retardation and mental illness have been used as excuses for sterilization of poverty level people where no such necessity existed; and the practice has been widespread." SPLC president Julian Bond told the *New York Times* that "sterilization of the retarded had its precedent in Nazi Germany. This whole thing is an attack on privacy, innocence, and the right of motherhood."[4]

Although the Relf sisters were sterilized amid liberalizing attitudes toward birth control and a surge in "voluntary" surgical sterilizations, a comparison between the Alabama and Minnesota sterilization programs is instructive. The racial and regional contexts were different, but both programs manifested depressingly similar attitudes about sex, welfare, and supposed mental deficiency. The (white) director of the Montgomery clinic sounded much like Mildred Thomson when she defended the decision to sterilize Minnie and Mary Alice. She said that child-rearing would place too great a burden on the mentally incapable girls (who were not even "disciplined enough" to take birth control pills), and there had been "no misunderstanding" about the operation. Mrs. Relf was fully informed about the nature of the surgery and gave her voluntary consent. In addition, the clinic director insisted, racism could not be a factor in the decision because the nurses who took the girls to the hospital were black. In Montgomery as in Minneapolis, nurses and social workers frustrated by their clients' persistent poverty and worried about the economic and social costs of out-of-wedlock births emphasized the connection between welfare dependency, sexual delinquency, and mental deficiency. They saw sterilization as a simple fix that would provide "protection" for poor, supposedly subnormal girls and taxpayers alike.[5]

What was different in the 1970s was the scale of the sterilization program, the juridical context, and the enormity of the public response. As many as 150,000 low-income persons were sterilized under federally funded programs in the early 1970s, and although specific sterilizations encountered little organized opposition in Mildred Thomson's day, the Relf sisters' sterilizations provoked an enormous response. Coming on the heels of the black freedom and feminist movements and a series of court decisions that affirmed reproduction as a basic privacy right, Judge Gerhard Gesell's 1974 decision in *Relf v. Weinberger* found "uncontroverted evidence" that minors and legal incompetents were being improperly sterilized and an "indefinite number" of people were coerced into consenting to sterilization by threats that their welfare benefits would be withdrawn. He placed an immediate prohibition on the use of federal funds for involuntary sterilizations and for the sterilizations of minors or mental incompetents, whose capacity for voluntary consent was in doubt. The judge also ordered the US Department of Health, Education, and Welfare (HEW) to establish new guidelines to ensure that federally funded family planning sterilizations were truly voluntary. Even if "irresponsible reproduction . . . places increasing numbers of unwanted or mentally defective children into tax-supported institutions," Gesell wrote, Congress and not individual social workers or physicians should determine sterilization policy. "The dividing line between family planning and eugenics is murky," and the country "should not drift into a policy" that deprives citizens of their procreative abilities without "adequate legal safeguards and a legislative determination of the appropriate standards in light of the general welfare and of individual rights."[6]

The Relf lawsuit inspired other sterilization survivors to come forward, and their stories revealed widespread sterilization abuse. Less than a month after the case became public in June 1973, sterilizations elsewhere in the South hit the news. First, a New York nurse named Nial Cox sued the state of North Carolina for sterilizing her under the state's eugenics statute when she was eighteen years old. The surgeon had characterized Cox as a "mentally defective Negro girl," but the American Civil Liberties Union contended that she was sterilized because she was "black, a member of a welfare family, and at the time of operation, a minor." Minors considered mentally defective could be sterilized under North Carolina's eugenics law if their parents gave consent, and Cox's mother had been told that her family of ten would lose their welfare benefits if she refused to consent to the surgery. A week after Cox brought her suit, a group of welfare mothers in Aiken County, South Carolina, complained about several local obstetricians who had refused to treat welfare mothers with three or more children unless they agreed to be sterilized; sixteen of the eighteen sterilized mothers were black. While one of the doctors justified his action by the "heavy tax burden welfare was causing," many African Americans saw unwanted sterilization as a form of genocide—and some whites agreed. One academic told the *New York Times* that many whites unconsciously saw birth control as a "way to save the white race from being overwhelmed."[7]

In October, Ralph Nader's Health Research Group issued a report on the "epidemic of sterilization" which brought further attention to the issue. One million vasectomies and one million female sterilizations were performed annually, the Nader group wrote, but there was "little evidence of informed consent." Doctors "cavalierly" subjected poor, black women to sterilization because doctors and teaching hospitals needed bodies on which to practice their surgical techniques, and they used "deceptive marketing practices" to "sell" the operations to consumers. "Almost every major teaching hospital had doubled the number of elective tubal ligations in the past two years," the Nader group observed, calling on the HEW to issue stringent guidelines to prevent further indiscriminate sterilizations.[8]

Despite their own state's history, most Minnesotans followed these stories of sterilization abuse with detachment. Even a 1974 report written for the state legislature, "Sterilization: Use, Misuse and Abuse," had remarkably little to say about Minnesota's past or present sterilization practice. Tricia Farris's report began with the story of the Relf sisters and then followed Nader's Health Research Group in describing the dramatic increase in voluntary sterilizations as a "dangerous epidemic of abuse rather than a clear-cut choice of sterilization as a form of contraception." Like the Nader group and Judge Gesell, Farris recognized that "many classes of persons" were "extremely susceptible to coercion" and stressed that legal consent must be "voluntary, competent, and knowing." Yet although Farris mentioned that Minnesota had a sterilization statute dating back to 1925, she did not discuss the state's once-aggressive eugenics program. Instead, she focused much of her energy on sterilization abuse among minors, women of color, and the poor. Regarding minors, Farris observed that Minnesota law and federal court decisions were contradictory and argued that safeguards should be established to ensure that consent was "truly informed and voluntary." On the sterilization of racial minorities and the poor, she took a stronger stand. She noted that despite the efforts of "civil libertarians and various 'pro-life groups'" that adamantly opposed public funding for sterilizations, a "growing minority" of states were contemplating legislation that would require unwed welfare mothers to undergo sterilization. Quoting four prominent female members of the Congressional Black Caucus, Farris wrote that the "heart of the issue" was the need to make family planning services universally available, while still ensuring that "no element of coercion creeps into programs which Congress has specifically mandated must be voluntary in nature." On this matter, Farris maintained, the law was clear: from *Skinner* to *Roe*, the courts repeatedly held that the right to privacy included the right to be "free from unwarranted government intrusion into matters so fundamentally affecting a person as the decision whether to bear or beget a child."[9]

Farris struggled to show the relevance of the national sterilization scandal to Minnesota, conceding in her report that "the existence and/or extent of such abuse in Minnesota is difficult to ascertain." A study by the Minnesota Civil Liberties Union had revealed no formal reports of sterilization abuse, although two sources indicated that "several welfare mothers" were coerced into sterilization during childbirth or legal abortion. Farris's unnamed sources "spoke favorably of DPW programs and personnel on the state level" and indicated that coercion was "least likely" to occur in the Twin Cities. However, they had "less confidence" in county programs, especially in rural areas. Remarkably, she had nothing to say about the sterilization of indigenous women.[10]

The sterilization of persons with intellectual disabilities presented Farris with a thorny problem. When she submitted her report, Minnesota's eugenic sterilization law was still on the books, and legal opinion about the "voluntary" sterilization of mentally retarded persons was divided. In *Relf v. Weinberger*, Judge Gesell had disputed the ability of mental incompetents to meet the standard of a truly voluntary consent and ordered a moratorium on federal funding for such sterilizations. However, several state courts upheld laws permitting the involuntary sterilization of persons with serious mental deficiencies. Compared to them, Minnesota's sterilization law looked enlightened. It applied "only" to mentally retarded wards of the state and mentally ill inmates of state hospitals and was "considered to be voluntary" because it required the written consent of kin (and personal consent in the case of the mentally ill). In addition, Farris pointed out, administrative regulations went further than the law in protecting a person who had become a ward of the state from being coerced. The Department of Public Welfare required the personal consent of the mentally deficient ward and explicitly rejected sterilization on "social management grounds."[11] (Farris seemed unaware that personal consent had been an administrative requirement since Thomson's day and made no reference to Robert Levy's scathing critique of Minnesota's guardianship program.) In any case, the number of sterilizations performed under the law seemed to be small. One sterilization was reported between 1964 and 1970 (on an institutionalized ward in 1969), and eighteen sterilizations performed on wards living in the community were reported between 1970 and 1973.[12]

While administrative regulations and the law provided some protection to state wards, medical decisions affecting mentally retarded persons not under public guardianship were "left to the arbitrary discretion of individual doctors and hospitals." There was nothing to prevent the sterilization of a non-ward on "social management grounds," and Farris said that two or three mentally retarded girls in early adolescence were given vaginal hysterectomies "to relieve them and their parents of ever having to deal with the girls' sexuality." In the absence of clear statutory guidelines, she wrote, it "appears hazardous" to rely on the good faith and sound judgment of individual doctors and welfare officials. A "clarification of legislative intent, a determination of state policy, and the implementation of adequate procedural safeguards" were "urgently needed."[13]

That clarification came in 1975 when the Minnesota legislature revised its eugenics-era guardianship and sterilization laws. Fifty years after legalizing eugenic sterilization, the state enacted the Minnesota Mental Retardation Protection Act, which placed significant limits on the state's authority over its mentally retarded citizens and affirmed a new policy of providing a "coordinated approach to [their] supervision, protection and habilitation." The vague outdated definition of a "mentally deficient person" (as someone "so mentally defective as to require treatment or supervision for his own or the public welfare") was replaced with an updated and supposedly more precise description. A "mentally retarded person," the new law stated, was someone who had been "diagnosed as having significantly subaverage intellectual functioning existing concurrently with demonstrated deficits in adaptive behavior such as to require supervision and protection for his welfare or the public welfare." The law also established a new category of conservatorship, which gave the commissioner of public welfare "some, but not all" of the powers of public guardian without depriving the person with an intellectual disability of the right to vote.[14]

The 1975 law aimed to protect mentally retarded Minnesotans from violations of their civil rights by strengthening the procedural safeguards of the commitment process and specifying the powers the commissioner held as guardian or conservator. The commissioner retained broad powers over the ward's residence, medical care, education, employment, property transactions, and ability to marry, but the new law also limited the state's power to institutionalize the ward by stipulating that supervisory authority should be exercised in a "manner which is least restrictive of the ward's personal freedom consistent with the need for supervision and protection."[15]

The new law also replaced Minnesota's fifty-year-old sterilization statute, adding new procedural safeguards and strengthening the role of the court. Adult conservatees who retained the right to consent to surgery could be sterilized only after providing their written consent and certifying that a doctor or nurse had given them a "full explanation" of the "nature and irreversible consequences of the sterilization operation." For those under full guardianship, the law required judicial determination that the surgery was in the "best interest" of the ward. Even more than in the past, expert testimony was central to this determination: a licensed physician, a psychologist with expertise in the area of mental retardation, and a social worker familiar with the specific case were required to submit written reports addressing the medical risks of surgery and whether "alternative methods of contraception" would be just as effective. Despite new safeguards, in other words, Minnesota continued to permit the surgical sterilization of young people and adults with intellectual disabilities, as long as there was a court order.[16]

Outside of Minnesota, the routine practice of and debate over contraceptive sterilization—now inextricably bound up with the battles over birth control, abortion, and welfare—continued to grow. By 1977, nearly 10 million Americans, and about 30 percent of married couples between the ages of fifteen and forty-four, had been surgically sterilized. Sterilization rates varied significantly by sex, race, income, and age, and while white married couples generally chose sterilization, many poor women did not. Low-income women of color were much more likely than affluent whites to be sterilized before the age of thirty-five. As before, welfare recipients were especially susceptible. According to one study, the sterilization rate of welfare recipients was 49 percent higher than nonrecipients, and 67 percent higher among those with three or more children. The statistical evidence of such disparities created a "suspicion of involuntariness," feminist sociologist and reproductive rights activist Rosalind Pollack Petchesky contended, and it raised troubling questions about the nature of "voluntary" sterilizations chosen in the context of "heavy structural constraints."[17]

While the specter of eugenics haunted the sterilization debate, the social and legal context in the 1970s was very different from fifty years earlier. Both sides now talked openly about sexuality and claimed to be champions of human rights. Family planning experts, advocates for the "retarded," and some feminists campaigned for easier access to contraceptive sterilization, while other feminists joined welfare activists and people of color in seeing "family planning" and "voluntary" sterilization as euphemisms for racial extermination and genocide. The two sides clashed over HEW's proposed sterilization guidelines, especially the requirement of a thirty-day waiting period, and took opposing positions in several lawsuits. Pro-sterilization groups argued that the waiting period and other HEW restrictions constituted a "barrier to access," especially in rural areas, and reduced poor women's reproductive freedom. They maintained that women with mild retardation had the capacity to understand that sterilization was irreversible, and the moratorium on federal funding for their sterilization was a paternalistic denial of their reproductive rights. Organizations more concerned about sterilization abuse, on the other hand, focused on racist power structures, a punitive welfare system, and the importance of ensuring noncoerced consent. By mid-decade, the *New York Times* reported, the sterilization issue had become just as volatile as abortion: "It has made adversaries out of longtime allies, it has pitted consumer, medical institution and government agency against one another; it has raised questions of economics, race and class."[18]

Always, the debate was framed in terms of racism, eugenics, and welfare. While population control lobbyists stoked fears of a population explosion and presented family planning and voluntary sterilization as solutions to rising welfare costs and the global "population bomb," women of color sought redress for unwanted surgeries and the denial of their reproductive rights. In Los Angeles in 1975, ten Mexican immigrant women filed a class action suit against a Los Angeles teaching hospital, charging that they were coerced into signing English-language sterilization consent forms, often during labor. In addition to financial compensation, they sought more stringent regulations to prevent further abuses, including Spanish-language counseling and consent forms. Although the women lost their case—the court ruled that there was a "communication breakdown" but that the doctors had acted in "good faith"—their efforts led to improved sterilization consent procedures and the creation of a Chicana movement for reproductive rights.[19]

Closer to Minnesota, Native American activists also fought against astonishingly high sterilization rates in their communities. At least 25 percent of indigenous women between the ages of fifteen and forty-four were reportedly sterilized in the early 1970s, and a Government Accountability Office investigation found an astonishing 3,406 sterilizations performed in four of the twelve Indian Health Service (IHS) program areas between 1973 and 1976. (Minnesota was not included in the study.) Thirty-six of the sterilized women were under the age of twenty-one, despite the HEW moratorium on the sterilization of minors. IHS record keeping was inadequate, the investigation concluded, and federal guidelines for soliciting consent were ignored. Some women were told they would lose welfare benefits or medical care if they did not agree to the surgery; others were misinformed about its permanence. One researcher told the story of twenty-eight-year-old Julie, who was sterilized against her will at an IHS facility in Minnesota. She signed the consent form during labor, thinking she was consenting to a painkiller. To many indigenous leaders, the sterilizations performed at IHS facilities were "an insidious scheme to get the Indians' land once and for all" or a modern form of genocide, "which has been going on for hundreds of years, to totally exterminate the Red man." But some activists also pointed to the economic-welfare aspects of the policy. Dr. Constance Pinkerton-Uri, the Choctaw–Cherokee doctor who brought the IHS sterilizations to light, critiqued "the warped thinking of doctors who think the solution to poverty is not to allow people to be born."[20]

The intensity of the sterilization debate—and the dramatic shift in attitudes about sexuality, disability, and individual reproductive rights—is revealed in a pioneering volume, *The Mentally Retarded Citizen and the Law*, published in 1976 by the President's Committee on Mental Retardation. Unlike President Kennedy's 1962 Panel on Mental Retardation, which did not question the need for restrictions on the marriage and childbearing of people with intellectual disabilities, the 1976 President's Committee stressed its commitment to civil rights. The committee acknowledged that poor people and racial minorities were often wrongly classified as mentally retarded, but it insisted that regardless of the accuracy of the label, individuals described in this manner should receive equal treatment under the law and the "full enjoyment" of their personal and civil rights. In her foreword to the volume, Eunice Kennedy Shriver was unequivocal in her defense of every citizen's right to a sexual and family life, including the right to have children. She described guardianship as "totally unjustified" for persons with mild retardation and asserted the need for a mentally retarded citizen's "bill of rights."[21]

The volume also contained a searing critique of third-party consent to medical procedures, such as that used for decades in Minnesota. Government control had become more "sophisticated and appealing—and more subtle" since the days when "fear of 'three generations of imbeciles'" justified compulsory sterilization, legal scholars Monroe Price and Robert Burt observed. Experts now talked "confidently about 'good parenting' or breaking the vicious cycle of three generations of welfare clients," but they still deprived persons designated mentally retarded of their constitutional rights. Price and Burt strongly denounced the doctrine of third-party consent, whereby legal consent was granted by a parent or public guardian instead of the person directly involved. Third-party consent made state intervention appear to be freely chosen, they cautioned, and it virtually erased the "always thin line between involuntary and voluntary action." In the era of community care and normalization, new legal measures to protect individual rights were needed.[22]

The urgent need for new civil rights protections was made clear in one of the few sterilization cases that the United States Supreme Court consented to hear, *Stump v. Sparkman* (1978). In 1971, an Indiana mother filed a petition in DeKalb County Circuit Court to sterilize her fifteen-year-old daughter Linda, who was described as "somewhat retarded" although she attended public school and was promoted each year with her class. The symptoms of Linda's mental retardation were that she was socializing and "staying overnight" with "older youth and young men." Judge Harold D. Stump approved the order without notifying Linda, appointing a guardian ad litem to represent the girl's interests, or holding a hearing. Linda was not told about the sterilization order (she was told she was having an appendectomy), and she did not learn she was sterilized until several years later, when she was married and trying to get pregnant. After learning she had been sterilized, Linda sued her mother, her mother's lawyer, the doctor who performed the operation, the hospital, and the judge. The court rejected her suit, stating that judges had immunity from damage suits and that the judge's order also gave the other defendants immunity. The case went to the United States Supreme Court, which ruled 5–3 that Judge Stump had absolute immunity and could not be sued. Writing for the majority, Justice Byron White explained that the fact that the judge's ruling in this case had "tragic consequences" was irrelevant; indeed, the controversy surrounding sterilization was "all the more reason that he should be able to act without fear of suit."[23]

In a blistering dissent, Justice Potter Stewart described Stump's actions as "beyond the pale." Yet because the majority chose not to comment on the violations of Linda Sparkman's due process or procreative rights, the case set no precedent on sterilization policy or procedures. It indirectly influenced the thinking of individual judges, however, by assuring them that there would be no penalty for a bad decision. After *Stump*, most judges held that the courts had jurisdiction to authorize sterilization for a mentally retarded person, even when they disagreed with the decision to sterilize Linda. One jurist wrote disapprovingly that *Stump* had a "catalytic effect" and provided a "de facto point of departure" for the nonconsensual court-ordered sterilization of persons with intellectual disabilities. *Stump* was a heartbreaking illustration of the terrible vulnerability of the poor and the young, another critic observed; "Several adults conspired to victimize a teenage girl, and no one was held responsible."[24]

While *Stump* opened the door for private sterilizations, the long-awaited publication of the HEW guidelines in 1978 established some restrictive parameters for federally funded sterilizations. HEW prohibited the use of federal funds to sterilize persons deemed incapable of providing informed consent, including minors, people in institutions, and the mentally incompetent. It also proscribed efforts to obtain consent during labor or abortion or by threatening to cut the welfare or Medicaid benefits of nonconsenting patients, and it mandated a thirty-day waiting period between the signing of a consent form and the actual surgery. In addition, the new guidelines standardized procedures to ensure that patients were informed about the risks and irreversibility of sterilization in their preferred language.[25] Privately funded sterilizations were unaffected by these rules, however, and judicial decisions varied.

Most courts tried to balance an opposition to eugenic coercion with the right to *choose* contraceptive surgery. A New Jersey case, *In the Matter of Lee Ann Grady* (1981), is just one example. Lee Ann Grady was a nineteen-year-old with "severe Down syndrome" who lived at home and attended special education classes. Her parents believed that sterilization would enhance their daughter's independence and ability to live a normal life as she grew older. When the hospital refused to perform the operation without court authorization, the Gradys asked the court to allow them, as her legal guardians, to provide proxy consent to sterilization. In ruling on the case, the New Jersey Supreme Court attempted to strike a balance between the right to be protected from coerced sterilization and the right to obtain sterilization voluntarily. The court emphasized that sterilization had "a sordid past in this country—especially from the viewpoint of the mentally retarded," but also stressed that reproductive autonomy was a constitutional right "personal to the individual," even if the individual were unable to exercise it, and (as *Stump* made clear) the interests of Lee Ann and her parents were not the same. For that reason, decisions about the sterilization of people with intellectual disabilities should always be made by the courts. Given the past history of sterilization abuse, however, the court spelled out strict procedural safeguards and a number of factors that judges should consider when determining whether someone like Lee Ann should be sterilized. These included appointing a guardian ad litem to represent the prospective patient's interests in court, receiving independent medical and psychological assessments of her condition, and meeting with the patient to determine whether sterilization was in her best interests. Despite these procedural safeguards, another court criticized *Grady* for effectively equating a court-ordered sterilization with the choice Lee Ann would have made. A court-ordered sterilization decision was "not a personal choice, and no amount of legal legerdemain can make it so," it observed, raising the question of how much had changed.[26]

Despite the impassioned debates over sterilization, most welfare officials and advocates for persons with intellectual disabilities in Minnesota were more absorbed by the continuing problems in the state's public institutions. The institutional population had declined sharply in the 1960s and early 1970s, as special education programs and community-based services enabled parents to care for their children at home, but conditions remained dire in spite of a decade of reform. Many reformers who had been optimistic about institutional reform in the early 1960s now saw the institutions themselves as the problem.[27]

Three events in 1972 signaled a change. In January, television reporter Geraldo Rivera took an early morning visit to New York's Willowbrook State School and exposed a large television audience to shocking images of emaciated people in dormitories and halls. Rivera described Willowbrook as a "leper colony" and charged that conditions at the school were worse than they had been when Senator Robert F. Kennedy, in 1965, had described it as a snake pit. The next month, family members filed a class action lawsuit, launching the process that would eventually lead to the school's closure. Three months later, US district court judge Frank M. Johnson Jr. of Alabama issued his landmark decision, *Wyatt v. Stickney*. Named for fifteen-year-old Ricky Wyatt, an unruly young offender who had been committed to a state psychiatric institution even though he showed no signs of mental illness, the class action suit focused on the inhumane conditions and lack of treatment in three Alabama state institutions. Judge Johnson ruled that depriving a human being of liberty and failing to provide treatment violated the due process clause of the Fourteenth Amendment. He laid out minimum standards on matters such as staff–patient ratios, sanitation, and nutrition and insisted on the preservation of basic patient rights, including the right to privacy, the right to communicate with outsiders, compensation for labor, and freedom from medical treatment or experimentation without informed consent.[28]

Then, in August, a career navy man named Richard Welsch filed a similar class action suit against Minnesota's commissioner of public welfare and six state institutions. Welsch's twenty-one-year-old daughter, Patty, had lived at the Cambridge State Hospital since she was a child, but had received no education or treatment for her autism. The hospital was essentially a warehouse, her mother later said. Patty was heavily medicated, and on one unannounced visit, Mr. Welsch found his daughter tied to a bed. A two-week trial in late 1973 focused on the gaping contrast between modern scientific research, which proved that people with severe intellectual disabilities had the capacity to develop and improve, and the inhumane living conditions in Minnesota public institutions. Judge Earl Larson was persuaded. In a historic 1974 decision, he ruled that there was "overwhelming and convincing" evidence that habilitative services could improve the lives of hospital residents, and that "everyone, no matter the degree or severity of retardation, is capable of growth and development if given adequate and suitable treatment." Without treatment, he said, being hospitalized for mental retardation was like being imprisoned indefinitely without being convicted of a crime. Judge Larson ordered a number of changes, including improvements in staff–resident ratios, based on the *Wyatt* standard.[29]

Despite Judge Larson's ruling, the state failed to appropriate the funds needed for compliance. It also appealed a series of enforcement orders. Finally, in 1980 the Welsch–Noot Consent Decree required the state to reduce the number of people living in Minnesota state institutions by one-third over a six-year period. Discharged residents were to be placed in community programs appropriate to their "individual needs." As a result, the institutionalized population declined. The Faribault Regional Center closed in 1998.[30]

While deinstitutionalization was under way, new federal legislation extended civil rights protections to people with developmental disabilities. In 1973, the Rehabilitation Act and the Developmental Disabilities Assistance and Bill of Rights Act prohibited discrimination in federally funded programs and services and authorized protection and advocacy programs to prevent exploitation, abuse, and human rights violations. The 1975 Education for All Handicapped Children Act (later the Individuals with Disabilities Education Act, or IDEA) established every child's right to a "free appropriate public education" designed to meet his or her unique needs. Former institution residents moved into the community, school-age children integrated into mainstream schools, and the independent living movement gained strength. Soon, the voices of people with intellectual disabilities—self-advocates—were heard in public for the first time. A generation earlier, parent activists spoke on behalf of retarded "children," but now self-advocates insisted that adults with developmental disabilities could speak and act for themselves. They challenged the stigma of being "retarded" and asserted the right to make their own life decisions without being unduly influenced or controlled by others. They were "people first."[31]

In telling their stories and asserting their own self-worth, self-advocates emphasized the importance of history. In 1994, several Minnesota disability rights organizations formed Remembering with Dignity to "honor people who lived and died in Minnesota's state institutions." The group's first major project, which began when institutions were closing, was to replace the anonymous numbered graves of people buried in institution cemeteries with proper gravestones that included each individual's name. The group also collected oral histories of institution survivors and sought a formal apology from the state. Importantly, Remembering with Dignity demanded redress for the whole range of abuses that Minnesotans identified as having developmental disabilities or mental illness had suffered, and not for sterilization alone. Since the opening of the Faribault School in 1879, Remembering with Dignity declared, tens of thousands of Minnesotans had been taken from their families and communities, forced to labor without compensation, and subjected to medical experiments and procedures without their consent—including shock treatments, frontal lobotomies, isolation, aversive drug therapies, pain-based treatment regimens, and "the routine subjection of women inmates to involuntary sterilizations." State officials had depicted their fellow Minnesotans as "subhuman organisms, as deviant individuals to be feared by society, and as eternal children unaccountable for their behavior and incapable of speaking for themselves or shaping their own lives, which greatly diminished their fellow citizens' ability and willingness to accept them for their own unique qualities."[32]

The state of Minnesota issued a formal apology for its past treatment of people with disabilities in 2010. After a long thirteen-year campaign and testimony by people who had spent part of their childhoods in the state institutions, both houses of the legislature voted unanimously to pass the apology resolution, which was signed by Governor Tim Pawlenty. The official apology was momentous for the individuals and families affected by institutionalization, but it was less robust than the original resolution written by Remembering with Dignity, and Governor Pawlenty qualified it further in a letter emphasizing that state employees were acting in good faith and according to the scientific understanding of the time. Worse, the formal apology coincided with deep cuts to social services for poor people and people with disabilities. The apology about past practices was "very powerful and meaningful" to the people affected by them, disability rights organizer Rick Cardenas told a reporter, "but I want to remind you that we'll probably have to apologize for practices we have in place now and some point in the future."[33]

It is a cruel irony that the important legal and symbolic gains for people with disabilities coincided with an increasingly punishing approach to welfare dependency and sexual delinquency. Since the 1980s, amid recurring moral panics about drug addiction, child abuse, and crime, the ever-present fissure between the rhetoric of human rights and the realities of fiscal politics has developed into an open sore. Despite the Americans with Disabilities Act, several formal apologies issued by state governors for their sterilization programs, and a general revulsion against "eugenics," eugenics-like welfare policies persist and may even be on the rise, albeit in a new form. Most warnings about the resurgence of eugenics point to the most extreme examples, such as the highly publicized Project Prevention (formerly CRACK), a private organization that offers cash incentives to drug- or alcohol-addicted women willing to use long-term birth control or get sterilized, or to new reproductive technologies, such as preimplantation genetic diagnosis, which raise the specter of human genetic engineering and "reprogenetics." Yet the vast majority of present-day eugenics strategies are bureaucratic and mundane, just as they were in the past. There is "little need" to resort to sterilization today, the President's Committee on Mental Retardation observed more than forty years ago, and society is "too sophisticated to talk eugenics, at least aloud." As a result, "more modern and more acceptable interventions," such as child neglect statutes and criminal incarceration, have stepped in to take sterilization's place.[34]

The child welfare and criminal justice systems have emerged as leading instruments of eugenics control in the twenty-first century in part because they are easily reconciled with religious qualms about abortion, sterilization, and reprogenetic technologies. Just as Minnesota's 1917 Children's Code ranked the seemingly innocent children of deserving mothers above the supposedly menacing offspring of so-called defectives, current economic and social policies encourage affluent Americans to have children, while deterring childbearing and child-rearing by low-income women and single mothers, especially women with disabilities, drug addicts, and poor women of color. Echoes of Progressive Era eugenic jurisprudence can be seen in the sentencing and probation conditions imposed by both civil and criminal courts, and Minnesota's interwar eugenics program of commitment, institutionalization, and sterilization bears no small resemblance to the aggressive child protection and prison systems operating today.[35]

Indeed, prisons today serve many of the same functions as public institutions for the insane and feebleminded during the heyday of eugenics: they break up troublesome families, reduce the number of babies born to the "defective, dependent, and delinquent" classes, and promise to protect society from danger by keeping people considered dark, oversexed, and menacing "out of sight and out of mind." The news that nearly 150 women were illegally sterilized in California prisons between 2006 and 2010 led to a flurry of warnings that eugenics was "alive and well in the United States," but more routine cruelties, such as the overzealous termination of parental rights and the surge in the number of mothers incarcerated for drug offenses and nonviolent crimes, remain underreported. Nor has there been much public attention to health conditions or the high rate of disability within the prison population, although disability is exceedingly high; in 2011–2012, about 40 percent of women and 31 percent of men in prison reported a disability, nearly three times as high as the general population. Thirty percent of female prisoners reported a cognitive disability. While disability may be a contributing factor leading to a prison sentence, conditions in federal and state prisons and local jails, and indeed the very fact of incarceration, can be dehumanizing and disabling.[36]

Outside of prison, the child welfare system gives renewed strength to a eugenics-like stratification of motherhood. The 1996 welfare reform bill, which ended the federal Aid to Families with Dependent Children program established as mothers' pensions by early twentieth-century maternalist reformers, instituted strict work requirements, lifetime limits on benefits, measures to reduce illegitimacy and promote marriage, and the restoration of local responsibility and control. The Adoption and Safe Families Act made it easier to remove "at risk" children from families thought to be abusive, fast-tracking the termination of their parental rights. As in the past, tax-cutting politicians, beleaguered social workers, and elected judges convinced themselves and a large part of the public that reducing child-rearing among the "unfit" would save tax dollars and solve a host of social problems. As historian Rickie Solinger warns, motherhood is becoming a "class privilege" in America.[37]

Obviously, the United States is not as far removed from its eugenicist past as many people would like to believe. If terms like "feebleminded" and "mental deficiency" have fallen into disrepute, the images of impairment which drove early eugenics policies are still deployed in punitive welfare, drug, and crime control policies. Yet these programs are rarely recognized as eugenics inspired, just as the social welfare orientation and "bureaucentricity" of America's eugenics past have been overlooked. Today, sophisticated psychiatric and biomedical diagnoses, rather than dubious theories of human heredity, justify a range of interventions to "fix" the poor and help us avoid taking a hard look at the structural causes of poverty and dependency. Yet, as Minnesota's history shows, eugenic sterilization was never only about "race betterment" or social engineering; from the beginning, state sterilization policies were rooted in a chronically underfunded and locally variable public welfare system that pathologized persistent poverty and disparaged welfare-dependent individuals as mentally incompetent and undeserving. Such a welfare system exists to this day. Only by recognizing these continuities and acknowledging the mundane and deeply gendered aspects of sterilization's history can we begin to construct a society that is truly resistant to eugenics abuse.

Sterilization Data

State sterilization statistics are exceedingly unreliable. Poor record keeping, differences in state laws and administrative procedures, and perhaps even the willful destruction of evidence make it difficult to measure the full impact of America's sterilization programs. Sterilizations were sometimes performed in states without a sterilization law or in hospitals lacking oversight from sterilization administrators. Clerical errors and inconsistencies in reporting methods compound the problem. Some states compiled statistics annually, while others published biennial reports. Some counted operations performed between January 1 and December 31, while others used July 1 to June 30 as the reporting period or based their official reports on operations authorized but not necessarily performed during the reporting period.

Even a seemingly simple question—what counts as a eugenic sterilization?—can be difficult to answer. Some statutes, including Minnesota's, specify the type of operation that could be legally performed (e.g., tubectomy or vasectomy). Others left the type of surgery to the discretion of a physician or administrator, thereby expanding the kind of procedures that could potentially be counted as eugenic sterilization. The difficulty of categorizing—and counting—eugenic sterilizations is illustrated in the 1942 biennial report of Minnesota's Rochester State Hospital. A detailed list of 77 minor operations and 116 major operations, including thirteen hysterectomies, nine hysterectomies with salpingectomies, and five other salpingectomies (three of them done with other operations), is followed by a simple statement: "2 women sterilization operations were performed."[1] When compiling sterilization statistics, I have adhered to official reports; therefore, table 4.3 lists two sterilizations (not twenty-seven) performed at Rochester in 1941–42 and generally excludes hysterectomies from the number of sterilizations reported for the other years as well. My reliance on official reporting clearly results in undercounting sterilization operations. It also privileges administrators' objectives over the patients' experience.

The sterilization data I used in this volume come from two very different sources: (1) national reports from the pro-sterilization Human Betterment Association, now part of the Association for Voluntary Sterilization (AVS) Records at the Social Welfare History Archives, and (2) the records of the Faribault State School and Hospital, where most eugenic sterilizations in Minnesota were performed. Although table 4.3 records the number of sterilizations listed in the biennial reports of the Rochester State Hospital, I found only scattered references to sterilization in other state hospitals. Faribault is the only Minnesota institution that has sufficient sterilization records for meaningful analysis.

The AVS sterilization statistics are based on surveys and questionnaires that Ezra S. Gosney's Human Betterment Foundation and, later, the Human Betterment Association (formerly known as Birthright and the Sterilization League of New Jersey) sent to institution superintendents and other state authorities. Only sterilizations "officially reported" in states having a sterilization law are included, and the data are biased toward institutionalized persons designated mentally deficient or mentally ill. The statistics from the interwar years are particularly unreliable. For example, in 1928 Gosney's foundation reported incorrectly that Minnesota had sterilized 214 men (it transposed the numbers of male and female sterilizations), but in 1930 it listed just thirty-two Minnesota men sterilized up to January 1 of that year. Moreover, the last AVS report is dated December 31, 1963, when a few southern states' sterilization programs were in full swing.[2]

As flawed as the AVS statistics are, they provide the fullest picture of Minnesota's sterilization program in relation to other states. They also have the advantage of distinguishing between sterilizations performed on women and those performed on men. Even though the AVS reports stop in 1963, they remain the principal source for most scholars' statistics on the "total" number of operations performed under US sterilization laws. Although other studies appear to use more recent data, table A.1 matches the total sterilizations reported by other scholars, with my lower numbers for North Carolina and Virginia the most important exceptions.[3] For consistency's sake, I have chosen to restrict my analysis of sterilization data to a single source, the AVS reports. One final note: in addition to the AVS statistics, table 4.2 uses recorded Census Bureau information to calculate the approximate size of each state at the midpoint between the years in which the census was taken, that is, 1935, 1945, and 1955. These dates were used to provide a more accurate picture of each decade's sterilization rate per 100,000 population.

The analysis in chapter 4 is based on a database of the first thousand sterilization operations performed at the Faribault State School and Hospital, which Liza Piper expertly compiled and analyzed in June 2002.[4] The original register, recorded by hand in a large, leather-bound book, lists the patient's name, birth date, place of residence, and IQ (occasionally recorded as "mental age"), along with the date and nature of the operation(s), "pathalogical [*sic*] condition" found, and information about discharge. Administrative matters, such as who authorized the operation, who provided legal consent, and when and to whom the person was discharged, were also recorded. Postoperative complications, escapes, readmissions, and deaths were also noted. Unfortunately, the last entry in the record book is April 16, 1937, when the sterilization program was at its peak. Readers are reminded, therefore, that the analysis of the database encompasses fewer than half of the 2,350 sterilizations reported in Minnesota.

TABLE A.1

Sterilizations performed under US state sterilization statutes [through December 31, 1963]

State	Date of enactment	Female	Male	Total
Alabama	1919	95	129	224
Arizona	1929	20	10	30
California	1909	9,956	10,152	20,108
Connecticut	1909	511	46	557
Delaware	1923	477	468	945
Georgia	1937	1,810	1,474	3,284
Idaho	1925	30	8	38
Indiana	1907	1,257	1,167	2,424[a]
Iowa	1911	1,365	545	1,910
Kansas	1913	1,269	1,763	3,032
Maine	1925	280	46	326
Michigan	1913	2,795	991	3,786
Minnesota	1925	1,831	519	2,350
Mississippi	1928	523	160	683
Montana	1923	184	72	256
Nebraska	1915	479	423	902
Nevada	1911	0	0	0
New Hampshire	1917	527	152	679
New Jersey	1911	0	0	0
New York	1912	41	1	42
North Carolina	1919	5,225	1,072	6,297[b]
North Dakota	1913	652	397	1,049
Oklahoma	1931	434	122	556
Oregon	1917	1,453	888	2,341[c]
South Carolina	1935	255	22	277
South Dakota	1917	506	283	789
Utah	1925	418	354	772
Vermont	1931	170	83	253
Virginia	1924	4,383	2,779	7,162[d]
Washington	1909	501	184	685
West Virginia	1929	83	15	98
Wisconsin	1913	1,432	391	1,823
Total		38,962	24,716	63,678

Source: Human Betterment Association, "Sterilizations Performed Under U.S. State Sterilization Statutes through December 31, 1963," Association for Voluntary Sterilization Records, Social Welfare History Archives, University of Minnesota.

[a] By 1974, 2,500 sterilizations may have been performed in Indiana. See Lutz Kaelber, "Eugenics: Compulsory Sterilization in 50 American States," University of Vermont, www.uvm.edu/~lkaelber/eugenics/, under "Indiana."

[b] By 1973, the number of sterilizations is estimated to be about 7,600. See Kaelber, "North Carolina."

[c] By 1983, the total number of sterilizations was 2,648. See Kaelber, "Oregon."

[d] A total of 7,325 sterilizations were performed by 1979, according to Kaelber, "Virginia."

Despite these limitations and other issues discussed below, the medical register provides valuable information about sterilization practices and "feebleminded" patients in the first years of the program. Piper transcribed the information discussed in the preceding paragraph into Microsoft Excel and Access and prepared five reports: "Personal Information," "Institutional Information," "Operations," "Consent," and "After Faribault." Three records out of the total sample of 1,000 were duplicates; *n* = 997 was used as the total sample value.

The conclusions in Piper's reports are based on evidence that represents over 90 percent of the sample. Nevertheless, there are a number of errors. First, there are several duplicates within the original record. In addition to the three duplicates excluded from the sample total, other duplicates were noted later. However, fewer than ten duplicates were identified overall. Second, the original record contains some gaps and errors, likely due to clerical errors. For example, twenty-three entries on two days (June 7, 1927, and September 23, 1927) listed consent as "unknown," suggesting that an error had been made when recording the data. Elsewhere illogical birth dates and ages were given. For example, seven subjects had no reported birth date, and eight had unlikely ages (five years old but with a husband, one month old, etc.) All told, however, the information was complete and logical for 980 patients. When errors were not obvious, they would have been incorporated into the reports. Third, errors in transcription must have occurred. At least three different people copied sterilization information onto paper and then into the spreadsheet and database. At each stage of transcription additional errors likely crept in, and where not obvious they would have been incorporated into the analyses. Nevertheless, because of the size of the sample, the occasional errors should not undermine the broader conclusions drawn from the data.

Abbreviations

APS	American Philosophical Society Library, Philadelphia, Pennsylvania
AVS	Association for Voluntary Sterilization
ERO	Eugenic Record Office
GPO	Government Printing Office
JPA	*Journal of Psycho-Asthenics*
NCCC	National Conference of Charities and Corrections
SWHA	Social Welfare History Archives, University of Minnesota Libraries, Minneapolis, Minnesota

RECORDS OF THE MINNESOTA HISTORICAL SOCIETY

MHS	Minnesota Historical Society, St. Paul, Minnesota
ADD	Minnesota State Reformatory for Men, Annex for Defective Delinquents
DPI	Minnesota Division of Public Institutions
DPI MHU	Minnesota Division of Public Institutions, Mental Health Unit
DPW	Minnesota Department of Public Welfare
DPW PSB	Minnesota Department of Welfare, Psychological Services Bureau
FSSH	Faribault State School and Hospital Records
FSSH SC	Faribault State School and Hospital, Superintendent Correspondence (correspondence with Board of Control unless otherwise noted)
HSG	Home School for Girls at Sauk Centre
WWL	Women's Welfare League of Minneapolis

Introduction

1. Meridel Le Sueur, "Sequel to Love," *Anvil* (Jan.–Feb. 1935): 3–4.

2. Human Betterment Association, "Sterilizations Performed under U.S. State Sterilization Statutes through December 31, 1963," Sterilization Statistics, AVS Records, SWHA; Warner quoted in Alexandra Minna Stern, "Eugenics and Historical Memory in America," *History Compass* 3 (Jan. 2005): 1. See Adam Cohen, *Imbeciles: The Supreme Court, American Eugenics, and the Sterilization of Carrie Buck* (New York: Penguin, 2016); Edwin Black, *War against the Weak: Eugenics and America's Campaign to Create a Master Race* (New York: Four Walls Eight Windows, 2003). See also Thomas C. Leonard, *Illiberal Reformers: Race, Eugenics, and American Economics in the Progressive Era* (Princeton, NJ: Princeton University Press, 2016).

3. Constance Coiner, *Better Red: The Writing and Resistance of Tillie Olsen and Meridel Le Sueur* (New York: Oxford University Press, 1995), 110.

4. "Price of freedom" is from Abraham Myerson et al., *Eugenical Sterilization: A Reorientation of the Problem* (1936; repr., New York: Arno, 1980); Michael L. Wehmeyer, "Eugenics and Sterilization in the Heartland," *Mental Retardation* 41 (2003): 60. The Minnesota apology is an important exception. See Laws of Minnesota 2010, Resolution 4—H. F. No. 1680.

5. See Wendy Kline, *Building a Better Race: Gender, Sexuality, and Eugenics from the Turn of the Century to the Baby Boom* (Berkeley: University of California Press, 2001). My analysis

has benefited from Douglas C. Baynton, "Disability and the Justification of Inequality in American History," in *The New Disability History: American Perspectives*, ed. Paul K. Longmore and Lauri Umansky (New York: New York University Press, 2001), 33–57; James W. Trent Jr., *Inventing the Feeble Mind: A History of Mental Retardation in the United States* (Berkeley: University of California Press, 1994).

6. Davenport quoted in Alexandra Minna Stern, *Eugenic Nation: Faults and Frontiers of Better Breeding in Modern America* (Berkeley: University of California Press, 2005), 11; Black, *War against the Weak*, xvi. See also Harry Bruinius, *Better for All the World: The Secret History of Forced Sterilization and America's Quest for Racial Purity* (New York: Knopf, 2006); Stefan Kühl, *The Nazi Connection: Eugenics, American Racism, and German National Socialism* (New York: Oxford University Press, 1994); Allan Chase, *The Legacy of Malthus: The Social Costs of the New Scientific Racism* (Urbana: University of Illinois Press, 1980).

7. Frank Dikötter, "Race Culture: Recent Perspectives on the History of Eugenics," *American Historical Review* 103 (Apr. 1998): 467. See also Nancy Leys Stepan, *The Hour of Eugenics: Race, Gender, and Nation in Latin America* (Ithaca, NY: Cornell University Press, 1991); Marius Turda, *Modernism and Eugenics* (New York: Palgrave Macmillan, 2010); Alison Bashford and Philippa Levine, eds., *The Oxford Handbook of the History of Eugenics* (New York: Oxford University Press, 2010).

8. Paul A. Lombardo, *Three Generations, No Imbeciles: Eugenics, the Supreme Court, and* Buck v. Bell (Baltimore: Johns Hopkins University Press, 2008), 51. On positive and negative eugenics, see Molly Ladd-Taylor, "Eugenics, Sterilisation, and Modern Marriage in the USA: The Strange Career of Paul Popenoe," *Gender and History* 13 (Aug. 2001): 298–327.

9. Mark A. Largent, *Breeding Contempt: The History of Coerced Sterilization in the United States* (New Brunswick, NJ: Rutgers University Press, 2008), 68, 26–27; Joel T. Braslow, *Mental Ills and Bodily Cures: Psychiatric Treatment in the First Half of the Twentieth Century* (Berkeley: University of California Press, 1997), 59–68; Rebecca M. Kluchin, *Fit to Be Tied: Sterilization and Reproductive Rights in America, 1950–1980* (New Brunswick, NJ: Rutgers University Press, 2011), 53–54; Johanna Schoen, "Between Choice and Coercion: Women and the Politics of Sterilization in North Carolina, 1929–1975," *Journal of Women's History* 13 (Spring 2001): 132–56; Molly Ladd-Taylor, "Contraception or Eugenics? Sterilization and 'Mental Retardation' in the 1970s and 1980s," *Canadian Bulletin of Medical History* 31, no. 1 (2014): 189–211; Trent, *Inventing the Feeble Mind*, 224.

10. Philip R. Reilly, *The Surgical Solution: A History of Involuntary Sterilization in the United States* (Baltimore: Johns Hopkins University Press, 1991), 54–55. See Mark Haller, *Eugenics: Hereditarian Attitudes in American Thought* (1963; repr., New Brunswick, NJ: Rutgers University Press, 1983); Daniel J. Kevles, *In the Name of Eugenics: Genetics and the Uses of Human Heredity* (1985; repr., Cambridge, MA: Harvard University Press, 1995); Diane B. Paul, *Controlling Human Heredity: 1865 to the Present* (Atlantic Highlands, NJ: Humanities Press International, 1995).

11. Lombardo, *Three Generations*, xii, 134; *Buck v. Bell*, 274 U.S. 200 (1927) at 207.

12. Cohen, *Imbeciles*, 10, 12, 7; Lombardo, *Three Generations*, xi; Stephen Jay Gould, *The Mismeasure of Man*, rev. ed. (New York: W. W. Norton, 1996), 366. See also Nancy Isenberg, *White Trash: The 400-Year Untold History of Class in America* (New York: Viking, 2016).

13. Angela Y. Davis, *Women, Race, and Class* (1981; repr., New York: Vintage, 1983); Kluchin, *Fit to Be Tied*, 3–5. See also Randall Hansen and Desmond King, *Sterilized by the State: Eugenics, Race, and the Population Scare in Twentieth-Century North America* (Cambridge: Cambridge University Press, 2013); Ian Dowbiggin, *The Sterilization Movement and*

Global Fertility in the Twentieth Century (New York: Oxford University Press, 2008); Donald T. Critchlow, *Intended Consequences: Birth Control, Abortion, and the Federal Government in Modern America* (New York: Oxford University Press, 1999); Dorothy Roberts, *Killing the Black Body: Race, Reproduction, and the Meaning of Liberty* (New York: Pantheon, 1997).

14. Susan K. Cahn, *Sexual Reckonings: Southern Girls in a Troubling Age* (Cambridge, MA: Harvard University Press, 2012), 163; Michael A. Rembis, *Defining Deviance: Sex, Science, and Delinquent Girls, 1890–1960* (Urbana: University of Illinois Press, 2011), 147; Schoen, "Between Choice and Coercion," 133–34. See also Elaine Tyler May, *Barren in the Promised Land: Childless Americans and the Pursuit of Happiness* (New York: Basic, 1995).

15. Similar themes are explored in Margaret D. Jacobs, *White Mother to a Dark Race: Settler Colonialism, Maternalism, and the Removal of Indigenous Children in the American West and Australia, 1880–1940* (Lincoln: University of Nebraska Press, 2011); Laura Briggs, *Somebody's Children: The Politics of Transracial and Transnational Adoption* (Durham, NC: Duke University Press, 2012).

16. Minnesota Governor's Council on Developmental Disabilities, "Ed Skarnulis Interviews Rosemary and Gunnar Dybwad," *Parallels in Time: A History of Developmental Disabilities* (1987), http://mn.gov/mnddc/parallels2/one/dybwad-parents/rosemaryGunnar02.html.

17. Véronique Mottier, "Eugenics and the State: Policy-Making in Comparative Perspective," in *Oxford Handbook of the History of Eugenics*, ed. Bashford and Levine, 134–53; Largent, *Breeding Contempt*, 79–80. See also Peter B. Evans, Dietrich Rueschemeyer, and Theda Skocpol, eds., *Bringing the State Back In* (New York: Cambridge University Press, 1985); Meg Jacobs, William J. Novak, and Julian E. Zelizer, eds., *The Democratic Experiment: New Directions in American Political History* (Princeton, NJ: Princeton University Press, 2009); Hansen and King, *Sterilized by the State*, 18, 77.

18. Cahn, *Sexual Reckonings*, 162, 177; Alexandra Minna Stern, "When California Sterilized 20,000 of Its Citizens," *Zócalo*, Jan. 6, 2016, www.zocalopublicsquare.org/2016/01/06/when-california-sterilized-20000-of-its-citizens/chronicles/who-we-were/; "Sterilizations Performed through 1963," AVS Records; Hansen and King, *Sterilized by the State*, 19–21; Mildred Thomson, *Prologue: A Minnesota Story of Mental Retardation* (Minneapolis: Gilbert, 1963), 89.

19. Gunnar Broberg and Nils Roll-Hansen, *Eugenics and the Welfare State: Sterilization Policy in Denmark, Sweden, Norway, and Finland* (East Lansing: Michigan State University Press, 2005), ix–x; Mottier, "Eugenics and the State," 142.

20. Michael B. Katz, *In the Shadow of the Poorhouse: A Social History of Welfare in America* (New York: Basic Books, 1986), ix–xi.

21. See Lizzie Seal, "Designating Dependency: The 'Socially Inadequate' in the United States, 1910–1940," *Journal of Historical Sociology* 26 (June 2013): 143–68; Michael B. Katz, *Poverty and Policy in American History* (New York: Academic Press, 1983); Nancy Fraser and Linda Gordon, "A Genealogy of Dependency: Tracing a Keyword of the U.S. Welfare State," *Signs* 19 (Winter 1994): 309–36.

22. Katz, *In the Shadow of the Poorhouse*, 25. See Walter Trattner, *From Poor Law to Welfare State: A History of Social Welfare in America*, 6th ed. (New York: Free Press, 1999); Susan M. Schweik, *The Ugly Laws: Disability in Public* (New York: New York University Press, 2009); Ethel McClure, *More Than a Roof: The Development of Minnesota Poor Farms and Homes for the Aged* (St. Paul: Minnesota Historical Society Press, 1968).

23. Gioh-Fang Dju Ma, *One Hundred Years of Public Services for Children in Minnesota* (Chicago: University of Chicago Press, 1949).

24. Michael B. Katz, *The Undeserving Poor: America's Enduring Confrontation with Poverty* (New York: Oxford University Press, 2013); Elof Axel Carlson, *The Unfit: A History of a Bad Idea* (Cold Spring Harbor, NY: Cold Spring Harbor Laboratory Press, 2001); Nicole Hahn Rafter, *Creating Born Criminals* (Urbana: University of Illinois Press, 1997).

25. Viviana Zelizer, *Pricing the Priceless Child: The Changing Social Value of Children* (1985; repr., Princeton, NJ: Princeton University Press, 1994), 3, 11. See also Steven Mintz, *Huck's Raft: A History of American Childhood* (Cambridge, MA: Belknap Press of Harvard University Press, 2004).

26. White House Conference on the Care of Dependent Children, *Proceedings of the Conference on the Care of Dependent Children Held at Washington, D.C., January 25, 26, 1909* (Washington, DC: GPO, 1909), 9–10. See Gwendolyn Mink, *The Wages of Motherhood: Inequality in the Welfare State, 1917–1942* (Ithaca, NY: Cornell University Press, 1995); Molly Ladd-Taylor, "What Child Left Behind? U.S. Social Policy and the Helpless Child," in *Lost Kids: Vulnerable Children and Youth in Twentieth-Century Canada and the United States*, ed. Mona Gleason et al. (Vancouver: University of British Columbia Press, 2009), 157–74.

27. Michael Willrich, "Home Slackers: Men, the State, and Welfare in Modern America," *Journal of American History* 87 (2000): 463; Michael Willrich, *City of Courts: Socializing Justice in Progressive Era Chicago* (Cambridge: Cambridge University Press, 2003), 243.

28. Largent, *Breeding Contempt*, 77–78; US Bureau of the Census, *Historical Statistics of the United States, Colonial Times to 1970*, pt. 1, chap. A (Washington, DC: GPO, 1973), 24–37. See also Cahn, *Sexual Reckonings*, 160.

29. Robert J. Levy, "Protecting the Mentally Retarded: An Empirical Survey and Evaluation of the Establishment of Guardianship in Minnesota," *Minnesota Law Review* 49 (1965): 822–23.

30. US Census Bureau, "Table 1: Urban and Rural Population of the United States: 1900–1990" (Oct. 1995), www.census.gov/population/censusdata/urpop0090.txt; History Matters, "The Omaha Platform: Launching the Populist Party" (1892), http://historymatters.gmu.edu/d/5361. On Minnesota history, see Theodore C. Blegen, *Minnesota: A History of the State* (1963; repr., Minneapolis: University of Minnesota Press, 1975).

31. Anna Stubblefield, "'Beyond the Pale': Tainted Whiteness, Cognitive Disability, and Eugenic Sterilization," *Hypatia* 22 (Spring 2007): 162–81; US Bureau of the Census, "Population—Minnesota," *Fifteenth Census of the United States: 1930*, vol. 3, pt. 1, table 2, 9 (Washington, DC: GPO, 1933), 1187, 1194; June Holmquist, *They Chose Minnesota: A Survey of the State's Ethnic Groups* (St. Paul: Minnesota Historical Society Press, 1981), 8.

32. Jennifer A. Delton, *Making Minnesota Liberal: Civil Rights and the Transformation of the Democratic Party* (Minneapolis: University of Minnesota Press, 2002), 47; Steven Keillor, *Shaping Minnesota's Identity: 150 Years of State History* (Lakeville, MN: Pogo, 2007).

33. Jane Lawrence, "The Indian Health Service and the Sterilization of Native American Women," *American Indian Quarterly* 24 (2000): 400–419; Brianna Theobald, "Nurse, Mother, Midwife: Susie Walking Bear Yellowtail and the Struggle for Crow Women's Reproductive Autonomy," *Montana Magazine of Western History* 66 (Fall 2016): 17–35. See also Cahn, *Sexual Reckonings*, 177; Erika Dyck, *Facing Eugenics: Reproduction, Sterilization, and the Politics of Choice* (Toronto: University of Toronto Press, 2013), 57–60.

34. Governor's Human Rights Commission, *Minnesota's Indian Citizens, Yesterday and Today* (St. Paul: State of Minnesota, 1965), 51; Barbara Gurr, *Reproductive Justice: The Politics of Health Care for Native American Women* (New Brunswick, NJ: Rutgers University Press, 2015).

35. Dyck, *Facing Eugenics*, chaps. 5 and 6; Kevin Begos et al., *Against Their Will: North Carolina's Sterilization Program* (Apalachicola, FL: Gray Oak Books, 2012).

36. For thoughtful discussions of the methodological challenges of studying sterilization, see Johanna Schoen, *Choice and Coercion: Birth Control, Sterilization, and Abortion in Public Health and Welfare in the Twentieth Century* (Chapel Hill: University of North Carolina Press, 2005), 13–19; Rebecca M. Kluchin, "Locating the Voices of the Sterilized," *Public Historian* 29 (Summer 2007): 131–44.

37. E-mail communication to author, Dec. 18, 2007. Name withheld by request.

38. Liat Ben-Moshe, Chris Chapman, and Allison C. Carey, eds., *Disability Incarcerated: Imprisonment and Disability in the United States and Canada* (New York: Palgrave Macmillan, 2014); Dorothy Roberts, *Shattered Bonds: The Color of Child Welfare* (New York: Basic Books, 2001).

Chapter One • The Feebleminded Menace and the Innocent Child

1. Mildred Thomson, *Prologue: A Minnesota Story of Mental Retardation* (Minneapolis: Gilbert, 1963), 17–19.

2. Thomas C. Leonard, *Illiberal Reformers: Race, Eugenics, and American Economics in the Progressive Era* (Princeton, NJ: Princeton University Press, 2016), xi, 191; Alexandra Minna Stern, "Making Better Babies: Public Health and Race Betterment in Indiana, 1920–1935," *American Journal of Public Health* 92 (May 2002): 742–52. On eugenics as a progressive movement, see Edward J. Larson, *Sex, Race, and Science: Eugenics in the Deep South* (Baltimore: Johns Hopkins University Press, 1995). For a right-wing critique of progressivism and eugenics, see Jonah Goldberg, *Liberal Fascism: The Secret History of the American Left, from Mussolini to the Politics of Meaning* (New York: Doubleday, 2007).

3. Michael B. Katz, *In the Shadow of the Poorhouse: A Social History of Welfare in America* (New York: Basic Books), 183; Michel Foucault, *Discipline and Punish: The Birth of the Prison* (1977; repr., New York: Vintage, 1995).

4. Viviana A. Zelizer, *Pricing the Priceless Child: The Changing Social Value of Children* (1985; repr., Princeton, NJ: Princeton University Press, 1994), 3; Robin Bernstein, *Racial Innocence: Performing American Childhood and Race from Slavery to Civil Rights* (New York: New York University Press, 2012), 4.

5. See Michael B. Katz, *Poverty and Policy in American History* (New York: Academic Press, 1983).

6. Katz, *In the Shadow of the Poorhouse*, 69–70; Walter I. Trattner, *From Poor Law to Welfare State: A History of Social Welfare in America*, 6th ed. (New York: Free Press, 1999), 87–103, 236–37. See also Brent Ruswick, *Almost Worthy: The Poor, Paupers, and the Science of Charity in America, 1877–1917* (Bloomington: Indiana University Press, 2013). For a different view, see Joel Schwartz, *Fighting Poverty with Virtue: Moral Reform and America's Urban Poor, 1825–2000* (Bloomington: Indiana University Press, 2000).

7. Theodore C. Blegen, *Minnesota: A History of the State* (1963; repr., Minneapolis: University of Minnesota Press, 1975), 303–13; William E. Lass, *Minnesota: A History* (New York: W. W. Norton, 1998); Steven Keillor, *Shaping Minnesota's Identity: 150 Years of State History* (Lakeville, MN: Pogo, 2007); June D. Holmquist, *They Chose Minnesota: A Survey of the State's Ethnic Groups* (St. Paul: Minnesota Historical Society Press, 1981).

8. Pillsbury quoted in Annette Atkins, *Harvest of Grief: Grasshopper Plagues and Public Assistance in Minnesota, 1873–78* (St. Paul: Minnesota Historical Society Press, 1984), 84; Hart

quoted in Esther Benson, "Organization of Public Welfare Activities in Minnesota" (MA thesis, University of Minnesota, 1941), 36.

9. History Matters, "The Omaha Platform: Launching the Populist Party (1892)," http://historymatters.gmu.edu/d/5361; Laura L. Lovett, *Conceiving the Future: Pronatalism, Reproduction, and the Family in the United States, 1890–1938* (Chapel Hill: University of North Carolina Press, 2007), 22.

10. Richard L. Dugdale, *"The Jukes": A Study in Crime, Pauperism, Disease and Heredity: Also Further Studies of Criminals* (New York: G. P. Putnam's, 1877), 65; Nicole Hahn Rafter, *Creating Born Criminals* (Urbana: University of Illinois Press, 1997), 38. See also Elof Axel Carlson, *The Unfit: A History of a Bad Idea* (Cold Spring Harbor, NY: Cold Spring Harbor Laboratory Press, 2001).

11. Frederick Howard Wines, *Report on the Defective, Dependent and Delinquent Classes of the Population of the United States, as Returned at the 10th Census (June 1, 1880)* (Washington, DC: GPO, 1888), xix, xxiii.

12. Ibid., x.

13. Ibid., x; Katz, *Poverty and Policy*, 156.

14. Charles Richmond Henderson, *Introduction to the Study of the Dependent, Defective and Delinquent Classes* (Boston: D. C. Heath, 1893), 5–6.

15. Benson, "Organization of Public Welfare Activities," 13–14, 27; Ethel McClure, *More Than a Roof: The Development of Minnesota Poor Farms and Homes for the Aged* (St. Paul: Minnesota Historical Society Press, 1968), chap. 2.

16. Gioh-Fang Dju Ma, *One Hundred Years of Public Services for Children in Minnesota* (Chicago: University of Chicago Press, 1949), 32–34.

17. Henderson, *Dependent, Defective and Delinquent Classes*, 69–70; Hastings H. Hart, "The Child-Saving Movement," *Bibliotecha Sacra* 58 (July 1901): 520–21.

18. Minnesota State Public School, *Report of the Board of Managers and Superintendent for the Biennial Period Ending July 31, 1908*; Matthew A. Crenson, *Building the Invisible Orphanage: A Prehistory of the American Welfare System* (Cambridge, MA: Harvard University Press, 1998), 55; Galen A. Merrill, "The Dependent Normal Child," typescript, n.d., Minnesota State Public School, Correspondence, Speeches, and Writings of Galen A. Merrill, MHS. See also Priscilla Ferguson Clement, "With Wise and Benevolent Purpose: Poor Children and the State Public School at Owatonna, 1885–1915," *Minnesota History* 49 (1984): 2–13.

19. The site of the State Public School is now a museum; see www.orphanagemuseum.com/.

20. Isaac Kerlin, "Provision for Idiots: Report of Standing Committee," in *Proceedings of the National Conference of Charities and Correction* (Boston: Geo. Ellis, 1885), 172; "Remarks of Hon. R. A. Mott, Faribault Meeting, 1890," in *Proceedings of the Association of Medical Officers of American Institutions for Idiotic and Feeble-Minded Persons, 1887–1895* (New York: Johnson Reprint, 1964), 117–18. See also "The Inheritance of Crime," *New York Times*, Mar. 8, 1875.

21. Fernald quoted in Mildred Thomson, *Dr. Arthur C. Rogers: Pioneer Leader in Minnesota's Program for the Mentally Retarded* (Minneapolis: Minnesota Association for Retarded Children, n.d. [1966]), 8; "Minutes," *JPA* 22 (Sept. 1917): 52.

22. "Editorial," *JPA* 3 (Mar. 1899): 144; Arnold Madow, "Brief History of Minnesota's Mental Retardation Institutions," typescript, 1977, FSSH, Historical Data Files. See James W. Trent Jr., *Inventing the Feeble Mind: A History of Mental Retardation in the United States*

(Berkeley: University of California Press, 1994); Peter L. Tyor and Leland V. Bell, *Caring for the Retarded in America: A History* (Westport, CT: Greenwood, 1984).

23. *Sixth Biennial Report of the Minnesota Institute for Defectives for the Period Ending July 31, 1890*, 93, 99; Admission Photographs, n.d., FSSH, Audio-Visual Materials; US Bureau of the Census, *Insane and Feeble-Minded in Institutions, 1910* (Washington, DC: GPO, 1914), 192.

24. Trent, *Inventing the Feeble Mind*, 79–84.

25. Thomson, *Dr. Arthur C. Rogers*, 16–22. See David Wallace Adams, *Education for Extinction: American Indians and the Boarding School Experience, 1875–1928* (Lawrence: University Press of Kansas, 1995); Brenda J. Child, *Boarding School Seasons: American Indian Families, 1900–1940* (Lincoln: University of Nebraska Press, 1998).

26. "Minutes, July 4, 1890," in *Proceedings of the Association of Medical Officers*, 90–91. See William W. Folwell, *A History of Minnesota*, vol. 4 (St. Paul: Minnesota Historical Society Press, 1930), 472–78.

27. James W. Trent Jr., "Defective's at the World's Fair: Constructing Disability in 1904," *Remedial and Special Education* 19 (July/Aug. 1998): 201–11. See Nancy J. Parezo and Don D. Fowler, *Anthropology Goes to the Fair: The 1904 Louisiana Purchase Exposition* (Lincoln: University of Nebraska Press, 2009).

28. William B. Fish, "Care of Feeble-Minded," in *Proceedings of the National Conference of Charities and Correction* (Boston: Geo. Ellis, 1891), 103; "Does the Education of the Feeble-Minded Pay?," *JPA* 2 (June 1898): 158.

29. A. C. Rogers, "Report of Five Cases of Mental and Moral Aberration among the Feeble-Minded at the Minnesota School for the Feeble-Minded" (1892), in *Proceedings of the Association of Medical Officers*, 325; "Sterilization of the Unfit," *JPA* 9 (June 1905): 128; FSSH, *Report of the Superintendent of the School for the Feeble-Minded and Colony for Epileptics for the Biennial Period Ending July 31, 1910*, 226. On the debate between Denmark's Christian Keller and Martin Barr, a key US proponent of sterilization, see Gunnar Broberg and Nils Roll-Hansen, *Eugenics and the Welfare State: Sterilization Policy in Denmark, Sweden, Norway, and Finland* (1997; repr., East Lansing: Michigan State University Press, 2005), 16–18.

30. "Editorial: As Others See Us," *JPA* 2 (Sept. 1897): 49; "Minutes of the 23rd Session," *JPA* 3 (Sept. 1898): 41; "Editorial," *JPA* 3 (Mar. 1899): 145.

31. A. C. Rogers, "Modern Studies in Heredity," *JPA* 14 (1909): 120; A. C. Rogers and Maud A. Merrill, *Dwellers in the Vale of Siddem: A True Story of the Social Aspect of Feeble-Mindedness* (Boston: Richard D. Badger, 1919), 13.

32. On the ERO, see Garland E. Allen, "The Eugenics Record Office at Cold Spring Harbor, 1910–1940: An Essay in Institutional History," *Osiris* 2 (1986): 225–64; Amy Sue Bix, "Experiences and Voices of Eugenics Field Workers: 'Women's Work' in Biology," *Social Studies of Science* 27 (1997): 625–68.

33. Nicole Hahn Rafter, *White Trash: The Eugenic Family Studies, 1877–1919* (Boston: Northeastern University Press, 1988), 341–43.

34. Rogers and Merrill, *Dwellers*, 15, 76, 11.

35. Charles B. Davenport et al., *The Study of Human Heredity*, Eugenics Record Office Bulletin no. 2 (Cold Spring Harbor, NY: Eugenics Record Office, 1911), 1. On fieldwork as "institutional extension work," see Frederick Kuhlmann to Bertha M. Luckey, Mar. 7, 1917, FSSH SC.

36. Elizabeth Kite, "Mental Defect as Found by the Field Worker [and discussion],"

JPA 18 (1913): 149. Historian Alice Wexler found a similar range of responses to the ERO investigations of Huntington's disease in New England and New York. Although the ERO's conclusions were useless from a genetic point of view, local people were active participants in the fieldwork process and conveyed their "local knowledge." Alice Wexler, *The Woman Who Walked into the Sea: Huntington's and the Making of a Genetic Disease* (New Haven, CT: Yale University Press, 2008), 134–50.

37. Laws of Minnesota 1907, chap. 292, sec. 1; Marie T. Curial to Rogers, Sept. 18, 1914, FSSH SC.

38. A. C. Rogers, "Mental Deficiency as Shown in Field Work [and discussion]," in *Proceedings of the Minnesota State Conference of Charities and Correction* (Stillwater, MN: Mirror Print, 1914), 33–34. On poor mothers turning to the state for assistance, see Linda Gordon, *Heroes of Their Own Lives: The Politics and History of Family Violence, Boston, 1880–1960* (New York: Viking, 1988); Mary E. Odem, *Delinquent Daughters: Protecting and Policing Adolescent Female Sexuality in the United States, 1885–1920* (Chapel Hill: University of North Carolina Press, 1995); Kathleen Jones, *Taming the Troublesome Child: American Families, Child Guidance, and the Limits of Psychiatric Authority* (Cambridge, MA: Harvard University Press, 1999).

39. FSSH, *Biennial Report for the Period Ending July 31, 1908*, 7.

40. See, e.g., E. W. Allen to Board of Control, Dec. 17, 1914; Mira Gray to Rogers, Jan. 20, 1915, FSSH SC.

41. Mira Gray to Rogers, Aug. 20, 1914; Rogers to Board of Control, Sept. 21, 1919, FSSH SC.

42. The first case prompted considerable discussion. The state attorney general ruled in 1907 that the woman could be held at Faribault against the wishes of her mother. Although other officials were sure his opinion would be overturned in court, they decided to keep the woman in the institution as long as they could. She was still listed as an inmate in the 1920 census. George Peterson to S. W. Leavitt, Oct. 17, 1907; O. B. Gould to Rogers, Feb. 17, 1906; Rogers to Board of Control, Feb. 15, 1913; Rogers to Board of Control, Mar. 22, 1915; Letter to Rogers, July 6, 1915; "Myrna Jones" to Board of Control, Apr. 7, 1916; "Erma Stewart" to Gov. A. O. Eberhart, Oct. 1, 1913, all in FSSH SC.

43. Letter to State Attorney, Aug. 19, 1907; Rogers to Board of Control, Aug. 8, 1913, FSSH SC.

44. Hart, "Child-Saving Movement," 520–23. See also Susan Tiffin, *In Whose Best Interest? Child Welfare Reform in the Progressive Era* (Westport, CT: Greenwood, 1982); Katz, *In the Shadow of the Poorhouse*, chap. 5.

45. Dorothy Ross, *G. Stanley Hall: The Psychologist as Prophet* (Chicago: University of Chicago Press, 1972); Theresa R. Richardson, *The Century of the Child: The Mental Hygiene Movement and Social Policy in the United States and Canada* (Albany, NY: SUNY Press, 1989); Josef Brožek, *Explorations in the History of Psychology in the United States* (Cranbury, NJ: Bucknell University Press, 1984), 248–52.

46. G. Stanley Hall, *Youth: Its Education, Regimen, and Hygiene* (New York: D. Appleton, 1906), 1–2; Ross, *G. Stanley Hall*, 312–15. See also Gail Bederman, *Manliness and Civilization: A Cultural History of Gender and Race in the United States, 1880–1917* (Chicago: University of Chicago Press, 1995), chap. 3.

47. A. C. Rogers, "The Juvenile Court," n.d. (ca. 1912), FSSH Reports and Miscellaneous Records.

48. Hastings H. Hart, "Distinctive Features of the Juvenile Court," *Annals of the American Academy of Political and Social Science* 36 (1910): 57. The literature on the juvenile court

is vast. Especially useful for this study were David Tanenhaus, *Juvenile Justice in the Making* (New York: Oxford University Press, 2004); Eric Schneider, *In the Web of Class: Delinquents and Reformers in Boston, 1810s–1930s* (New York: New York University Press, 1992).

49. Ma, *One Hundred Years*, 68–69. Minnesota courts already had the power to remove children under the age of ten from negligent or abusive parents, but the new law expanded the court's jurisdiction to children under seventeen and centralized it under one judge. See also Edward F. Waite, *The Origin and Development of the Minnesota Juvenile Court: Address before the Minnesota Association of Probate Judges, January 15, 1920* (St. Paul: State Board of Control, 1920), MHS.

50. General Laws of Minnesota 1905, chap. 285; Ma, *One Hundred Years*, 72–73. See also David S. Tanenhaus, "Growing Up Dependent: Family Preservation in Early Twentieth-Century Chicago," *Law and History Review* 19 (Fall 2001): 547–82.

51. Waite, *Origin and Development*, 10. See also Ma, *One Hundred Years*, 76–80. Historical studies of mothers' pensions include Joanne Goodwin, *Gender and the Politics of Welfare Reform: Mothers' Pensions in Chicago, 1911–1929* (Chicago: University of Chicago Press, 1997); Molly Ladd-Taylor, *Mother-Work: Women, Child Welfare, and the State, 1890–1930* (Urbana: University of Illinois Press, 1994); Theda Skocpol, *Protecting Soldiers and Mothers: The Political Origins of Social Policy in the United States* (Cambridge, MA: Belknap Press of Harvard University Press, 1992); Linda Gordon, *Pitied but Not Entitled: Single Mothers and the History of Welfare* (New York: Free Press, 1994).

52. Michael J. Willrich, *City of Courts: Socializing Justice in Progressive Era Chicago* (New York: Cambridge University Press, 2003); Michael J. Willrich, "The Case for Courts: Law and Political Development in the Progressive Era," in *The Democratic Experiment: New Directions in American Political History*, ed. Meg Jacobs, William J. Novak, and Julian E. Zelizer (Princeton, NJ: Princeton University Press, 2003), 198–221; Edward F. Waite, *Juvenile Court in the Rural Community: An Address Delivered at the Regional Conference of the Minnesota State Conference of Social Work on June 11, 1932*, MHS.

53. Edward F. Waite, "How Far Can Court Procedure Be Socialized without Impairing Individual Rights?," *Journal of the American Institution of Criminal Law and Criminology* 12 (1921): 344.

54. Roy Lubove, *The Professional Altruist: The Emergence of Social Work as a Career, 1880–1930* (Cambridge, MA: Harvard University Press, 1965), 66. On Healy, see Jones, *Taming the Troublesome Child*, 38–50.

55. Mrs. Frederick W. Reed, "Research Work in the Minneapolis Juvenile Court," *American Review of Reviews* 48 (1913): 216–17.

56. Edward F. Waite, "The Physical Bases of Crime: From the Standpoint of the Judge of a Juvenile Court," *Bulletin of the American Academy of Medicine* 14 (1913): 393, 392.

57. Ibid., 395.

58. "Edward Waite, Retired District Judges, Dies at 98," *Minneapolis Morning Tribune*, Apr. 28, 1958; Walter Fernald, "The Burden of Feeble-Mindedness," *JPA* 17 (1912): 87–99; Thomson, *Dr. Arthur C. Rogers*, 26; Editorial, *Survey* 33 (Oct. 31, 1914): 115–16. See also Anne Meis Knupfer, *Reform and Resistance: Gender, Delinquency, and America's First Juvenile Court* (New York: Routledge, 2013), Tamara Myers, *Caught: Montreal's Modern Girls and the Law, 1869–1945* (Toronto: University of Toronto Press, 2006); Wendy Kline, *Building a Better Race: Gender, Sexuality, and Eugenics from the Turn of the Century to the Baby Boom* (Berkeley: University of California Press, 2005).

59. Michael A. Rembis, *Defining Deviance: Sex, Science, and Delinquent Girls, 1890–1960* (Urbana: University of Illinois Press, 2011), 14; Nancy Freeman Rohde, "Gratia Alta Countryman," in *Women of Minnesota: Selected Biographical Essays*, ed. Barbara Stuhler and Gretchen Kreuter (St. Paul: Minnesota Historical Society Press, 1977), 187. See also Leigh Ann Wheeler, *Against Obscenity: Reform and the Politics of Womanhood in America, 1873–1935* (Baltimore: Johns Hopkins University Press, 2004), 31–35.

60. Lynn Weiner, "'Our Sister's Keepers': The Minneapolis Woman's Christian Association and Housing for Working Women," *Minnesota History* 46 (Spring 1979): 189–90; Elizabeth Faue, *Writing the Wrongs: Eva Valesh and the Rise of Labor Journalism* (Ithaca, NY: Cornell University Press, 2002). See also Mari Jo Buhle, *Women and American Socialism, 1870–1920* (Urbana: University of Illinois Press, 1983), 82–89.

61. Vice Commission of Minneapolis, *Report of the Vice Commission of Minneapolis to His Honor, James C. Haynes, Mayor* (Minneapolis: H. M. Hall, 1911), 104, 132. Vice commissions are the subject of an extensive literature. See esp. Mara L. Keire, "The Vice Trust: A Reinterpretation of the White Slavery Scare in the United States, 1907–1917," *Journal of Social History* 35 (Fall 2001): 5–41; Barbara Meil Hobson, *Uneasy Virtue: The Politics of Prostitution and the American Reform Tradition* (New York: Basic Books, 1987), 142–45.

62. Mary M. Bartelme, "The Girls Today and Juvenile Court Methods [and discussion]," *Quarterly Representing the Minnesota Educational, Philanthropic, Correctional and Penal Institutions under the State Board of Control* 21 (Aug. 2, 1921): 8–26; Ma, *One Hundred Years*, 43–46.

63. Legislative Committee Minutes, Nov. 14, 1912; Minutes of Executive Meeting, Jan. 17, 1913, WWL; "Gets License to Marry," *St. Paul Dispatch*, Dec. 3, 1912.

64. *Unpublished Facts and Letters of the 'Uncle Ned' nee Joseph W. Bragdon: Exploits and Trials, 1916–1917* (Minneapolis: J. M. Near and J. D. Bevans, 1917), MHS; "Bragdon's Appeal Denied; He Must Serve Sentence," *Minneapolis Morning Tribune*, Apr. 28, 1917. See also Wheeler, *Against Obscenity*, 46–47.

65. "Hundred Women Offer City Help in Vice Crusade," *Minneapolis Morning Tribune*, Mar. 18, 1916.

66. US Children's Bureau, *State Commissions for the Study and Revision of Child Welfare Laws* (Washington, DC: GPO, 1924), 7–8. See Ma, *One Hundred Years*, 79, 83.

67. Edward MacGaffey, "A Pattern for Progress: the Minnesota Children's Code," *Minnesota History* 41 (Spring 1969): 229–36. See the obituaries of Rogers in *The National Cyclopaedia of American Biography* 17 (New York: James T. White, 1927), 248, and *Survey* 37 (Feb. 24, 1917): 619. On the fracturing of the progressive coalition, see Keillor, *Shaping Minnesota's Identity*, 136–42.

68. "Report of Minnesota Child Welfare Commission Appointed by the Governor to Revise and Codify the Laws of Minnesota Relating to Children," Dec. 16, 1916, enclosed in J. A. A. Burnquist, Inaugural Message of Governor, 1917, J. A. A. Burnquist Papers, MHS; Edward F. Waite, "New Laws for Minnesota Children," *Minnesota Law Review* 1 (1917): 48–62.

69. Minnesota Child Welfare Commission, *Report of the Minnesota Child Welfare Commission* (St. Paul: Office of the Commission, 1917), 9; "Delay of Marriage License Issue Asked by Welfare Report," *Minneapolis Journal*, Feb. 18, 1917.

70. *Report of the Minnesota Child Welfare Commission*, 10–11.

71. Ibid., 14. On modern adoption and the Minnesota law, see Ellen Herman, *Kinship by Design: A History of Adoption in the Modern United States* (Chicago: University of Chicago

Press, 2008); E. Wayne Carp, *Family Matters: Secrecy and Disclosure in the History of Adoption* (Cambridge, MA: Harvard University Press, 1998).

72. Ma, *One Hundred Years*, 111; *Report of the Minnesota Child Welfare Commission*, 13, 42.

73. *Report of the Minnesota Child Welfare Commission*, 11–12, 26.

74. Ibid., 12–13, 18.

75. W. W. Hodson, "The Minnesota Child Welfare Commission [and discussion]," in US Children's Bureau, *Standards of Child Welfare: A Report of the Children's Bureau Conferences, May and June 1919* (Washington, DC: GPO, 1919), 422, 426.

76. Ma, *One Hundred Years*, 90; MacGaffey, "Pattern for Progress," 230.

Chapter Two · *Two Roads to Sterilization*

1. Edward F. Waite, "The Next Step in Child Welfare in Minnesota," in *Proceedings of the Minnesota State Conference of Charities and Correction* (Stillwater, MN: Mirror Print, 1917), 64.

2. Sharon M. Leon, *An Image of God: The Catholic Struggle with Eugenics* (Chicago: University of Chicago Press, 2013), 36. On the post–World War I eugenics movement and sterilization, see Philip R. Reilly, *The Surgical Solution: A History of Involuntary Sterilization in the United States* (Baltimore: Johns Hopkins University Press, 1991); Daniel J. Kevles, *In the Name of Eugenics: Genetics and the Uses of Human Heredity* (Cambridge, MA: Harvard University Press, 1995); Paul A. Lombardo, *Three Generations, No Imbeciles: Eugenics, the Supreme Court, and* Buck v. Bell (Baltimore: Johns Hopkins University Press, 2008).

3. Walter I. Trattner, *From Poor Law to Welfare State: A History of Social Welfare in America*, 6th ed. (New York: Free Press, 1998), chap. 12.

4. See, e.g., David M. Kennedy, *Over Here: The First World War and American Society* (New York: Oxford University Press, 1980); Alan Dawley, *Struggles for Justice: Social Responsibility and the Liberal State* (Cambridge, MA: Belknap Press of Harvard University Press, 1991).

5. Carl H. Chrislock, *Watchdog of Loyalty: The Minnesota Commission on Public Safety during World War I* (St. Paul: Minnesota Historical Society Press, 1991), chap. 11; Theodore C. Blegen, *Minnesota: A History of the State* (1963; repr., Minneapolis: University of Minnesota Press, 1975), 470–73; Steven Keillor, *Shaping Minnesota's Identity: 150 Years of State Identity* (Lakeville, MN: Pogo, 2007), 140–59.

6. Michael A. Rembis, *Defining Deviance: Sex, Science, and Delinquent Girls, 1890–1960* (Urbana: University of Illinois Press, 2011), 59–64; Dawley, *Struggles for Justice*, 212–17.

7. Kennedy, *Over Here*, 187–89; Mark H. Haller, *Eugenics: Hereditarian Attitudes in American Thought* (1963; repr., New Brunswick, NJ: Rutgers University Press, 1984), 113–14. See also Kevles, *In the Name of Eugenics*, 80–83.

8. Randall Hansen and Desmond King, *Sterilized by the State: Eugenics, Race, and the Population Scare in Twentieth-Century North America* (Cambridge: Cambridge University Press, 2013), 17–18.

9. On the idea that new policies create new politics, or policy feedback, see Theda Skocpol, *Protecting Soldiers and Mothers: The Political Origins of Social Policy in the United States* (Cambridge, MA: Belknap Press of Harvard University Press, 1992), 57–60.

10. Gioh-Fang Dju Ma, *One Hundred Years of Public Services for Children in Minnesota* (Chicago: University of Chicago Press, 1948), 94–95. In counties with large cities, the Board of Control appointed five members for a seven-person board.

11. Laws of Minnesota 1917, chap. 194, secs. 1–2 and 5–6; Laws of Minnesota 1917, chap. 344.

12. William Hodson, "A State Program for Child Welfare," *Annals of the American Academy of Political and Social Science* 98 (Nov. 1921): 165; H. Ida Curry, *Public Child-Caring Work in Certain Counties of Minnesota, North Carolina, and New York* (Washington, DC: GPO, 1927), 13.

13. Jerome Tweton, *Depression: Minnesota in the Thirties* (Fargo: North Dakota Institute for Regional Studies, 1981), 9; Ma, *One Hundred Years*, 190–92.

14. Mildred Thomson, *Prologue: A Minnesota Story of Mental Retardation* (Minneapolis: Gilbert, 1963), 19.

15. William Hodson to Guy C. Hanna, Feb. 20, 1918, FSSH SC; FSSH, *Report of the Superintendent of the School for the Feeble-Minded and Colony for Epileptics for the Biennial Period Ending June 30, 1920*, 51–52.

16. Laws of Minnesota 1917, chap. 344, secs. 2 and 3; William Hodson, "What Minnesota Has Done and Should Do for the Feeble-Minded," *Quarterly Conference of the Executive Officers of State Institutions with the State Board of Control*, Aug. 6, 1918, 5–12.

17. Ma, *One Hundred Years*, 95–99; Curry, *Public Child-Caring Work*, 10–12.

18. On the House of the Good Shepherd, see Bluestem Heritage Group, *Frogtown Park and Farm History* (St. Paul, 2014), www.stpaul.gov/DocumentCenter/View2/74315.pdf; see also the correspondence between FSSH and the Board of Control. On Ojibwe girls and the House of the Good Shepherd, see Social Worker's Yearly Report, Aug. 10, 1936, to June 30, 1937, Records of the Health Division, Bureau of Indian Affairs, National Archives. See also Regina G. Kunzel, *Fallen Women, Problem Girls: Unmarried Mothers and the Professionalization of Social Work, 1890–1945* (New Haven, CT: Yale University Press, 1995); Marian J. Morton, *And Sin No More: Social Policy and Unwed Mothers in Cleveland, 1855–1990* (Columbus: Ohio State University Press, 1993).

19. Curry, *Public Child-Caring Work*, 15–24; Ma, *One Hundred Years*, 111–30.

20. Curry, *Public Child-Caring Work*, 17, 19; Charlotte Lowe, "The Intelligence and Social Background of the Unmarried Mother," *Mental Hygiene* 11 (1927): 793.

21. Laws of Minnesota 1917, chap. 211; Laws of Minnesota 1919, chap. 193, sec. 1; Curry, *Public Child-Caring Work*, 22–24. See also Mildred Dennett Mudgett, *Results of Minnesota's Laws for Protection of Children Born Out of Wedlock* (Washington, DC: GPO, 1924), 193–94.

22. Mudgett, *Results of Minnesota's Laws*, 192; Curry, *Public Child-Caring Work*, 21.

23. Kunzel, *Fallen Women, Problem Girls*, 54; Mudgett, *Results of Minnesota's Laws*, 202, 213.

24. Mudgett, *Results of Minnesota's Laws*, 212, 236.

25. Ibid., 213–14.

26. Walter E. Fernald, "The Burden of Feeble-Mindedness," *JPA* 17 (Mar. 1912): 87–111; Hodson, "What Minnesota Has Done," 6.

27. Minnesota State Board of Control, *Biennial Report of the State Board of Control of Minnesota for the Period Ending June 30, 1922*, 18.

28. Mildred Thomson, Memo to Members of the Child Welfare Boards of Minnesota, n.d., Gilman (Robbins and Family) Papers, MHS.

29. Blanche La Du, "Treatment of the Social Offender from the Standpoint of the State," in *Proceedings of the Minnesota State Conference and Institute of Social Work* (St. Paul: State Board of Control, 1925), 73, 67.

30. "The Loyalist Waggoners of Vermont: Information about Blanche L. Waggoner," www.genealogy.com/ftm/w/a/g/Linda-Waggoner-CA/WEBSITE-0001/UHP-0225.html.

31. Secretary's Report for 1920; "Eleven years ago this month" (untitled Secretary's Report

for 1922); Secretary's Annual Report for 1923; Regular Meeting, Nov. 14, 1924; Annual Report of the Secretary—1924, all in WWL.

32. Thomson, *Prologue*, 23, 50–51. On Bernstein, see James W. Trent Jr., *Inventing the Feeble Mind: A History of Mental Retardation in the United States* (Berkeley: University of California Press, 1994), 207–15.

33. Hodson, "What Minnesota Has Done," 6; Thomson, *Prologue*, 49–50.

34. Minnesota State Board of Control, *Biennial Report of the State Board of Control for the Period Ending June 30, 1924*, 18–19; Annual Report of the Secretary—1924, WWL.

35. Thomson, *Prologue*, 53; G. C. Hanna, "The Menace of the Feebleminded [and discussion]," in Minnesota State Board of Control, *Quarterly Conference Representing the Minnesota Educational, Philanthropic Correctional and Penal Institutions* 24 (Feb. 10, 1925): 48.

36. Thomson, *Prologue*, 55.

37. Ibid., 6–13.

38. FSSH, *Report of the Superintendent of the School for Feeble-Minded and Colony for Epileptics for the Biennial Period Ending June 30, 1922*, 19, 24.

39. Thomson, *Prologue*, 27, 51; G. C. Hanna to Agnes Crowley, Jan. 11, 1924, FSSH SC.

40. Thomson, *Prologue*, 51, 63.

41. G. C. Hanna to Mildred Thomson, Nov. 5, 1924; "List of Cases Recommended by Mr. Hanna for the Club House," enclosed in Mildred Thomson to G. C. Hanna, Nov. 21, 1924, FSSH SC; Case no. 35, Record of Sterilization Cases, 1916–1937, FSSH. For Devitt's report on "Greta Acker," see S. C. Devitt (June 1914), ser. 7, Field Worker Files, ERO Records, APS.

42. Hanna, "Menace of the Feebleminded [and discussion]," 21, 39, 27, 43. Thomson discusses her reaction to Hanna's paper in *Prologue*, 63–64.

43. Hanna, "Menace of the Feebleminded [and discussion]," 46; A. L. Beier, "The Operation of the Wisconsin Sterilization Law [and discussion]," *Quarterly Conference Representing the Minnesota Educational, Philanthropic Correctional and Penal Institutions* 19 (May 1920): 16.

44. *Casti Connubii* quoted in Leon, *Image of God*, 61; Beier, "Wisconsin Sterilization Law [and discussion]," 14–15, 21.

45. Hanna, "Menace of the Feebleminded [and discussion]," 44–45.

46. Hodson, "What Minnesota Has Done [and discussion]," 21.

47. Hanna, "Menace of the Feebleminded [and discussion]," 53, 46. Vasaly remained "utterly opposed" to sterilization.

48. Charles Dight, *History of the Early Stages of the Organized Eugenics Movement* (Minneapolis: Minnesota Eugenics Society, 1935), 8, MHS. For a fuller account of the origins of the MES, see Neal Ross Holtan, "From Eugenics to Public Health Genetics in Mid-Twentieth Century Minnesota" (PhD diss., University of Minnesota, 2011).

49. Dight, *History of the Early Stages*, 9–11. On Catheryne Cooke Gilman, see Elizabeth Gilman, "Catheryne Cooke Gilman: Social Worker," in *Women of Minnesota: Selected Biographical Essays*, ed. Barbara Stuhler and Gretchen Kreuter (St. Paul: Minnesota Historical Society Press, 1977), 190–207; Cynthia A. Hanson, "Catheryne Cooke Gilman and the Minneapolis Better Movie Movement," *Minnesota History* 51 (Summer 1989): 202–16; Leigh Ann Wheeler, *Against Obscenity: Reform and the Politics of Womanhood in America, 1873–1935* (Baltimore: Johns Hopkins University Press, 2007). On Victoria McAlmon, see Elaine Showalter, *These Modern Women: Autobiographical Essays from the Twenties* (New York: Feminist Press, 1989), 109–15. See also Daniel E. Bender, *American Abyss: Savagery and Civilization in the Age

of Industry (Ithaca, NY: Cornell University Press, 2009); Howard Jacob Karger, *The Sentinels of Order: A Study of Social Control and the Minneapolis Settlement House Movement, 1915–1950* (Lanham, MD: University Press of America, 1987).

50. Holtan, "From Eugenics to Public Health Genetics," 46–52; Gary Phelps, "The Eugenics Crusade of Charles Dight," *Minnesota History* 49 (Fall 1984): 99–108; Evadene Burris Swanson, "Some Sources for Northwest History," *Minnesota History* 25 (1944): 62–64.

51. Charles F. Dight, "Human Thoroughbreds—Why Not?" (1922), iii, 27, Charles Fremont Dight Papers, MHS; Charles F. Dight, "The American Beet Sugar Company," typescript, n.d. (1925), Dight Papers. See also Mark Soderstrom, "Family Trees and Timber Rights: Albert E. Jenks, Americanization, and the Rise of Anthropology at the University of Minnesota," *Journal of the Gilded Age and Progressive Era* 3 (Apr. 2004): 176–204.

52. Dight, *History of the Early Stages*, 43, 46–47.

53. "Preamble" [to typescript on resolution to form a eugenics association], 2, Dight Papers.

54. Dight, "Human Thoroughbreds," 32–33.

55. George Sparks to Dight, Oct. 4, 1922; Thomas Canfield to Dight, Feb. 4, 1924, Dight Papers; Dight, *History of the Early Stages*, 9.

56. Harry H. Laughlin, *Eugenical Sterilization in the United States* (Chicago: Psychopathic Laboratory of the Municipal Court of Chicago, 1922), 446–47; Harry H. Laughlin, "The Socially Inadequate: How Shall We Designate and Sort Them?," *American Journal of Sociology* 27 (July 1921): 54–70; Holtan, "From Eugenics to Public Health Genetics," 40. See also Lizzie Seal, "Designating Dependency: The 'Socially Inadequate' in the United States, 1910–1940," *Journal of Historical Sociology* 26 (June 2013): 143–68. Dight had a copy of Laughlin's book.

57. Laws of Minnesota 1925, chap. 154, secs. 1 and 2; James E. Hughes, *Eugenic Sterilization in the United States: A Comparative Summary of Statutes and Review of Court Decisions* (Washington, DC: GPO, 1940), 2–3. The other state was Vermont.

58. Phelps, "Eugenics Crusade," 103; Frederick Kuhlmann to Dight, Jan. 9, 1925, Dight Papers.

59. Minnesota House of Representatives, Committee Meeting Minutes, Public Welfare and Social Legislation, Jan. 28–Feb. 5, 1925. Two amendments were made from the floor, both of which applied only to "insane" persons: the patient had to be hospitalized for "at least six consecutive months," and the surgery had to be performed by a "competent surgeon." See Minnesota House Journal, 44th legislature, regular session (Feb. 25, 1925); Dight, *History of the Early Stages*, 9.

60. "Report to the Executive of the Minnesota Eugenics Society," typescript, n.d. [1925], Dight Papers; Phelps, "Eugenics Crusade," 103–4.

61. C. F. Dight, "The Outcome of This Endeavor," untitled typescript, n.d. [Mar. 1926], Dight Papers; Thomson, *Prologue*, 55.

62. C. F. Dight, "Increase of the Unfit a Social Menace: Facts Which Call for Enactment of an Adequate Eugenics Law for Human Betterment, Opposition to It by the Minnesota State Board of Control," n.d. [1930], Dight Papers; Dight, *History of the Early Stages*, 34, 5, 38.

63. C. F. Dight, "Handwritten Notes Regarding the State Board of Control," n.d. [1929], Dight Papers.

64. Mrs. Maude B. Arney to Dight, Feb. 19, 1930, and Mar. 16, 1930; Edward C. Baumann to Dight, Mar. 29, 1930, Dight Papers; Dight, *History of the Early Stages*, 15.

65. Dight, "Increase of the Unfit a Social Menace," and related correspondence, Dight Papers.

66. Dight to Adolf Hitler, Aug. 1, 1933; printed postcard from Hitler to Dight, Aug. 23, 1933, Dight Papers.

Chapter Three • Who Was Feebleminded?

1. Adam Cohen, *Imbeciles: The Supreme Court, American Eugenics, and the Sterilization of Carrie Buck* (New York: Penguin, 2016), 16; Edwin Black, *War against the Weak: Eugenics and America's Campaign to Create a Master Race* (New York: Four Walls Eight Windows, 2003), 77–79. The phrase "catchall term" was probably first used by Daniel J. Kevles, *In the Name of Eugenics: Genetics and the Uses of Human Heredity* (Cambridge, MA: Harvard University Press, 1995), 46.

2. Paul Popenoe and Roswell H. Johnson, *Applied Eugenics* (New York: Macmillan, 1918), 439. See James W. Trent Jr., *Inventing the Feeble Mind: A History of Mental Retardation in the United States* (Berkeley: University of California Press, 1994).

3. Henry Herbert Goddard, "The Elimination of Feeble-Mindedness," *Annals of the American Academy of Political and Social Science* 37 (Mar. 1911): 261, 506; A. C. Rogers and Maud A. Merrill, *Dwellers in the Vale of Siddem: A True Story of the Social Aspect of Feeble-Mindedness* (Boston: Richard D. Badger, 1919), 10; Nancy Ordover, *American Eugenics: Race, Queer Anatomy, and the Science of Nationalism* (Minneapolis: University of Minnesota Press, 2003), 12. See also Gerald V. O'Brien, *Framing the Moron: The Social Construction of Feeble-Mindedness in the American Eugenic Era* (Manchester: Manchester University Press, 2013).

4. See Ian Haney López, *White by Law: The Legal Construction of Race* (New York: New York University Press, 2006), 7–8. An astute analysis of a different type of incompetency proceeding can be found in Kim E. Nielsen, "Property, Disability, and the Making of the Incompetent Citizen in the United States, 1860s–1940s," in *Disability Histories*, ed. Susan Burch and Michael Rembis (Urbana: University of Illinois Press, 2014), 308–20.

5. Laws of Minnesota 1917, chap. 344, secs. 4–7.

6. Frederick Kuhlmann, "The New Law for the Feeble-Minded," in *Proceedings of the Minnesota State Conference of Charities and Correction* (Stillwater, MN: Mirror Print, 1918), 130.

7. Laws of Minnesota 1917, chap. 344, sec. 1. This uncertainty is documented in the proceedings of the Minnesota State Conference on Social Work and the quarterly conferences of the Board of Control.

8. Mildred Thomson, *Dr. Arthur C. Rogers: Pioneer Leader in Minnesota's Program for the Mentally Retarded* (Minneapolis: Minnesota Association for Retarded Children, n.d. [1966]), 36.

9. Leila Zenderland, *Measuring Minds: Henry Herbert Goddard and the Origins of American Intelligence Testing* (New York: Cambridge University Press, 1997), 80.

10. Susan M. Schweik, *The Ugly Laws: Disability in Public* (New York: New York University Press, 2010), 67; Martin W. Barr, *Mental Defectives: Their History, Treatment, and Training* (Philadelphia: Blakiston's, 1904), 23, 126; Frederick Kuhlmann, "What Constitutes Feeble-Mindedness?," *JPA* 19 (June 1915): 217. See also Zenderland, *Measuring Minds*, 74–81; Martin A. Elks, "Believing Is Seeing: Visual Conventions in Barr's Classification of the 'Feeble-Minded,'" *Mental Retardation* 42 (Oct. 2004): 371–82.

11. Kuhlmann, "What Constitutes Feeble-Mindedness?," 217–18.

12. Rogers and Merrill, *Dwellers in the Vale of Siddem*, 10–11, 43.

13. Goddard, "Elimination of Feeble-Mindedness," 266; A. C. Rogers to State Board of Control, June 28, 1910, FSSH SC; Kuhlmann, "What Constitutes Feeble-Mindedness?" 234.

14. A. C. Rogers, "Report of Committee of Research [and discussion]," *Quarterly Conference of the Executive Officers of State Institutions with the State Board of Control*, Feb. 2, 1912, 68.

15. Rogers, "Report of Committee," 66; FSSH, *Report of Superintendent Minnesota School for the Feeble-Minded and Colony for Epileptics, for the Biennial Period Ending July 31, 1912*, 220; Thomson, *Dr. Arthur C. Rogers*, 34–35.

16. This discussion is based on Saidee Devitt's and Marie Curial's folders in ser. 7, Field Worker Files, 1911–1926, ERO Records, APS.

17. Saidee Devitt, "Timber Rats," 8–10, in S. C. Devitt no. 2, Field Worker Files, ERO.

18. Ibid., 13–15.

19. Devitt, "Timber Rats," 42. See K. Kris Hirst, "Dugout Dwellings: Pioneer Housing in 19th Century Minnesota," http://archaeology.about.com/od/ancienthouses/a/dugouts.htm.

20. "Mary Schmidt," Data Collected by Miss Devitt, 4, 11, Sept. 1916, Devitt Files, ERO; Carl Henry Chrislock, *The Progressive Era in Minnesota, 1899–1918* (St. Paul: Minnesota Historical Society, 1971).

21. "Susan Herman," Mar. 1914, Devitt Files, ERO.

22. Ibid.

23. "Greta Acker," June 1914, Devitt Files, ERO; Case no. 35, Record of Sterilization Cases, 1916–1937, FSSH Miscellaneous Medical Records, MHS.

24. Saidee Devitt to A. C. Rogers, received June 2, 1915, Research Department, FSSH SC.

25. A. C. Rogers, "Editorial: The New Classification (Tentative) of the Feeble-Minded," *JPA* 15 (Sept.–Dec. 1910): 70; "Report on Committee of Classification of Feeble-Minded," *JPA* 15 (Sept.–Dec. 1910): 61.

26. Zenderland, *Measuring Minds*, 98–104; JoAnne Brown, *The Definition of a Profession: The Authority of Metaphor in the History of Intelligence Testing, 1890–1930* (Princeton, NJ: Princeton University Press, 1992), chap. 5.

27. A. C. Rogers, "President's Address, Faribault Meeting, 1890," in *Proceedings of the Association of Medical Officers of American Institutions for Idiotic and Feeble-Minded Persons, 1887–1895* (New York: Johnson Reprint, 1964), 29; Frederick Kuhlmann, "Distribution of Feeble-Minded in Society," *Journal of Criminal Law and Criminology* 7 (May 1916–Mar. 1917): 206; Henry Herbert Goddard, *Feeble-Mindedness: Its Causes and Consequences* (New York: Macmillan, 1914), 9, 15, 17; Alexander W. Pisciotta, *Benevolent Repression: Social Control and the American Reformatory-Prison Movement* (New York: New York University Press, 1996), 117.

28. Mark Haller, *Eugenics: Hereditarian Attitudes in American Thought* (New Brunswick, NJ: Rutgers University Press, 1963), 100; Michael A. Rembis, *Defining Deviance: Sex, Science, and Delinquent Girls, 1890–1960* (Urbana: University of Illinois Press, 2011), 59–61. See also Douglas C. Baynton, *Defectives in the Land: Disability and Immigration in the Age of Eugenics* (Chicago: University of Chicago Press, 2016); Steven A. Gelb, "Henry H. Goddard and the Immigrants, 1910–1917: The Studies and Their Social Context," *Journal of the History of the Behavioral Sciences* 22 (Oct. 1986): 324–32. Population statistics are from US Census Bureau, "Population-Minnesota," *Fourteenth Census of the United States* (1920), vol. 3, 504.

29. Mildred Thomson, *Prologue: A Minnesota Story of Mental Retardation* (Minneapolis: Gilbert, 1963), 62–63; Josef Brožek, *Explorations in the History of Psychology in the United States* (Cranbury, NJ: Bucknell University Press, 1984), 231–33.

30. Mildred Thomson, "Problems Relating to the Work of the Feeble-Minded," in *Proceedings of the Minnesota State Conference and Institute of Social Work* (St. Paul: State Board of Control, 1926), 305; Robert J. Levy, "Protecting the Mentally Retarded: An Empirical Survey and Evaluation of the Establishment of Guardianship in Minnesota," *Minnesota Law Review* 49 (1965): 842.

31. Laws of Minnesota 1917, chap. 344, sec. 14; Mildred Thomson, "My Thirty-Five Years with the Mentally Retarded in Minnesota," 133, typescript, n.d. [1962], MHS.

32. "Agnes Ogden," Home School for Girls, Case Files, MHS. The literature on IQ testing is vast. See, e.g., Stephen Jay Gould, *The Mismeasure of Man* (New York: W. W. Norton, 1981).

33. "Vera Hardy," HSG Case Files; Frederick Kuhlmann, "The State's Program for the Feeble-Minded," in *Proceedings of the Minnesota State Conference and Institute of Social Work* (St. Paul: State Board of Control, 1927), 156. Vera's sister was FSSH Sterilization Case no. 781.

34. Kuhlmann, "State's Program for the Feeble-Minded," 156.

35. Quoted in Levy, "Protecting the Mentally Retarded," 842.

36. Rogers, "Report of Committee," 69; Hennepin County Child Welfare Board, *Annual Report for 1927*, 14, Hennepin County Welfare Department, MHS.

37. "Edna Collins" and "Lillian Green," HSG Case Files; FSSH Sterilization Case no. 382.

38. "Edna Collins" and "Lillian Green," HSG Case Files; FSSH Sterilization Case no. 382; Mildred Thomson, "Supervision of the Feeble-Minded by County Welfare Boards," paper given to the American Association of Mental Deficiency, May 1940, DPW Library, MHS. On sexual rebelliousness and the feebleminded label, see Mary Odem, *Delinquent Daughters: Protecting and Policing Adolescent Female Sexuality in the United States, 1885–1920* (Chapel Hill: University of North Carolina Press, 1995), 98; Wendy Kline, *Building a Better Race: Gender, Sexuality, and Eugenics from the Turn of the Century to the Baby Boom* (Berkeley: University of California Press, 2001), 20.

39. "Rachel Kopf" and "Sarah Berger," HSG Case Files.

40. Thomson, *Prologue*, 72–73.

41. Walter Fernald, "The Burden of Feeble-Mindedness," *JPA* 17 (Mar. 1912): 87–99; Helen Ross Nelson, "A Study of the Social Background of Delinquent Girls in Juvenile Court of Minneapolis" (MA thesis, University of Minnesota, 1926), 49–50; "Possibilities for Clubhouse (Sterilized 9/29/28)," enclosed in J. M. Murdoch to Mildred Thomson, Nov. 13, 1928, "Parole Cases II," typescript, 1934, FSSH SC. See also Lynn Sacco, *Unspeakable: Father–Daughter Incest in American History* (Baltimore: Johns Hopkins University Press, 2009); Hughes Evans, "The Discovery of Child Sexual Abuse in America," in *Formative Years: Children's Health in the United States, 1880–2000*, ed. Alexandra Minna Stern and Howard Markel (Ann Arbor: University of Michigan Press, 2002), 233–59.

42. FSSH Admissions Records, vol. G, MHS.

43. My interpretation is based on the Red Lake and Consolidated Chippewa Indian Agencies Social Worker's Reports, Records of the Health Division, Bureau of Indian Affairs, National Archives, and the *Proceedings of the Minnesota State Conference and Institute of Social Work*. See also Margaret D. Jacobs, "Diverted Mothering among American Indian Domestic Servants, 1920–1940," in *Indigenous Women's Work: From Labor to Activism*, ed. Carol Williams (Urbana: University of Illinois Press, 2012), 179–92.

44. Thomson, *Prologue*, 88–89.

45. Licia Carlson, *The Faces of Intellectual Disability: Philosophical Reflections* (Blooming-

ton: Indiana University Press, 2010), 68–71; Molly Ladd-Taylor and Lauri Umansky, *"Bad" Mothers: The Politics of Blame in Twentieth-Century America* (New York: New York University Press, 1998).

46. "Girls who could be considered for sterilization," typescript, May 10, 1933, FSSH SC.

47. Kathleen Jones, *Taming the Troublesome Child: American Families, Child Guidance, and the Limits of Psychiatric Authority* (Cambridge, MA: Harvard University Press, 1999); Ladd-Taylor and Umansky, *"Bad" Mothers*, 1–28.

48. Florence S. Davis, "The Neglect of Children as Related to Feeble-Mindedness," typescript, Sept. 21, 1934, DPW Library; Florence Goodenough, "Education of the Feebleminded in the Home," typescript, 1935, DPW Library, MHS.

49. "Parole Cases IV," typescript, 1934, FSSH SC.

50. Medical Staff Minutes, Jan. 18, 1937, and Sept. 28, 1936, FSSH; Sterilization Case nos. 995 and 946.

51. Chas. E. Dow, "The Problem of the Feeble-Minded III," typescript, Aug. 9, 1934, DPW Library.

52. Davis, "Neglect of Children."

53. Ibid.; Goodenough, "Education of the Feebleminded." For a powerful discussion of the removal of indigenous children in the same period, see Margaret D. Jacobs, *White Mother to a Dark Race: Settler Colonialism, Maternalism, and the Removal of Indigenous Children in the American West and Australia, 1880–1940* (Lincoln: University of Nebraska Press, 2011).

54. Margot Canaday, *The Straight State: Sexuality and Citizenship in Twentieth-Century America* (Princeton, NJ: Princeton University Press, 2009), 95–108.

55. Mildred Thomson to J. M. Murdoch, Apr. 16, 1935, FSSH SC; "Record of Eleven Patients Who Escaped from the Main Boys' Annex," Oct. 1, 1938, in Edward J. Engberg to State Board of Control, Dec. 1, 1938, FSSH SC; Summary of Case Record, June 24, 1939, FSSH SC.

56. Engberg to Board of Control, Dec. 1, 1938.

57. "Edward Wood," Inmate Case Files, Annex for Defective Delinquents, 1945–1961, Minnesota State Reformatory for Men, MHS. On eugenics laws targeting gay men, see Peter Boag, *Same-Sex Affairs: Constructing and Controlling Homosexuality in the Pacific Northwest* (Berkeley: University of California Press, 2003), chap. 6; Mark A. Largent, *Breeding Contempt: The History of Coerced Sterilization in the United States* (New Brunswick, NJ: Rutgers University Press, 2008), 94–95.

58. Enclosed in Mildred Thomson to J. M. Murdoch, Sept. 8, 1932, FSSH SC. Genealogical sources suggest that Brian eventually married and moved out of state.

59. State Board of Control v. Herman Fechner, 192 Minn. 412, 256 N.W. 662 (1934); State ex rel. Fechner v. Carlgren, 296 N.W. 573, 209 Minn., 362 (1941).

60. Trial Transcript, Rice County 5th Judicial District Court, 28–29, Case no. 30054, Minnesota State Supreme Court, Case Files, MHS.

61. Ibid.

62. Ibid., 83–84.

63. Ibid.

64. *Board of Control v. Fechner.*

65. *State ex rel. Fechner v. Carlgren*; Minnesota Death Certificate, Feb. 28, 1946, ID no. 1946-MN-009608, MHS.

66. FSSH, *Report of Superintendents to the State Board of Control for the Period Ending*

June 30, 1930, 16; FSSH, *Report of Superintendents to the State Board of Control for the Period Ending June 30, 1934*, 17.

67. Engberg to Board of Control, Dec. 1, 1938, FSSH SC; Mildred Thomson to O. J. Anderson, Dec. 18, 1951, ADD, St. Cloud Reformatory, Miscellaneous Subject Files, MHS.

68. Engberg to Board of Control, Dec. 1, 1938.

69. Walter Fernald, "The Imbecile with Criminal Instincts," *JPA* 14 (Apr. 1909): 35; Walter Fernald, "Remarks," *JPA* 23 (1918–1919): 98–99, quoted in Nicole Hahn Rafter, *Creating Born Criminals* (Urbana: University of Illinois Press, 1997), 190; Arthur E. Westwell, "The Defective Delinquent," *American Journal of Mental Deficiency* 56 (1951): 283.

70. "60 Defective Delinquents Better Off at St. Cloud," *Minneapolis Star Journal*, July 4, 1945. See Molly Ladd-Taylor, " 'Ravished by Some Moron': Panic, Politics, and the Minnesota Psychopathic Personalities Law of 1939" (unpublished paper, presented at University of Lethbridge, Aug. 2015).

71. Thomson to Anderson, Dec. 18, 1951.

Chapter Four • The Price of Freedom

1. Philip R. Reilly, *The Surgical Solution: A History of Involuntary Sterilization in the United States* (Baltimore: Johns Hopkins University Press, 1991), 88; FSSH, *Record of Sterilization Cases*, 1916–1937, MHS.

2. Mark H. Haller, *Eugenics: Hereditarian Attitudes in American Thought* (1963; repr., New Brunswick, NJ: Rutgers University Press, 1984), 140; Randall Hansen and Desmond King, *Sterilized by the State: Eugenics, Race, and the Population Scare in Twentieth-Century North America* (Cambridge: Cambridge University Press, 2013), 18.

3. Buck v. Bell, 274 U.S. 200 (1927) at 206.

4. James W. Trent Jr., *Inventing the Feeble Mind: A History of Mental Retardation in the United States* (Berkeley: University of California Press, 1994), 198–99.

5. Laws of Minnesota 1925, chap. 154, secs. 1 and 2.

6. Mildred Thomson, *Prologue: A Minnesota Story of Mental Retardation* (Minneapolis: Gilbert, 1963), 71. This correspondence is located in FSSH SC.

7. James E. Hughes, *Eugenic Sterilization in the United States: A Comparative Summary of Statutes and Review of Court Decisions* (Washington, DC: GPO, 1940), 3–4.

8. Ibid., 16–17; Harry H. Laughlin, *Eugenical Sterilization in the United States* (Chicago: Psychopathic Library of the Municipal Court of Chicago, 1922), 96. For an exceptionally insightful analysis of gender and sterilization, see Allison C. Carey, "Gender and Compulsory Sterilization Programs in America: 1907–1950," *Journal of Historical Sociology* 11 (Mar. 1998): 74–105.

9. FSSH, *Report of the Superintendents to the State Board of Control for the Biennial Period Ending June 30, 1928*, 13; E. J. Engberg to Carl Swanson, June 22, 1946, FSSH SC; Liza Piper, "Analysis of Sterilization Records: Personal Information" (unpublished report in author's possession); Mildred Thomson, "Memo to Child Welfare Boards and Others Concerned with Carrying Out the Sterilization Law," Dec. 12, 1934, DPW PSB.

10. Piper, "Personal Information."

11. Trent, *Inventing the Feeble Mind*, 194–96; FSSH Sterilization Case nos. 1–3.

12. Mark A. Largent, *Breeding Contempt: The History of Coerced Sterilization in the United States* (New Brunswick, NJ: Rutgers University Press, 2008), chap. 1.

13. Angela Gugliotta, "'Dr. Sharp with His Little Knife': Therapeutic and Eugenic Origins of Eugenic Vasectomy—Indiana, 1892–1911," *Journal of the History of Medicine and Allied Sciences* 53 (Oct. 1998): 371–406; Paul A. Lombardo, ed., *A Century of Eugenics in America: From the Indiana Experiment to the Human Genome Era* (Bloomington: Indiana University Press, 2011); Human Betterment Foundation, "Operations for Eugenic Sterilization Performed in State Institutions under State Laws up to January 1, 1930," Sterilization Statistics, AVS Records.

14. Neal Holtan, "The Eitels and Their Hospital," *Minnesota Medicine* 86 (Sept. 2003): 52–54; Neal Holtan, "Breeding to Brains: Eugenics, Physicians, and Politics in Minnesota in the 1920s" (MA thesis, University of Minnesota, 2000), 64–65.

15. Thomson, *Prologue*, 56; Liza Piper, "Analysis of Sterilization Records: After Faribault" (unpublished report in author's possession).

16. FSSH Sterilization Case nos. 749, 641, 720, 345, 735; Liza Piper, "Analysis of Sterilization Records: Operations" (unpublished report in author's possession).

17. FSSH Sterilization Case nos. 67, 749, 90, 338, 140, 151, 23.

18. The literature on this topic is vast. See, e.g., Regina Morantz-Sanchez, *Conduct Unbecoming a Woman: Medicine on Trial in Turn-of-the-Century Brooklyn* (New York: Oxford University Press, 1999); Harriet A. Washington, *Medical Apartheid: The Dark History of Medical Experimentation on Black Americans from Colonial Times to the Present* (New York: Broadway Books, 2008); Barron H. Lerner, "Constructing Medical Indications: The Sterilization of Women with Heart Disease and Tuberculosis, 1905–1935," *Journal of the History of Medicine and Allied Sciences* 49 (1994): 362–79.

19. Piper, "Operations."

20. FSSH Sterilization Case nos. 21 and 24; Blanche La Du to G. C. Hanna, Dec. 9, 1926; Hanna to La Du, Dec. 11, 1926, FSSH SC.

21. Human Betterment Foundation, "Table of Sterilizations Done in State Institutions under State Laws up to and Including the Year 1937," Sterilization Statistics, AVS Records; G. C. Hanna, "The Menace of the Feebleminded [and discussion]," *Quarterly Representing the Minnesota Educational, Philanthropic Correctional and Penal Institutions under the State Board of Control* 25 (Feb. 10, 1925): 48.

22. Compare Rochester State Hospital's *Biennial Report for the Period Ending June 30, 1928*, MHS, with the Minnesota State Board of Control Minutes, MHS, from the same period. See Birthright, Inc., "Sterilizations Officially Reported from States Having a Sterilization Law up to January 1, 1945," Sterilization Statistics, AVS Records.

23. Laws of Minnesota 1925, chap. 154, sec. 2; Minnesota House of Representatives, Committee Meeting Minutes, Public Welfare and Social Legislation, Jan. 28–Feb. 5, 1925.

24. Joel Braslow, *Mental Ills and Bodily Cures: Psychiatric Treatment in the First Half of the Twentieth Century* (Berkeley: University of California Press, 1997), 55–57.

25. Rochester State Hospital, *Biennial Report for the Period Ending June 30, 1946*. This analysis is based on a review of the biennial reports from 1928 to 1952.

26. Piper, "After Faribault"; Minnesota State Board of Control, Department for the Feeble-Minded, *Biennial Report for the Period Ending June 30, 1926*, 15.

27. Board of Control, *Biennial Report for 1926*, 13–15.

28. Thomson, *Prologue*, 55; Minnesota State Board of Control, Department for the Feeble-Minded, *Biennial Report for the Period Ending June 30, 1928*, 19.

29. Thomson, *Prologue*, 55, 70.

30. Mildred Thomson, "Problems Relating to the Work of the Feeble-Minded," in *Proceedings of the Minnesota State Conference and Institute of Social Work* (St. Paul: State Board of Control, 1926), 303–4; Mildred Thomson, Memo to Members of the Child Welfare Boards of Minnesota, n.d., Robbins Gilman and Family Papers, MHS.

31. Secretary's Report for 1926; Annual Report of Secretary—1924, WWL.

32. Secretary's Annual Report (1929), WWL.

33. Mildred Thomson to G. C. Hanna, Aug. 4, 1927, and Aug. 8, 1927, FSSH SC; Thomson, *Prologue*, 70.

34. "Girls sterilized and available for parole, 11/19/27," in J. M. Murdoch to Mildred Thomson, FSSH SC.

35. "Girls sterilized and available, 11/19/27"; FSSH Sterilization Case no. 119.

36. Thomson, *Prologue*, 75; Mildred Thomson to G. C. Hanna, Jan. 6, 1927; Thomson to Hanna, July 29, 1927, FSSH SC.

37. Thomson, *Prologue*, 74–75; J. M. Murdoch to Thomson, Sept. 28, 1929, FSSH SC; FSSH Sterilization Case no. 575.

38. Piper, "After Faribault"; Thomson, *Prologue*, 72.

39. Secretary's Report for Year 1930, WWL; Board of Control, *Biennial Report for 1926*, 14–15; Thomson, *Prologue*, 53–55, 70.

40. Piper, "After Faribault."

41. St. Peter State Hospital, Jan. 27, 1930, Minnesota State Board of Control, *Visitation Reports*, 1928–1930, MHS; FSSH, Sterilization Case no. 42.

42. St. Peter State Hospital, Oct. 24, 1928, Dec. 18, 1929; Feb. 22, 1929, Board of Control, *Visitation Reports*. Death information from www.findagrave.com/.

43. Thomson, *Prologue*, 55.

44. For a thoughtful analysis of sterilization consent in Alberta, see Erika Dyck, *Facing Eugenics: Reproduction, Sterilization, and the Politics of Choice* (Toronto: University of Toronto Press, 2013). See also Jordan Goodman, Anthony McElligott, and Lara Marks, eds., *Useful Bodies: Humans in the Service of Medical Science in the Twentieth Century* (Baltimore: Johns Hopkins University Press, 2004).

45. Liza Piper, "Analysis of Sterilization Records: Consent" (unpublished paper in author's possession).

46. Ibid.

47. Mildred Thomson, Memo to Child Welfare Board Members and Others Concerned with Carrying Out the Sterilization Law," Dec. 12, 1934, DPW PSB; "History of the Sterilization of the Feeble-Minded," typescript, n.d., DPW PSB.

48. "Consideration of Inmates Sterilized March 8, 1929," enclosed in J. M. Murdoch to Mildred Thomson, Apr. 13, 1929; "Paroled to Club Houses during the period 7-1-28 to 7-1-30," typescript, FSSH SC; FSSH Sterilization Case no. 205.

49. Fergus Falls State Hospital, May 17, 1929, and June 14, 1930, Minnesota State Board of Control, Visitation Reports, MHS; Fergus Falls State Hospital, *Biennial Report for the Period Ending June 30, 1930*, 21, MHS.

50. Mildred Thomson to J. M. Murdoch, Sept. 29, 1927, FSSH SC; Juliane Muus to Stuart Cook, Mar. 27, 1942; Muus to Cook, May 11, 1942, Follow-up of Psychological Study, DPW PSB.

51. Charles E. Dow, "The Problem of the Feeble-Minded III," typescript, Aug. 9, 1934, DPW Library.

52. Stella Hanson, "Outside Supervision of the Feebleminded," typescript, ca. 1940, DPW PSB.

53. Johanna Schoen, "Between Choice and Coercion: Women and the Politics of Sterilization in North Carolina, 1929–1975," *Journal of Women's History* 13 (Spring 2001): 133; FSSH Medical Staff Minutes, May 10, 1937, MHS; FSSH Admissions Records, vol. I, no. 311, 287, MHS; FSSH Sterilization Case nos. 414, 381. On birth control in Minnesota, see Mary Losure, "'Motherhood Protection' and the Minnesota Birth Control League," *Minnesota History* 54 (Winter 1995): 359–70.

54. Mildred Thomson to J. M. Murdoch, Feb. 23, 1933, FSSH SC; FSSH Sterilization Case no. 485.

55. Mrs. —— to Sir, Sept. [20], 1926, FSSH SC.

56. Mildred Thomson to J. M. Murdoch, Nov. 15, 1927; Thomson to Murdoch, Apr. 27, 1928, FSSH SC; Thomson, *Prologue*, 71.

57. Regular Meeting, June 8, 1928, WWL; Annual Meeting Report 1931, WWL; Thomson, *Prologue*, 74.

58. Thomson, *Prologue*, 85; Secretary's Report for Year 1930, WWL.

59. Secretary's Annual Report (1929); Regular Meeting, Dec. 11, 1931, WWL.

60. Mildred Thomson, "My Thirty-Five Years of Work with the Mentally Retarded in Minnesota," typescript, 1961–1962, 20, MHS.

Chapter Five · Sterilization and Welfare in Depression and War

1. Mildred Thomson, "Supervision of the Feeble-Minded by County Welfare Boards," paper presented to the American Association on Mental Deficiency, May 1940, DPW PSB.

2. Ibid.; "History of the Sterilization of the Feeble-Minded," typescript, n.d. [1939], DPW PSB.

3. E. J. Engberg to Carl Swanson, June 22, 1946, FSSH SC.

4. Charles F. Dight, "First Radio Talk," Sept. 29, 1933, "A Series of Twelve Radio Talks on Heredity and Eugenics," Charles Fremont Dight Papers, MHS; Mildred Thomson, *Prologue: A Minnesota Story of Mental Retardation* (Minneapolis: Gilbert, 1963), 83. On sterilization in the 1930s, see Diane B. Paul, *Controlling Human Heredity: 1865 to the Present* (Atlantic Highlands, NJ: Humanities Press International, 1995); Philip Reilly, *The Surgical Solution: A History of Involuntary Sterilization in the United States* (Baltimore: Johns Hopkins University Press, 1991); Susan Currell and Christina Cogdell, eds., *Popular Eugenics: National Efficiency and American Mass Culture in the 1930s* (Athens: Ohio University Press, 2006).

5. Michael B. Katz, *In the Shadow of the Poorhouse: A Social History of Welfare in America* (New York: Basic Books, 1986), 226.

6. D. Jerome Tweton, *The New Deal at the Grassroots: Programs for the People in Otter Tail County, Minnesota* (St. Paul: Minnesota Historical Society Press, 1988), 167, 21; Mildred Thomson, "One of the most serious welfare problems presented by the changing social order of to-day," typescript, n.d. [Jan. 1, 1937], 16, DPW Library. For a powerful recent argument about the limitations of the New Deal, see Ira Katznelson, *Fear Itself: The New Deal and the Origins of Our Time* (New York: W. W. Norton, 2013).

7. Alice Kessler-Harris, *In Pursuit of Equity: Women, Men and the Quest for Economic Citizenship in 20th-Century America* (New York: Oxford University Press, 2002), 3–18; Roosevelt quoted in Katz, *In the Shadow of the Poorhouse*, 226. On gender and the two-track welfare

state, see esp. Linda Gordon, *Women, the State, and Welfare* (Madison: University of Wisconsin Press, 1991); Nancy Fraser and Linda Gordon, "A Genealogy of Dependency: Tracing a Keyword of the U.S. Welfare State," *Signs* 19 (Winter 1994): 309–36. On disability, see Paul K. Longmore and David Goldberger, "The League of the Physically Handicapped and the Great Depression: A Case Study in the New Disability History," *Journal of American History* 87 (Dec. 2000): 888–922; Deborah A. Stone, *The Disabled State* (Philadelphia: Temple University Press, 1984).

8. Ira Katznelson, *When Affirmative Action Was White: An Untold History of Racial Inequality in Twentieth-Century America* (New York: W. W. Norton, 2006), 29. See also Cybelle Fox, *Three Worlds of Relief: Race, Immigration, and the American Welfare State from the Progressive Era to the New Deal* (Princeton, NJ: Princeton University Press, 2012).

9. D. Jerome Tweton, *Depression: Minnesota in the Thirties* (Fargo: North Dakota Institute for Regional Studies, 1981), 9; Meridel Le Sueur, "Cows and Horses are Hungry (1934)," in *Ripening: Selected Work, 1927–1980* (Old Westbury, NY: Feminist Press, 1982), 167–68.

10. Elizabeth Faue, *Community of Suffering and Struggle: Women, Men and the Labor Movement in Minneapolis, 1915–1945* (Chapel Hill: University of North Carolina Press, 1991), 58–59; Thomson, *Prologue*, 79; Meridel Le Sueur, "Women on the Breadlines (1932)," in *Ripening*, 142.

11. Blanche La Du, "A Picture of Minnesota in 1932," in *Proceedings of the Minnesota State Conference and Institute of Social Work* (St. Paul: State Board of Control, 1932), 3, 6.

12. Mildred Thomson to J. M. Murdoch, Jan. 11, 1930, FSSH SC; Case no. 60, FSSH, *Record of Sterilization Cases*, 1916–1937, MHS.

13. Thomson, *Prologue*, 85.

14. George H. Mayer, *The Political Career of Floyd B. Olson* (Minneapolis: University of Minnesota Press, 1951), 108.

15. Thomson, *Prologue*, 76–78. See Raymond L. Koch, "The Development of Public Relief Programs in Minnesota, 1929–1941" (PhD diss., University of Minnesota, 1967).

16. Tweton, *New Deal at the Grassroots*, 15, 40; La Du, "Picture of Minnesota," 9–10.

17. Since allotted lands were subdivided into tiny and unworkable fractions and subject to taxation, many families were forced to sell. In contrast to White Earth, the Red Lake Band voted against allotment and held their remaining lands in common. See Melissa L. Meyer, *The White Earth Tragedy: Ethnicity and Dispossession at a Minnesota Anishinaabe Reservation, 1889–1920* (Lincoln: University of Nebraska Press, 1999); Chantal Norrgard, *Seasons of Change: Labor, Treaty Rights, and Ojibwe Nationhood* (Chapel Hill: University of North Carolina Press, 2014); Brenda J. Child, *My Grandfather's Knocking Sticks: Ojibwe Family Life and Labor on the Reservation* (St. Paul: Minnesota Historical Society Press, 2014); M. Inez Hilger, *Chippewa Families: A Social Study of White Earth Reservation, 1938* (1939; repr., St. Paul: Minnesota Historical Society Press, 1998).

18. Lewis Meriam, *The Problem of Indian Administration* (Baltimore: Johns Hopkins University Press, 1928), 2, 548, 7; Robert T. Lansdale, "The Place of the Social Worker in the Indian Service Problem," in *Proceedings of the National Conference of Social Work, 1932* (Chicago: University of Chicago Press, 1933), 611. On children, see Marilyn Irvin Holt, *Indian Orphanages* (Lawrence: University Press of Kansas, 2001); Brenda J. Child, *Boarding School Seasons: American Indian Families, 1900–1940* (Lincoln: University of Nebraska Press, 1998). On family strategies, see Child, *My Grandfather's Knocking Sticks*, 11.

19. Blanche L. La Du, "What Minnesota Is Doing for the Indians," 627, 635, and Lewis Meriam, "Cooperation in Work for Indians," 612, both in *Proceedings of the National Conference of Social Work, 1931* (Chicago: University of Chicago Press, 1931).

20. See Koch, "Development of Public Relief," 101–10; Barbara W. Sommer, *Hard Work and a Good Deal: The Civilian Conservation Corps in Minnesota* (St. Paul: Minnesota Historical Society Press, 2008); Calvin W. Gower, "The CCC Indian Division: Aid for Depressed Americans, 1933–1942," *Minnesota History* 43 (Apr. 1972): 3–13.

21. Lorena Hickok quoted in Linda Gordon, *Pitied but Not Entitled: Single Mothers and the History of Welfare* (New York: Free Press, 1994), 192; Koch, "Development of Public Relief," 70.

22. Koch, "Development of Public Relief," 244–45. See also Raymond L. Koch, "Politics and Relief in Minneapolis during the 1930s," *Minnesota History* 41 (Winter 1968): 153–70; Elizabeth Faue, "Farmer–Labor Women and Social Policy in the Great Depression," in *Women, Politics and Change*, ed. Louise Tilly and Pat Gurin (New York: Russell Sage Foundation, 1992), 436–56.

23. Richard Lowitt and Murine Beasley, eds., *One Third of a Nation: Lorena Hickock Reports on the Great Depression* (Urbana: University of Illinois Press, 1981), 123–26.

24. Ibid., 125, 131, 134–36. Other New Dealers were more impressed. A FERA field representative wrote Hopkins that Olson "deserves a great deal of credit" for his efforts to overcome local obstructionism and depoliticize relief. William R. Brock, *Welfare, Democracy, and the New Deal* (Cambridge: Cambridge University Press, 1988), 223.

25. Minnesota State Conference of Social Work, *A Study of Mothers' Allowance in Minnesota: 1935*, 19, in Minnesota Social Service Association Records, SWHA; Frederick Kuhlmann to Judge K. G. Brill, Dec. 17, 1930, DPW PSB. See also Gioh-Fang Dju Ma, *One Hundred Years of Public Services for Children in Minnesota* (Chicago: University of Chicago Press, 1948), 192–96.

26. Chisago County Child Welfare Board, Minutes, 1924–1937, Chisago County (Minn.) Health and Human Services Board, MHS.

27. The Chisago board discussed the "Lidstrom" case between Apr. 4, 1935, and Jan. 11, 1938 (quotation from July 8, 1937). See also Minnesota State Board of Control, Minutes, bk. I, June 8, 1938, MHS.

28. Mildred Thomson, "Social Aspects of Minnesota's Program for the Feebleminded," *Proceedings from the American Association on Mental Deficiency* 44, no. 1 (1939): 239.

29. FSSH Sterilization Case nos. 84, 170, 369, 521, 544, 577, 866, 915, 958; Special Folder on Indians, 1931–1934, 1937, FSSH SC.

30. Red Lake Indian Agency [Mary Kirkland], "Annual Narrative Report," n.d. (received Nov. 11, 1937), and Mary M. Kirkland, "Quarterly Report of School Social Worker for Period Ending Dec. 30, 1937," Social Workers' Reports, 1932–1942, Welfare Branch [Records of Health Division], Bureau of Indian Affairs, National Archives and Record Administration, Washington, DC. I am grateful to Brianna Theobald for the reference.

31. M. Manifold, "The Problem of the Feeble-Minded II," typescript, Aug. 9, 1934; Fern Chase, "The Care and Social Control of the Feebleminded in Minnesota," Minutes, First Meeting of the Committee to Discuss Problems of the Feebleminded, Mar. 7, 1934; Miss Bowman, Minutes, Fourth Meeting, May 2, 1934, all in DPW Library, MHS.

32. Thomson, *Prologue*, 79–80.

33. Thomson, "Social Aspects of Minnesota's Program," 240.

34. Thomson, "One of the most serious welfare problems," 14–16; Louise M. Clevenger, "The problem of feeblemindedness as a whole," typescript, Mar. 1, 1935, DPW Library. See also Holly Allen, *Forgotten Men and Fallen Women: The Cultural Politics of New Deal Narratives* (Ithaca, NY: Cornell University Press, 2015); Margot Canaday, *The Straight State: Sexuality and Citizenship in Twentieth-Century America* (Princeton, NJ: Princeton University Press, 2009).

35. John Rockwell, "A Few of the Problems That Must Be Faced in the Consideration of the Feebleminded," Minutes, First Meeting, Mar. 7, 1934.

36. Clevenger, "Problem of feeblemindedness," 3.

37. Laws of Minnesota 1935, chap. 364; Thomson, *Prologue*, 95.

38. Frederick Kuhlmann, "Report on Census of the Feeble-Minded," typescript, n.d., DPW PSB; Thomson, *Prologue*, 94–95.

39. Laws of Minnesota 1935, chap. 72, sec. 174. A statutory definition of "feebleminded person" was partially restored in 1945. See Robert J. Levy, "Protecting the Mentally Retarded: An Empirical Survey and Evaluation of the Establishment of Guardianship in Minnesota," *Minnesota Law Review* 49 (1965): 826–28.

40. Roy C. Frank to Downer Mullen, Dec. 18, 1936, and "Opinion of Attorney General William S. Ervin," Dec. 18, 1936, and Apr. 7, 1937, enclosed in Mildred Thomson to Carl Swanson, June 10, 1947, ADD Records, MHS.

41. Thomson, *Prologue*, 109.

42. The literature on this episode of Minnesota's political history is large and quite partisan. See John Earl Haynes, *Dubious Alliance: The Making of Minnesota's DFL Party* (Minneapolis: University of Minnesota Press, 1984); Richard M. Valelly, *Radicalism in the States: The Minnesota Farmer–Labor Party and the American Political Economy* (Chicago: University of Chicago Press, 1989); James M. Shields, *Mr. Progressive: A Biography of Elmer Austin Benson* (Minneapolis: T. S. Denison, 1971); Steven J. Keillor, *Hjalmar Petersen of Minnesota: The Politics of Provincial Independence* (St. Paul: Minnesota Historical Society Press, 1987); Millard L. Gieske, *Minnesota Farmer–Laborism: The Third-Party Alternative* (Minneapolis: University of Minnesota Press, 1979). On anti-Semitism, see Hyman Berman, "Political Antisemitism in Minnesota during the Great Depression," *Jewish Social Studies* 38 (Summer–Fall 1976): 247–64.

43. Thomson, *Prologue*, 102, 35, 107.

44. Anna Determan to Edward J. Engberg, Sept. 9, 1938; Gale Plagman to Board of Control, Dec. 5, 1938, FSSH SC.

45. Ma, *One Hundred Years*, 228.

46. Ibid., chap. 11; Thomson, *Prologue*, 130.

47. Thomson, *Prologue*, 119; "15% of State Employes Out in Job Purge," *Minneapolis Journal*, July 28, 1939. See also Koch, "Development of Public Relief," 432–39.

48. See, e.g., "History of the Sterilization of the Feeble-Minded."

49. Jacob Landman, *Human Sterilization: The History of the Sexual Sterilization Movement* (New York: Macmillan, 1932), 469–70; Abraham Myerson et al., *Eugenical Sterilization: A Reorientation of the Problem* (1936; repr., New York: Arno, 1980), 14–15, 178–80; "Against Sterilization," *New York Times*, Jan. 26, 1936.

50. Meridel Le Sueur, "Women Are Hungry (1934)," in *Ripening*, 149.

51. Meridel Le Sueur, *The Girl*, rev. ed. (1978; repr., Albuquerque, NM: West End Press, 1990), 1, 114, 124; italics in the original. See Paula Rabinowitz, *Labor and Desire: Women's*

Revolutionary Fiction in Depression America (Chapel Hill: University of North Carolina Press, 1991).

52. Frederick Kuhlmann to Walter Finke, Oct. 17, 1939; Mildred Thomson to J. A. A. Burnquist, Feb. 9, 1940, DPW PSB.

53. Minnesota Legislature Joint Committee on Acts and Activities of the Various Governmental Departments and Agencies, *Report from the Joint Senate and House Investigating Committee Covering the Acts and Activities of the Various Governmental Departments and Agencies of the State of Minnesota, 1939–40 Interim* (St. Paul, 1941), MHS.

54. Joint Committee, *Report from the Joint Investing Committee*; A. L. Haynes, Statement on Miss Blanche Harkner, June 19, 1939; Edward J. Engberg to Charles E. Houston, June 24, 1939, FSSH SC.

55. E. J. Engberg to Carl Swanson, June 22, 1946, FSSH SC; "Six Employes of State School in City Lose Jobs," *Faribault Daily News*, July 25, 1939.

56. Grover A. Kempf and Samuel W. Hamilton, "Section X of a Survey of the State Hospitals of Minnesota, Section I," United States Public Health Service Report (Washington, DC, 1939), typescript, DPW PSB.

57. Milton Kirkpatrick, "From Supplementary Report on the Mental Health Program in Minnesota by the American Public Welfare Association," typescript, n.d., DPW PSB; Thomson, *Prologue*, 125–30.

58. Kirkpatrick, "Supplementary Report on the Mental Health Program."

59. Thomson, *Prologue*, 127–28, 134, 126; Minnesota Division of Public Institutions, *Ninth Biennial Report for the Biennial Period Ending June 30, 1942*, 20–21.

60. In re Masters, 216 Minn. 553, 13 N.W.2d 487 (1944). My analysis of this case is based on the Minnesota Supreme Court decision and supporting materials, including the transcript of the trial in district court and the minutes of the Martin County Welfare Board. See Minnesota Supreme Court Case File no. 33719, and Martin County (Minn.) Welfare Board Minutes, 1937–1978, both in MHS.

61. "Report of Data and Evidence Presented in Hearing on Feeble-mindedness or Epilepsy," n.d.; "Petition for Restoration to Capacity of Rose Masters," in Minnesota Supreme Court Case File no. 33719.

62. *In re Masters*, 216 Minn. at 490, 489, 494.

63. "Petition of Rose Masters," transcript, May 4, 1943, 69, 41, 47–48.

64. *In re Masters*, 216 Minn. at 490; "Petition of Rose Masters," 36.

65. *In re Masters*, 216 Minn. at 493.

66. *In re Masters*, 216 Minn. at 493, 492.

67. Minnesota Division of Public Institutions, *Manual for Welfare Boards* (1943), 13–14, MHS; Minnesota Division of Public Institutions, *Tenth Biennial Report for the Biennial Period Ending June 30, 1944*, 23; Division of Public Institutions, *Biennial Report for 1942*, 122; Minnesota Division of Public Institutions, *Eleventh Biennial Report for the Biennial Period Ending 1946*, 108.

68. Division of Public Institutions, *Biennial Report for 1944*, 23; Mildred Thomson to Tom White, Apr. 11, 1945; Tom White to Mildred Thomson, Apr. 4, 1945, DPW PSB; Mary Losure, " 'Motherhood Protection' and the Minnesota Birth Control League," *Minnesota History* 54 (Winter 1995): 359–70.

69. Rickie Solinger, *Wake Up Little Susie: Single Pregnancy and Race before* Roe v. Wade (New York: Routledge, 1991); Regina G. Kunzel, "White Neurosis, Black Pathology: Con-

structing Out-of-Wedlock Pregnancy in the Wartime and Postwar United States," in *Not June Cleaver: Women and Gender in Postwar America, 1945–1960*, ed. Joanne Meyerowitz (Philadelphia: Temple University Press, 1994), 304–31.

70. Thomson, *Prologue*, 143. See Steven A. Gelb, "'Mental Deficients' Fighting Fascism: The Unplanned Normalization of World War II," in *Mental Retardation in America: A Historical Reader*, ed. Steven Noll and James W. Trent Jr. (New York: New York University Press, 2004), 308–21.

71. Thomson, *Prologue*, 142–43; Division of Public Institutions, *Biennial Report for 1944*, 111.

72. Thomson, *Prologue*, 140–42; Minnesota Division of Public Institutions, *Twelfth Biennial Report for the Biennial Period Ending June 30, 1948*, 156–57.

73. "Cruelty in State School Charged," *Veterans' News*, June 19, 1946, in Political Campaign—H. Peterson Folder, Minnesota, Legislature, House of Representatives, Journal of the House of Representatives, 1947, MHS; "Petersen Asks Investigation of School Here," *Faribault Daily News*, June 11, 1946; "State School Probe Report Is Filed: Thye Asks Investigation of State News Charges," *Faribault Daily News*, June 28, 1946.

74. Cruelty in State School Charged"; "State School Here Is Cleared by Grand Jury of Charges of Cruelty," *Faribault Daily News*, Nov. 16, 1946; "As Expected," *Faribault Daily News*, Nov. 20, 1946. See also Thomson, *Prologue*, 147–48.

75. Donald H. Berglund, foreword to Thomson, *Prologue*.

Chapter Six · From Fixing the Poor to Fixing the System?

1. Birthright, Inc., "Sterilizations Officially Reported from States Having a Sterilization Law up to January 1, 1947," and Birthright, Inc., "Sterilizations Officially Reported up to January 1, 1949," Sterilization Statistics, AVS Records, SWHA. On Minnesota's changing politics, see Jennifer A. Delton, *Making Minnesota Liberal: Civil Rights and the Transformation of the Democratic Party* (Minneapolis: University of Minnesota Press, 2002).

2. Mark Haller, *Eugenics: Hereditarian Attitudes in American Thought* (New Brunswick, NJ: Rutgers University Press, 1963), 180; Edwin Black, *War against the Weak: Eugenics and America's Campaign to Create a Master Race* (New York: Four Walls Eight Windows, 2003), 418; Harry Bruinius, *Better for All the World: The Secret History of Forced Sterilization and America's Quest for Racial Purity* (New York: Vintage, 2007), 361.

3. Birthright, Inc., "Sterilizations Officially Reported from States Having a Sterilization Law up to January 1, 1946"; Human Betterment Association, "Sterilizations Performed under U.S. State Sterilization Statutes through December 31, 1963," AVS Records. On postwar eugenics, see Randall Hansen and Desmond King, *Sterilized by the State: Eugenics, Race, and the Population Scare in Twentieth-Century North America* (Cambridge: Cambridge University Press, 2013); Matthew Connelly, *Fatal Misconception: The Struggle to Control World Population* (Cambridge, MA: Belknap Press of Harvard University Press), 2008; Ian Dowbiggin, *The Sterilization Movement and Global Fertility in the Twentieth Century* (New York: Oxford University Press, 2008); Wendy Kline, *Building a Better Race: Gender, Sexuality and Eugenics from the Turn of the Century to the Baby Boom* (Berkeley: University of California Press, 2001).

4. Skinner v. Oklahoma, 316 U.S. 535 (1942). See also Molly Ladd-Taylor, "'Ravished by Some Moron': Panic, Politics, and the Minnesota Psychopathic Personalities Law of 1939," paper presented to the Conference on Controlling Sexuality and Reproduction: Past and Present, University of Lethbridge, Aug. 2015.

5. Gunnar Myrdal, *An American Dilemma: The Negro Problem and American Democracy*

(New York: Harper, 1944), 928. See Carl Degler, *In Search of Human Nature: The Decline and Revival of Darwinism in American Social Thought* (New York: Oxford University Press, 1992).

6. Daniel Kevles, *In the Name of Eugenics: Genetics and the Uses of Human Heredity* (Cambridge, MA: Harvard University Press, 1995), 164; Michelle Brattain, "Race, Racism, and Antiracism: UNESCO and the Politics of Presenting Science to the Postwar Public," *American Historical Review* 112 (Dec. 2007): 1386–413; Nathaniel Comfort, *The Science of Human Perfection: How Genes Became the Heart of American Medicine* (New Haven, CT: Yale University Press, 2012).

7. Frederick Osborn, *Preface to Eugenics* (New York: Harper, 1940); Kevles, *In the Name of Eugenics*, chap. 11.

8. Mildred Thomson, *Prologue: A Minnesota Story of Mental Retardation* (Minneapolis: Gilbert, 1963), 146.

9. Delton, *Making Minnesota Liberal*, chap. 2; Alan Brinkley, *The End of Reform: New Deal Liberalism in Recession and War* (New York: Vintage, 1996), 269–71.

10. Delton, *Making Minnesota Liberal*, 134; Robert Esbjornson, *A Christian in Politics, Luther W. Youngdahl* (Minneapolis: T. S. Denison, 1955), 173; "DFL Backs Mental Aid," *Minneapolis Morning Tribune*, June 15, 1948.

11. Delton, *Making Minnesota Liberal*, 41.

12. Albert Q. Maisel, "Bedlam 1946: Most U.S. Mental Hospitals Are a Shame and a Disgrace," *Life*, May 6, 1946; Albert Deutsch, *The Shame of the States* (1948; repr., New York: Arno, 1973), 96.

13. Minnesota Unitarian Conference Committee, "A Summary of Conditions in Minnesota State Hospitals for the Mentally Ill: A Report to Governor Luther W. Youngdahl," n.d. [1948], 5, https://mn.gov/mnddc/past/pdf/40s/47/47-mn-dpw-summ-conditions.pdf.

14. Unitarian Conference Committee, "Summary of Conditions," 1; Geri Hoffner, "Improved Mental Hospitals Urged: Youngdahl Asks New 'Attitude,'" *Minneapolis Morning Tribune*, May 6, 1948.

15. Geri Hoffner, "Minnesota Bedlam: Mentally Ill Need Care, Get Little Besides Custody," *Minneapolis Morning Tribune*, May 13, 1948; Geri Hoffner, "State 'Bad Girls' Lead Dull, Hard Lives at 'School,'" *Minneapolis Morning Tribune*, Dec. 27, 1948.

16. Royal Gray, Memo on "Bridget O'Grady," Nov. 3, 1948, DPI MHU, Correspondence, 1941–1950, MHS.

17. Royal Gray to Edward J. Engberg, Sept. 9, 1946; Gray to Engberg, Feb. 28, 1945; Gray to Engberg, Aug. 7, 1946, DPI MHU.

18. Mr. and Mrs. —— to Governor Luther Youngdahl, n.d. [1948]; Royal Gray, Memo on "Astrid Helsin," July 16, 1946, DPI MHU.

19. "Mental Health Programs," *St. Paul Dispatch*, Mar. 14, 1949; Youngdahl quoted in Gunnar Dybward, paper presented at the National Association for Retarded Children, Oct. 26, 1963, www.disabilitymuseum.org/dhm/lib/detail.html?id=2233.

20. Geri Hoffner, "Minnesota Bedlam Revisited—State Has No More 'Incurable' Patients," *Minneapolis Morning Tribune*, Jan. 5, 1951; Geri Hoffner, "Minnesota Bedlam Revisited—Mental Patients Get Better Food Now," *Minneapolis Morning Tribune*, Jan. 2, 1951; Arthur Hager, "Much Remains to Be Done in State Mental Hospitals," *Minneapolis Morning Tribune*, Jan. 5, 1951.

21. Thomson, *Prologue*, 157, 160–61. On Rossen as visionary, see Minnesota Governor's

Council on Developmental Disabilities, "With an Eye to the Past—1940s to 50s: Lighting the Fire," www.mncdd.org/past/1940-50/1940s-6.html.

22. Mildred Thomson to Ralph Rossen, and enclosures, May 29, 1950, DPI MHU.

23. Sheldon C. Reed to Mrs. Ernest J. Schrader, Jan. 16, 1951, Dight Institute Records, University Archives, University of Minnesota, Twin Cities; Thomson, *Prologue*, 182–83.

24. Thomson, *Prologue*, 139; Phyllis Mickelson, "The Feebleminded Parent: A Study of 90 Family Cases; an Attempt to Isolate Those Factors Associated with Their Successful or Unsuccessful Parenthood," *American Journal of Mental Deficiency* 51 (1947): 644–53.

25. A. A. Heckman to Sheldon C. Reed, Oct. 10, 1952, Dight Institute Records.

26. For the history of ARC in Minnesota, see the Minnesota Governor's Council on Developmental Disabilities, "With an Eye to the Past," http://mn.gov/mnddc/past/index.html. On parent activism, see Kathleen W. Jones, "Education for Children with Mental Retardation: Parent Activism, Public Policy, and Family Ideology in the 1950s," 322–50; Katherine Castles, " 'Nice, Average Americans': Postwar Parents' Groups and the Defense of the Normal Family," in *Mental Retardation in America: A Historical Reader*, ed. Steven Noll and James W. Trent Jr. (New York: New York University Press, 2004), 351–70; Melanie Panitch, *Disability, Mothers, and Organization: Accidental Activists* (New York: Routledge, 2007).

27. Thomson, *Prologue*, 170–71, 191–92.

28. Ibid., 150; University of Minnesota Dight Institute, "The Biennial Report of the Dight Institute for 1946–48," Dight Institute Records. See Molly Ladd-Taylor, " A Kind of Genetic Social Work," in *Women, Health and Nation: Canada and the United States since 1945*, ed. Georgina Feldberg et al. (Montreal: McGill-Queen's University Press, 2003), 67–84.

29. V. Elving Anderson, "Sheldon C. Reed, Nov. 7, 1910–Feb. 1, 2003: Genetic Counseling, Behavioral Genetics," *American Journal of Human Genetics* 73 (July 2003): 1–4; Sheldon C. Reed, "Heredity Counseling," *Eugenics Quarterly* 1 (1954): 48–49. See also Diane Paul, "The Eugenic Origins of Medical Genetics," in *The Politics of Heredity: Essays on Eugenics, Biomedicine, and the Nature–Nurture Debate* (Albany, NY: SUNY Press), 133–56; Neal Holtan, "From Eugenics to Public Health Genetics in Mid-Twentieth Century Minnesota" (PhD diss., University of Minnesota, 2011).

30. Sheldon C. Reed, "All Men Are Brothers Under the Skin," Address at Annual Race Relations Day Observance, Feb. 11, 1951; Reed to Mrs. C. H. Chalmers, Nov. 1, 1949; Reed to Roscoe C. Brown, Nov. 3, 1952; Sheldon C. Reed, "Color of the U.S.A.—3000 A. D.," typescript, Dight Lectures, all in Dight Institute Records. See also Alexandra Minna Stern, *Telling Genes: The Story of Genetic Counseling in America* (Baltimore: Johns Hopkins University Press, 2012), chap. 3.

31. Sheldon C. Reed to Ralph Hayes, Mar. 25, 1949; S. C. Reed, "Toward a New Eugenics: the Importance of Differential Reproduction," n.d. [1965], both in Dight Institute Records.

32. Elizabeth W. Reed and Sheldon C. Reed, *Mental Retardation: A Family Study* (Philadelphia: Saunders, 1965), 77–78.

33. Sheldon C. Reed, *Counseling for Medical Genetics* (Philadelphia: Saunders, 1955), 92–93.

34. Eunice Kennedy Shriver, "Hope for Retarded Children (1962)," in *Mental Retardation in America*, 304, 307; James W. Trent Jr., *Inventing the Feeble Mind: A History of Mental Retardation in the United States* (Berkeley: University of California Press, 1995), 230–43.

35. The records of ARC Minnesota and ARC Greater Twin Cities are held in MHS.

36. Allison C. Carey, *On the Margins of Citizenship: Intellectual Disability and Civil Rights in Twentieth-Century America* (Philadelphia: Temple University Press, 2010), 105; John L. Holahan, "A Study of the Institutional Needs for the Mentally Retarded in the State of Minnesota," 1952, ARC Greater Twin Cities Records, MHS.

37. Castles, "Nice, Average Americans," 355.

38. Minnesota DPW, *You Are Not Alone: Information Helpful to Parents of Retarded Children* (St. Paul: DPW, 1954), 7, 10, 13.

39. Minnesota DPW, *Looking Ahead: Suggestions for Parents of Retarded Children* (St. Paul: DPW, 1956), 17–18.

40. In re Wretlind, 225 Minn. 554, 32 N.W.2d 161 (1948).

41. Thomson, *Prologue*, 177.

42. Legislative Committee and Institutional Committee of the Minnesota Association for Retarded Children, *Study of the Needs of Institutions for Mentally Retarded in Minnesota* (Minneapolis: MARC, 1959), http://mn.gov/mnddc/past/pdf/50s/59/59-SNI-LCI.pdf.

43. "Dr. David J. Vail, 45, State Welfare Official, Dies," *Minneapolis Tribune*, Oct. 22, 1971; David J. Vail to Superintendents, "A Statement of Expectations," July 26, 1960, https://mn.gov/mnddc/past/pdf/60s/60/60-ASE-DJV.pdf.

44. Frances Coakley, "New Concepts in Mental Retardation," Minutes, Inter-institutional Meeting, Feb. 19, 1960, FSSH Superintendent, Subject Files.

45. Philip R. Reilly, *The Surgical Solution: A History of Involuntary Sterilization in the United States* (Baltimore: Johns Hopkins University Press, 1991), 142.

46. Minutes, Inter-institutional Meeting, Nov. 21, 1960, FSSH Superintendent, Subject Files.

47. Ibid.

48. Ibid. See also Reilly, *Surgical Solution*, 142.

49. G. Sabagh and R. B. Edgerton, "Sterilized Mental Defectives Look at Eugenic Sterilization," *Eugenics Quarterly* 9 (1962): 218.

50. See Edward Shorter, *The Kennedy Family and the Story of Mental Retardation* (Philadelphia: Temple University Press, 2000); Kate Clifford Larson, *Rosemary: The Hidden Kennedy Daughter* (New York: Houghton Mifflin Harcourt, 2015).

51. United States, President's Panel on Mental Retardation, *Report to the President: A Proposed Program for National Action to Combat Mental Retardation* (Washington, DC: GPO, 1962), 8.

52. President's Panel, *Proposed Program*, 2, 66, 150, 13–14. My analysis of the panel's report has benefited from Edward D. Berkowitz, "The Politics of Mental Retardation during the Kennedy Administration," *Social Science Quarterly* 61 (June 1980): 128–42; Carey, *On the Margins of Citizenship*, 127–30.

53. Minnesota Governor's Council on Developmental Disabilities, "With an Eye to the Past—1960s: Building the Momentum," www.mncdd.org/past/1960/1960s-8.html.

54. President's Panel, *Proposed Program*, 14; United States, President's Panel on Mental Retardation, *Report of the Task Force on Law* (Washington, DC: GPO, 1963), 6, 11–12.

55. President's Panel, *Task Force on Law*, 21–23.

56. Julius Paul, "' . . . Three Generations of Imbeciles Are Enough . . . ': State Eugenic Sterilization Laws in American Thought and Practice" (1965), *Buck v. Bell Documents*, Paper 95, http://readingroom.law.gsu.edu/buckvbell/95; President's Panel, *Task Force on Law*, 19; President's Panel, *Proposed Program*, 94, 152.

57. Minutes, Inter-institutional Meeting, Apr. 22, 1960, FSSH Superintendent, Subject Files; Elizabeth M. Boggs, "Legal Aspects of Mental Retardation," in *Prevention and Treatment of Mental Retardation*, ed. Irving Philips (New York: Basic Books, 1966), 424–25.

58. Oscar Lewis, "The Culture of Poverty," *Scientific American* 215 (1966): 19–25; Mollie Orshansky, "Children of the Poor," *Social Security Bulletin* 26 (July 1963): 3. On the culture of poverty and the undeserving poor, see esp. Michael B. Katz, *The Undeserving Poor: From the War on Poverty to the War on Welfare* (New York: Pantheon, 1989); Michael B. Katz, ed., *The "Underclass" Debate: Views from History* (Princeton, NJ: Princeton University Press, 1993); Alice O'Connor, *Poverty Knowledge: Social Science, Social Policy, and the Poor in Twentieth-Century U.S. History* (Princeton, NJ: Princeton University Press, 2002).

59. Mical Raz, *What's Wrong with the Poor? Psychiatry, Race, and the War on Poverty* (Chapel Hill: University of North Carolina Press, 2013), chap. 4.

60. Ibid., 140; Molly Ladd-Taylor, "What Child Left Behind? U.S. Social Policy and the Hopeless Child," in *Lost Kids: Vulnerable Children and Youth in Twentieth-Century Canada and the United States*, ed. Mona Gleason et al. (Vancouver: University of British Columbia Press, 2010), 157–74.

61. David J. Vail, *Dehumanization and the Institutional Career* (Springfield, IL: Charles C. Thomas, 1966).

62. Wolf Wolfensberger, "A Contribution to the History of Normalization," in *A Quarter-Century of Normalization and Social Role Valorization: Evolution and Impact*, ed. Robert J. Flynn and Raymond A. Lemay (Ottawa: University of Ottawa Press, 1999), 59–60; Trent, *Inventing the Feeble Mind*, 250–52. For a powerful portrait of dehumanization in practice, see Claudia Malacrida, *A Special Hell: Institutional Life in Alberta's Eugenic Years* (Toronto: University of Toronto Press, 2015).

63. Sam Newlund, "Some at Faribault Live Like Animals," *Minneapolis Tribune*, Jan. 10, 1965.

64. "Medical Director Comments," *Minneapolis Tribune*, Jan. 31, 1965; "More Readers Comment on Faribault State Mental Hospital Article," *Minneapolis Tribune*, Jan. 24, 1965; "Readers Praise Article on Faribault School, Hospital," *Minneapolis Tribune*, Feb. 7, 1965; Vail, *Dehumanization*, 41–42.

65. Jean T. Brust, "Toward an Ethnography of the Mentally Retarded in a State Institution" (MA thesis, University of Minnesota, 1969).

66. Ibid., 3, 46, 60–61.

67. Ibid., 95.

68. Bengt Nirje, "How I Came to Formulate the Normalization Principle," in *A Quarter-Century of Normalization*, 33; Gerald F. Walsh, "Has the Role of Our State Institutions Changed?," presentation to the 1964 Convention of the Minnesota Association for Retarded Children, June 5, 1964, http://mn.gov/mnddc/past/pdf/60s/64/64-HRO-GFW.pdf.

69. Vail, *Dehumanization*, 38–40, 44.

70. Robert J. Levy, "Protecting the Mentally Retarded: An Empirical Survey and Evaluation of the Establishment of Guardianship in Minnesota," *Minnesota Law Review* 49 (1965): 821–87.

71. Ibid., 881. The year was 1963.

72. Ibid., 854.

73. Ibid., 832.

74. Ibid., 874–76.

75. Ibid., 876. She remained an epileptic ward, however, and the commissioner kept her at Faribault until the medical staff approved her release. The juvenile court ruled against the termination of her parental rights.

76. Ibid., 853, 868, 877–78.

77. Samuel Brachel and Ronald Rock, *The Mentally Disabled and the Law*, rev. ed. (Chicago: University of Chicago Press, 1971), 209; Reilly, *Surgical Solution*, 142–43. See Donald T. Critchlow, *Intended Consequences: Birth Control, Abortion, and the Federal Government in Modern America* (Oxford: Oxford University Press, 2001), chap 2.

78. Reilly, *Surgical Solution*, 128; Rebecca M. Kluchin, *Fit to Be Tied: Sterilization and Reproductive Rights in America, 1950–1980* (New Brunswick, NJ: Rutgers University Press, 2009), 78–80, 93; Randall Hansen and Desmond King, *Sterilized by the State: Eugenics, Race, and the Population Scare in Twentieth-Century North America* (Cambridge: Cambridge University Press, 2013), chap. 13.

79. Julius Paul, "The Return of Punitive Sterilization Proposals: Current Attacks on Illegitimacy and the AFDC Program," *Law and Society Review* 3 (Aug. 1968): 100–101.

Conclusion

1. "Agency Sued for Sterilizing 2 Girls," *Minneapolis Tribune*, June 28, 1973.

2. B. Drummond Ayres Jr., "Exploring Motives and Methods," *New York Times*, July 8, 1973. The best analysis of the *Relf* case is Gregory Michael Dorr, "Protection or Control? Women's Health, Sterilization Abuse, and *Relf v. Weinberger*," in *A Century of Eugenics in America: From the Indiana Experiment to the Human Genome Era*, ed. Paul A. Lombardo (Bloomington: Indiana University Press, 2011), 161–90. See also Lisa C. Ikemoto, "Infertile by Force and Federal Complicity: The Story of *Relf v. Weinberger*," in *Women and the Law Stories*, ed. Elizabeth Schneider and Stephanie Wildman (New York: Foundation Press, 2010), 179–206. On the Tuskegee Study, see Susan M. Reverby, *Examining Tuskegee: The Infamous Syphilis Study and Its Legacy* (Chapel Hill: University of North Carolina Press, 2009); James H. Jones, *Bad Blood: The Tuskegee Syphilis Experiment*, rev. ed. (1981; repr., New York: Free Press, 1993).

3. Robert G. Weisbord, *Genocide? Birth Control and the Black American* (Westport, CT: Greenwood, 1975), 169–70; Dorothy Roberts, *Killing the Black Body: Race, Reproduction, and the Meaning of Liberty* (New York: Pantheon, 1997), 93; Angela Y. Davis, *Women, Race, and Class* (1981; repr., New York: Vintage, 1983), 215–16.

4. Ayres, "Exploring Motives and Methods"; B. Drummond Ayres Jr., "Racism, Ethics and Rights at Issue in Sterilization Case," *New York Times*, July 2, 1973.

5. Ayres, "Exploring Motives and Methods." The Relf girls could no longer receive injections of Depo-Provera because the substance had recently been banned.

6. Relf v. Weinberger, 372 F. Supp. 1196 (D.D.C. 1974).

7. Edward Hudson, "Suit Seeks to Void Sterilization Law: A.C.L.U. Asks $1-Million for North Carolina Woman," *New York Times*, July 13, 1973; Nancy Hicks, "Sterilization of Black Mother of 3 Stirs Aiken, S.C.," *New York Times*, Aug. 1, 1973.

8. Bernard Rosenfeld, Sidney M. Wolfe, and Robert E. McGarrah Jr., *A Health Research Group Study on Surgical Sterilization: Present Abuses and Proposed Regulations* (Washington, DC: Health Research Group, 1973), 1–2, 8.

9. Tricia Farris, "Sterilization: Use, Misuse and Abuse" (St. Paul: State of Minnesota House Research Department, 1974), 1, ii, 2, 7. The final quotation is from *Eisenstadt v. Baird*,

405 U.S. 438 (1972), which struck down a Massachusetts law prohibiting the distribution of contraceptives to unmarried persons.

10. Farris, "Sterilization," 7–8.

11. In the case of a hereditary condition, a sterilization request had to be accompanied by a genetic report from the Human Genetics Unit of the Minnesota Department of Health. Ibid., 13.

12. Ibid., 13. The increase in the early 1970s coincided with a national increase in surgical sterilizations, increased opportunities for living outside the institution, and the death of David Vail.

13. Ibid., 1, 13–14, 16–17.

14. Laws of Minnesota 1975, chap. 208, sec. 2, subd. 2, 8.

15. Laws of Minnesota 1975, chap. 208, sec. 11, subd. 5.

16. Laws of Minnesota 1975, chap. 208, sec. 13. The requirement of written consent could be waived if there was sworn confirmation by an interested person of nonwritten consent.

17. Thomas M. Shapiro, *Population Control Politics: Women, Sterilization, and Reproductive Choice* (Philadelphia: Temple University Press, 1985), 103–4; Rosalind Pollack Petchesky, "Reproduction, Ethics, and Public Policy: The Federal Sterilization Regulations," *Hastings Center Report* 9 (Oct. 1979): 30–31.

18. Nadine Brozan, "The Volatile Issue of Sterilization Abuse: A Tangle of Accusations and Remedies," *New York Times*, Dec. 9, 1977. The debate over the guidelines is discussed in Rebecca M. Kluchin, *Fit to Be Tied: Sterilization and Reproductive Rights in America, 1950–1980* (New Brunswick, NJ: Rutgers University Press, 2009), 203–11.

19. Elena R. Gutiérrez, "Policing 'Pregnant Pilgrims': Situating the Sterilization Abuse of Mexican-Origin Women in Los Angeles County," in *Women, Health and Nation: Canada and the United States since 1945*, ed. Georgina Feldberg et al. (Montreal: McGill-Queen's University Press, 2003), 379–403.

20. Comptroller General of the United States, "Report to Senator James G. Abourezk: Investigation of Allegations Concerning Indian Health Service" (Washington, DC: Government Accountability Office, 1976); Jane Lawrence, "The Indian Health Service and the Sterilization of Native American Women," *American Indian Quarterly* 24 (2000): 411–12. The four program areas studied by the Government Accountability Office were in South Dakota, New Mexico, Oklahoma, and Arizona. Although an IHS program area was located in Bemidji, Minnesota, and the American Indian Movement was headquartered in Minneapolis, I found little direct information about IHS sterilizations in Minnesota. See Kluchin, *Fit to Be Tied*, 108–11; Sally J. Torpy, "Native American Women and Coerced Sterilization: On the Trail of Tears in the 1970s," *American Indian Culture and Research Journal* 24 (2000): 1–22; Katsi Cook interview, Voices of Feminism Oral History Project, Sophia Smith Collection, Smith College, Northampton, MA. Thanks to Brianna Theobald for the last reference.

21. Michael Kindred, ed., *The Mentally Retarded Citizen and the Law: The President's Committee on Mental Retardation* (New York: Free Press, 1976), xx, xxix. See also Allison C. Carey, *On the Margins of Citizenship: Intellectual Disability and Civil Rights in Twentieth-Century America* (Philadelphia: Temple University Press, 2009), chap. 7.

22. Monroe E. Price and Robert A. Burt, "Nonconsensual Medical Procedures and the Right to Privacy," in *The Mentally Retarded Citizen and the Law*, 95–96, 101–2. Price and Burt specifically criticized the Minnesota statute, which empowered the commissioner of public welfare to consent to sterilization when no relative was available.

23. Stump v. Sparkman, 435 U.S. 349 (1978). Linda tells her own story in Jamie Renee Coleman and Paula Bateman Headley, *The Blanket She Carried* (Bloomington, IN: Authorhouse, 2003). Most scholarship on the case has focused on the precedent for judicial immunity. A recent exception is Laura T. Kessler, "'A Sordid Case': *Stump v. Sparkman*, Judicial Immunity, and the Other Side of Reproductive Rights," *Maryland Law Review* 74 (2015): 833–920.

24. *Stump v. Sparkman*, 435 U.S. at 435; E. (Mrs.) v. Eve, 2 S.C.R. 388 (1986) at 62; Judith A. Baer, *Women in American Law: The Struggle toward Equality from the New Deal to the Present*, 2nd ed. (New York: Holmes & Meier, 1996), 186. That the Supreme Court of Canada commented on *Stump* in its landmark ruling against the nontherapeutic sterilization of persons with intellectual disabilities reveals the decision's importance. See Molly Ladd-Taylor, "Contraception or Eugenics? Sterilization and 'Mental Retardation' in the 1970s and 1980s," *Canadian Bulletin of Medical History* 31 (2014): 189–211.

25. Kluchin, *Fit to Be Tied*, 203–11.

26. In re Grady, 85 N.J. 235, 426 A.2d. 467 (1981); In re Eberhardy, 102 Wis. 2d 539, 307 N.W.2d. 881 (1981). See Ladd-Taylor, "Contraception or Eugenics?," 203–20; Philip R. Reilly, *The Surgical Solution: A History of Involuntary Sterilization in the United States* (Baltimore: Johns Hopkins University Press, 1991), 155–56. My interpretation has benefited from Martha A. Field and Valerie A. Sanchez, *Equal Treatment for People with Mental Retardation: Having and Raising Children* (Cambridge, MA: Harvard University Press, 2000); Ellen Brantlinger, *Sterilization of People with Mental Disabilities: Issues, Perspectives, and Cases* (Westport, CT: Auburn House, 1995).

27. For example, sterilization is not a major topic in the excellent historical archives section of the website of the Minnesota Governor's Council on Developmental Disabilities, http://mn.gov/mnddc/, nor is it discussed in histories of the welfare rights movement in Minnesota. See, e.g., Susan Handley Hertz, "The Politics of the Welfare Mothers Movement: A Case Study," *Signs* 2 (Spring 1977): 600–611.

28. David J. Rothman and Sheila M. Rothman, *The Willowbrook Wars* (New York: Harper & Row, 1984); *Wyatt v. Stickney*, 325 F. Supp. 781 (M.D. Ala. 1971).

29. Luther Granquist, "A Brief History of the Welsch Case," paper presented at the Meeting of the American Association on Mental Deficiency, Boston, MA, 1982. This and other documents pertaining to the case are posted at http://mn.gov/mnddc/past/pdf/pdf-index_st-inst-welsch.html.

30. Ibid.

31. Joseph P. Shapiro, *No Pity: People with Disabilities Forging a New Civil Rights Movement* (New York: Times Books, 1994), 184–92; Carey, *On the Margins of Citizenship*, 154–58.

32. *PBS NewsHour*, "Returning Dignity in Death to Those Who Were Forgotten during Their Lives," December 2013, www.pbs.org/newshour/bb/nation-july-dec13-graves_12-26/; Advocating Change Together, "Remembering with Dignity Apology Resolution" (2007), typescript in author's possession.

33. Laws of Minnesota 2010, Resolution 4—H. F. No. 1680; Doug Grow, "Minnesota Finally Apologies to Thousands of Mentally Disabled," *MinnPost*, June 3, 2010, www.minnpost.com/politics-policy/2010/06/minnesota-finally-apologizes-thousands-mentally-disabled.

34. Price and Burt, "Nonconsensual Medical Procedures," 107.

35. See, e.g., Jeanne Flavin, *Our Bodies, Our Crimes: The Policing of Women's Reproduction in America* (New York: New York University Press, 2009); Rachel Roth, "'No New Babies?'

Gender Inequality and Reproductive Control in the Criminal Justice and Prison Systems," *Journal of Gender, Social Policy and the Law* 12 (2005): 391–425.

36. Paul Campos, "Eugenics Are Alive and Well in the United States," *Time*, July 10, 2013, http://ideas.time.com/2013/07/10/eugenics-are-alive-and-well-in-the-united-states/; US Department of Justice, Bureau of Justice Statistics, *Special Report: Disabilities among Prison and Jail Inmates, 2011–12*, by Jennifer Bronson, Laura M. Maruschak, and Marcus Berzofsky, NCJ 249151 (Washington, DC: Bureau of Justice Statistics, December 2015), www.bjs.gov/content/pub/pdf/dpji1112.pdf. See Liat Ben-Moshe, Chris Chapman, and Allison C. Carey, *Disability Incarcerated: Imprisonment and Disability in the United States and Canada* (Basingstoke, UK: Palgrave Macmillan, 2014); Dorothy E. Roberts, "The Social and Moral Cost of Mass Incarceration in African American Communities," *Stanford Law Review* 56 (2004): 1271–305.

37. Rickie Solinger, *Beggars and Choosers: How the Politics of Choice Shapes Adoption, Abortion, and Welfare in the United States* (New York: Hill & Wang, 2002). See also Dorothy Roberts, *Shattered Bonds: The Color of Child Welfare* (New York: Basic Civitas, 2003); Michael B. Katz, *The Price of Citizenship: Redefining the American Welfare State* (New York: Metropolitan Books, 2001); Laura Briggs, *Somebody's Children: The Politics of Transracial and Transnational Adoption* (Durham, NC: Duke University Press, 2012).

Appendix

1. Rochester State Hospital, *Biennial Report of the Rochester State Hospital for the Period Ending June 30, 1942*, 2–3.

2. E. S. Gosney, "Operations for Eugenic Sterilization Performed in State Institutions under State Laws up to January 1, 1928"; Human Betterment Foundation, "Operations for Eugenic Sterilization Performed in State Institutions under State Laws up to January 1, 1930"; "Sterilizations Performed under U.S. State Sterilization Statutes through December 31, 1963," Sterilizaton Statistics, AVS Records, SWHA.

3. Compare "Sterilizations Performed through December 31, 1963" to Lutz Kaelber, "Eugenics: Compulsory Sterilization in 50 American States," www.uvm.edu/~lkaelber/eugenics/; Mark A. Largent, *Breeding Contempt: The History of Coerced Sterilization in the United States* (New Brunswick, NJ: Rutgers University Press, 2008), 79–80; Randall Hansen and Desmond King, *Sterilized by the State: Eugenics, Race, and the Population Scare in Twentieth-Century North America* (Cambridge: Cambridge University Press, 2013), 77; Paul A. Lombardo, *Three Generations, No Imbeciles: Eugenics, the Supreme Court, and* Buck v. Bell (Baltimore: Johns Hopkins University Press, 2008), 294; Jonas Robitscher, *Eugenic Sterilization* (Springfield, IL: Thomas, 1973), 118–19; Julius Paul, " ' . . . Three Generations of Imbeciles Are Enough . . . ': State Eugenic Sterilization in American Thought and Practice" (1965), *Buck v. Bell Documents*, Paper 95, http://readingroom.law.gsu.edu/buckvbell/95.

4. FSSH, *Record of Sterilization Cases*, 1916–1937, MHS; Liza Piper, "Analysis of Sterilization Records" (2002; unpublished report in author's possession).

Page numbers in *italics* refer to tables and illustrations.